P. J. Frosch · J. D. Johansen · I. R. White (Eds.)

Fragrances: Beneficial and Adverse Effects

Springer
Berlin
Heidelberg
New York
Barcelona
Budapest
Hong Kong
London
Milan
Paris
Santa Clara
Singapore
Tokyo

P. J. Frosch · J. D. Johansen · I. R. White (Eds.)

FRAGRANCES

Beneficial and Adverse Effects

With Foreword by H. Möller

With 33 Figures (Some in Colour)
and 42 Tables

Springer

Prof. Dr. med. PETER J. FROSCH
Städtische Kliniken Dortmund, Hautklinik
and Department of Dermatology,
University of Witten/Herdecke
Beurhausstraße 40, D-44137 Dortmund, Germany

Dr. JEANNE DUUS JOHANSEN
University of Copenhagen
Gentofte Hospital, Department of Dermatology
Niels Andersen Vej 65, DK-2900 Hellerup, Denmark

Dr. IAN R. WHITE
St. John's Institute of Dermatology
St. Thomas' Hospital
London SEI 7EH, England

ISBN-13: 978-3-642-80342-0 e-ISBN-13: 978-3-642-80340-6
DOI: 10.1007/978-3-642-80340-6

Library of Congress Catalogin-in-Publication Data
Fragrances : beneficial and adverse effects / P. J. Frosch, J. D.
Johansen, I. R. White (eds.).
p. cm.
Includes bibliographical references and index.

1. Perfumes – Toxicology. 2. Perefumes. I. Frosch, Peter J.
II. Johansen, J. D. (Jeanne Duus) III. White, I. R. (Ian R.)
RA 1270.P37F73 1998
615.9'51 -- dc21

Cover design: Design & Production, Heidelberg
Typesetting: Fotosatz-Service Köhler OHG, Würzburg
The text printed in this book was taken directly from data supplied by the editors.
SPIN: 10545329 23/3134 – 5 4 3 2 1 0 – Printed on acid-free paper

Foreword

Satellite symposia of a commercial nature are frequent additions to scientific meetings. The organisers of the Jadassohn Centenary Congress (a joint meeting of the European Society of Contact Dermatitis and the American Contact Dermatitis Society, London, October 1996) chose to start their meeting with a thematic symposium independent of any drug or cosmetic promotion. Doing this, and taking "Fragrances" as a theme, was motivated by the need for informed debate on an important medical and environmental issue without the bias that sponsorship brings.

That time is now remote when perfumes were applied exclusively as such on the skin in order to attain a specific odour for the purpose of increasing the powers of attraction and self-esteem, in many cases also with the aim of covering a malodour. The next stage of the evolution of fragrance use was their addition to skin care products such as cleansers and emollients. Today, fragrance use is ubiquitous and they are present in a multitude of products not primarily designed for skin contact. Because of these many uses contact may occur from airborne perfumes and by daily social interaction. Consequently, in modern society nobody can avoid exposure to fragrances.

The present volume demonstrates that the reported adverse effects of fragrance compounds are relatively few in relation to the vast amounts used. However, irritant and allergic skin reactions do occur and many of these are not reported to manufacturers and physicians. Nevertheless, those reactions investigated by dermatologists and diagnosed by patch testing constitute a very substantial part of all contact allergies seen in dermatological practice. In females, contact allergy to fragrances is usually second in frequency after nickel allergy; in males, in many laboratories fragrance has become number 1!

The above leads to a need for a much increased understanding of the biology and chemistry of fragrance materials. Also required are improved methods to diagnose skin disease induced by fragrances: irritant and phototoxic reactions, contact and photocontact allergy as well as contact urticaria. The medical community and the fragrance industry are very interested in the prevention of skin damage caused by fragrance compounds. Therefore, predictive testing of fragrance materials, a politically somewhat debated issue, is covered in the present volume.

Being comprehensive, the symposium also discussed the beneficial effects of fragrances, primarily as psychosocial means of interpersonal communication. Also, we learnt of the importance of fragrance signals in the insect kingdom.

Quite clearly, this book covers an essential area of dermatology. It certainly needs no scented cover to attract readers!

Malmö 1997

HALVOR MÖLLER
President, European Society of Contact Dermatitis

Preface

We all agree that the use of fragrances enriches our lives. Who does not like the marvellous bouquet of fragrances emanating from fresh flowers? Youth and beauty are associated with a refreshing odour but death and decay with a bad smell.

Man's use of perfumes can be traced back to ancient times. Beautiful glass flasks bear witness that the Romans produced a large variety of scented materials. Oils extracted from fruits and plants were used for baths and emollients; fine perfumes were kept in valuable flacons.

The art of perfumery has come a long way since. Nowadays it is a worldwide multibillion dollar business. Fragrances are ubiquitous. Advertising has created a fascinating world where dreams come true and youth, power and sexual success are directly linked to specific products. Famous designers have developed their own lines of after shave, perfume, body lotion, and deodorant. Today, it is rare to find a person who does not regularly use any perfumed article. There are now "special" fragrances for children.

The editors of this volume observe the side effects of fragrances in use. The well-known "Berloque Dermatitis" resulting from phototoxic furocoumarins in oil of bergamot presents with an acute inflammatory reaction and an often longstanding hyperpigmentation. Although this complication is now uncommon due to purification methods by manufacturers, dermatologists continue to diagnose allergic contact dermatitis to fragrances. Fragrances are the most frequent single cause of cosmetic allergy according to recent studies. Allergic reactions to the "fragrance mix" – a screening tool used for patch testing – are among the leading contact allergens, in most studies only surpassed by nickel in women. Dermatological patients in a patch test clinic show a frequency of positive reactions to the fragrance mix in the range of 5% to 11%. In the general population this figure may be 1%–2% according to a Danish study. Although not all of these reactions are clinically meaningful, adverse reactions to scented materials are by no means rare. They often cause considerable discomfort, require medical attention and are a burden for the highly sensitised patient. Individuals may react after airborne contact and may have to avoid elevators or shopping areas where perfumery is on display.

There are publications regarding the chemistry and methods of producing perfumes. They are primarily directed towards cosmetic manufacturers. This book is intended to fill the painful gap with regard to clinical aspects. For the first time a series of chapters by renowned experts covers important research areas in the field of fragrances, with molecular aspects of sensitization, frequency and clinical picture, diagnostic methods, and new and old sensitizers discussed. Special emphasis is placed on safety aspects regarding absorption in humans and various in vivo and in vitro techniques for predicting the irritating, sensitizing and phototoxic potential of fragrance materials. The musk fragrances have caused considerable concern regrading accumulation in animal tissue and the environment. The producers and their self-monitoring institutions (RIFM, IFRA) have also contributed. It becomes clear that their effort has been substantial: guidelines for safe use have been suggested based on numerous animal and human studies. Some compounds have been banned because of the high risk of sensitization or neurotoxic hazards; others now cause fewer adverse effects after purification or concentration limits have been followed.

There is no doubt that progress has been made in improving the safety standards of fragrances. However, the figures on adverse effects reported by dermatologists worldwide suggest that the safety procedures employed so far are not sufficient. Some fragrances are produced in thousands of tons each year and they are applied by millions of people, often for many years. Materials with a very low potential for adverse effects escape the laboratory screening methods available today. A close surveillance system with full cooperation of manufacturers, dermatologists, pharmacologists, toxicologists, epidemiologists and consumer agencies is overdue. Only a combined effort will lead to a decrease of the "fragrance problem". A good example of successful cooperation between dermatologists and manufacturers is the story of "pigmented cosmetic dermatitis" in Japan. In the 1960s an epidemic occcurred among women who presented with bizarre hyperpigmentations of the face. Ingredients of cosmetics were finally discovered as the culprit: coal-tar-derived dyes and various fragrances. On the basis of extensive patch test studies, Nakayama and colleagues developed the "allergen control system" (ACS) for the production of safer cosmetics. After major cosmetic companies in Japan avoided or reduced the concentration of these chemicals the number of patients suffering from this disfiguring condition sharply declined.

Legislation is still very "generous" about fragrances as important ingredients of cosmetics. We need global regulations for materials which are distributed worldwide in large quantities. It can no longer be tolerated that some manufacturers sell their perfume as an artful creation but as a "black box" regarding the constituents and safety data. Some of them do not even respect the safety recommendations of their own industry.

To increase the safety standard of fragrance compounds and provide more transparency in the data was the consensus of a 1-day symposium held in London, October 9, 1996, on the occasion of the Jadassohn Centenary Congress of the European Society of Contact Dermatitis. During the preparation of this symposium the organizers came to realize that the role of fragrances is under intensive research in other biological areas such as neurophysiological mechanisms and psychological aspects – finally, structures have been identified in human body secretions which might be a key for the attractiveness of sexual partners. The saying "I cannot stand the smell of him" might have a real biological odoriferous basis!

A new fascinating research area is the use of fragrances in the control of insects as a "biological weapon" in vineyards and other agricultural areas. The basis for this is the discovery of fragrances as an important communication tool among insects, bees and many other animals. It is therefore a pleasure to the editors that a few papers deal with effects which definitely can be termed "beneficial".

The editors wish to express their gratitude to Springer-Verlag, particularly to Dr. W. Wiegers and Mrs. B. Fingerhuth, for supporting the project and facilitating publication without delay.

Dortmund/Copenhagen/London

P. J. Frosch
J. D. Johansen
I. White

Contents

Part I: The Basics 1

The Art of Creating a Perfume 3
U. Harder

Cerebral Representation of Odour Perception 6
G. Kobal and B. Kettenmann

Part II: Beneficial Biological Effects 19

The Structure, Origin and Function of Human Axillary Odours 21
G. Preti, A. I. Spielman and J. J. Leyden

Communication by Odour – The Influence of Body Odour
on the Attractiveness of Men 28
R. E. Maiworm and W. U. Langthaler

Orientation of Insects in a Multitrophic System:
The Role of Fragrances 36
P. Christiansen-Weniger, N. Siri and S. G. Micha

Chemical Signals During Raids by the Robber Bee *Lestrimelitta limao*
on Other Stingless Bee Nests (Hymenoptera, Apidae, Meliponinae) . . 43
R. Radtke

Part III: Adverse Effects in Humans 47

Molecular Aspects of Fragrance Sensitisation 49
J. P. Lepoittevin and V. Mutterer

Identification of Fragrance Sensitizers by QSAR 57
J. J. Hostýnek, P. S. Magee and H. I. Maibach

Fragrances as a Cause of Contact Dermatitis in Cosmetics: Clinical Aspects and Epidemiological Data 66
A.C. de Groot and P.J. Frosch

How Do We Test for Fragrance Allergy? 76
W.G. Larsen

Fragrance Hypersensitivity and Its Control 83
H. Nakayama

Are Major Components of Fragrances a Problem? 92
P.J. Frosch, on behalf of the European Environmental and Contact Dermatitis Research Group (EECDRG)

Quantitative Aspects in Patch Testing and Usage Tests 100
J.D. Johansen

d-Limonene – An Old Perfume Ingredient Introduced as a "Natural" Solvent in Industry: Is There a Risk of Sensitization? 106
A.-T. Karlberg

Contents of Sensitizing Fragrance Materials in Natural Ingredient Based Cosmetics 113
S.C. Rastogi

RIFM Activities in the Safety Assessment of Systemic Effects of Fragrance Materials 121
E.A. Pfitzer

Absorption of Fragrance Ingredients Using In Vitro Models with Human Skin 125
S.A.M. Hotchkiss

Synthetic Musk Fragrances in Human Fat and Their Potential Uptake by Dermal Resorption 136
G.G. Rimkus

Part IV: Safety Assessment – Predictive Assays for Irritation and Sensitization 151

A Reappraisal of the Guinea Pig Maximization Test 153
A.M. Kligman

The Hydroxycitronellal Story: What Can We Learn from It? 159
R. R. Suskind

The Value of Animal Assays and the Quenching Phenomenon 166
D. Basketter

In Vitro Phototoxicity Tests for Fragrances 175
W. W. Lovell

RIFM Activities in the Safety Assessment of the Dermal Effects
of Fragrance Materials 182
R. A. Ford

Part V: The Producer's View 191

The Producer's View: Do We Worry About Adverse Effects? 193
P. Cadby

The IFRA Guidelines 197
F. Grundschober

Fragrances and Environmental Issues: A Case Example
of Environmental Risk Assessments of Ingredients 206
W. de Wolf and P. J. Kloepper-Sams

Fragrances – Future Aspects 216
I. R. White

Subject Index 225

List of Contributors

DAVID BASKETTER
Unilever Environmental Safety Laboratory
Colworth House,
Sharnbrook, Bedford, MK44 1LQ, U.K.

Dr. PETER CADBY
Firmenich SA
Route des Jeunes 1
CH-1211 Genève 8, Switzerland

Dr. PETRA CHRISTIANSEN-WENIGER
Borbyhof
D-23340 Eckernförde, Germany

ANTON C. DE GROOT, MD, PhD
Department of Dermatology
Carolus-Liduina Hospital
P.O. Box 1101
52 BD 's-Hertogenbosch,
The Netherlands

WATZE DE WOLF
N.V. Procter & Gamble
European Technical Center S.A.
Temselaan 100
B-1853 Strombeek-Bever, Belgium

RICHARD A. FORD, Ph.D.
Vice-President International Research Institute for Fragrance Materials, Inc.
Two University Plaza, Suite 406
Hackensack, N.J. 07601, U.S.A.

Prof. Dr. med. PETER J. FROSCH
Städtische Kliniken Dortmund
and Department of Dermatology,
University of Witten/Herdecke
Beurhausstraße 40
D-44137 Dortmund, Germany

FRIEDRICH GRUNDSCHOBER,
Dr. sc. techn.
International Fragrance Association
IFRA/IOFI
8, Rue Charles-Humbert
CH-1205 Genève 8, Switzerland

Dr. U. HARDER
Haarmann & Reimer
Rumohrtalstraße 1
D-377601 Holzminden, Germany

JURIJ J. HOSTÝNEK, M.D.
Department of Dermatology
School of Medicine
University of California
San Francisco, CA 94143-0980, U.S.A.

Dr. SHARON A. M. HOTCHKISS
Imperial College School of Medicine
at St. Marys
Norfolk Place
London W2 1PG, U.K.

Dr. JEANNE DUUS JOHANSEN
Department of Dermatology
Gentofte Hospital
University of Copenhagen
DK-2900 Hellerup, Denmark

Prof. ANN-THÉRESE KARLBERG
Dermatology Division
Department of Occupational Health
National Institute for Working Life
S-17184 Sollna, Sweden

Dr. BIRGIT KETTENMANN
Department of Experimental and
Clinical Pharmacology
University of Erlangen-Nuremberg
Krankenhausstraße 9
D-91054 Erlangen, Germany

A. M. KLIGMAN, M. D., Ph. D.
Department of Dermatology
University of Pennsylvania
226 Curie Boulevard
Philadelphia, PA 19104-61423, U.S.A.

Dr. PAMELA J. KLOEPPER-SAMS
Procter & Gamble
Sharon Woods Technical Center
Cincinnaty, OH, U.S.A.

Prof. Dr. G. KOBAL
Friedrich-Alexander-Universität
Institut für Pharmakologie und
Toxikologie
Arbeitsgruppe Physiologische
Pharmakologie
Krankenhausstraße 9
D-91054 Erlangen, Germany

Prof. Dr. WERNER U. LANGTHALER
Westfälische Wilhelms-Universität
Psychologisches Institut II
Fliednerstraße 21
D-48149 Münster, Germany

WALTER G. LARSEN, M. D.
Portland Dermatology Clinic
2250 N. W. Flanders, Suite 205
Portland, OR 97210-3488, U.S.A.

JAMES J. LEYDEN, M. D.
Department of Dermatology
School of Medicine
University of Pennsylvania
Philadelphia, PA, U.S.A.

JEAN-PIERRE LEPOITTEVIN, D. Sc.
Laboratoire de Dermatochimie
Université Louis Pasteur
Clinique Dermatologique, CHU
F-67091 Strasbourg Cedex, France

WILLIAM W. LOVELL
Unilever
Environmental Safety Laboratory
Colworth House, Sharnbrook
Bedford MK44 1LQ, U.K.

PHILIP S. MAGEE, M.D.
UCSF School of Medicine
Department of Dermatology
San Francisco, Ca 94143, U.S.A.

HOWARD I. MAIBACH, M.D.
Department of Dermatology
School of Medicine
University of California
San Francisco, CA 94143-0980, U.S.A.

Dr. REGINA E. MAIWORM
Westfälische Wilhelms-Universität
Psychologisches Institut II
Fliednerstraße 21
D-48149 Münster, Germany

Dr. STEPHAN G. MICHA
University of Kiel
Institut für Phytopathologie
D-24118 Kiel, Germany

Dr. VINCENT MUTTERER
Laboratoire de Dermatochimie
associé au CNRS
Université Louis Pasteur
Clinique Dermatologique, CHU
F-67091 Strasbourg Cedex, France

HIDEO NAKAYAMA, M.D.
Nakayama Dermatology Clinic
Shinyo CK Building 6F
3-3-5, Kami-Ohsaki
Shinagawaku, Tokyo 141, Japan

EMIL A. PFITZER, Sc. D.
President
Research Institute for Fragrance
Materials, Inc.
Two University Plaza, Suite 406
Hackensack, N.J. 07601, U.S.A.

GEORGE PRETI, Ph.D.
Monell Chemical Senses Center
3500 Market Street
Philadelphia, PA 19104, U.S.A.
and
Department of Dermatology
School of Medicine
University of Pennsylvania
Philadelphia, PA, U.S.A.

Dr. RAINER RADTKE
vorm. Zoologisches Institut
Universität Tübingen
Hagellocher Weg 74/1
D-72070 Tübingen, Germany

SURESH C. RASTOGI
Ministry of Environment and Energy
National Environmental Research
Institute
Frederiksborgvey 358
P.O. Box 358
DK-4000 Riskilde, Denmark

GERHARD G. RIMKUS
Food and Veterinary Institute (LVUA)
Schleswig-Holstein
Department of Redisue
and Contamination Analysis
Max-Eyth-Straße 5
D-24537 Neumünster, Germany

Dr. NUTCHAREE SIRI
Khon Kaen University
Department of Entomology
400 Khon Kaen, Thailand

Andrew I. Spielman, D. M. D. Ph. D.
New York University
College of Dentistry
Division of Basic Science
345 E. 24th Street
New York, NY 10010-4086, U.S.A.

Raymond R. Suskind, MD
Professor and Director Emeritus
Department fo Environmental Health
University of Cincinnati
P.O. Box 6700056
Cincinnaty, Ohio 45267-0056, U.S.A.

Dr. Ian R. White
St. John's Institute of Dermatology
St. Thomas' Hospital
London SEI 7EH, England

Part I
The Basics

The Art of Creating a Perfume

U. Harder

A perfume is a composition of odorous ingredients generally diluted with ethyl alcohol and experienced over a certain time frame. To bear an artistic and aesthetic value its constituents must be selected and quantified deliberately to form a specific olfactory shape which should be recognizable, interesting and harmonious. The aim of a perfume is to improve the quality of life by underlining the personality, attractiveness and well-being of its bearers.

The history of perfumery goes back to the early days of civilized man. For approximately 3000 years perfumers have been creating fragrances. Over the centuries the role of fragrance in society has blossomed. As the level of technology has developed, the perfumers have refined their skills. Today, the occupation of the perfumer is a well-established, but rather rare profession. Worldwide there exist less than 1000 professional perfumers. The prerequisites for this profession include the following skills: memory for odours and their characteristics and an artistic talent.

The perfumer's talent in designing a perfume can be seen in the ability to combine the diverse range of fragrance ingredients into complex fragrances. In order to create a modern perfume the perfumer carries out hundreds of experiments to determine the optimal balance of the ingredients. In a finished fragrance the number of ingredients can reach into the hundreds – including the components of complex natural products and pre-fabricated "bases". A modern collection of raw materials contains 1000–3000 ingredients. In a well-balanced and constructed fragrance the materials have been arranged by the perfumer in a way that they interact and develop in a continuous and harmonious order.

Since a fragrance character evolves over time, the volatility of all raw materials play a decisive role. The most volatile ingredients are called "top notes" (citrus, green-leafy, herbaceous, aldehydic, fruity and spicy); this is then followed by the "bouquet" or "heart note" built up by floral accords, forming the most essential part of the perfume; the long-lasting materials must be learned as "bottom" or "dry-down" notes. These include woody, moss-like and sweet vanilla-like ingredients together with animal elements, mostly of musky character.

The talent of a perfumer in designing a perfume can be seen in his ability to combine components from different odour families and of different volatility in a way that a continuous development of the fragrance without fractures is achieved – with the aim to evoke emotions and passions.

Since ancient times there have been certain fundamental rules concerning the structure of a perfume. The framework is built up by ingredients reminiscent of our natural environment; these mostly belong to the floral, balsamic and woody family. To make the perfume sensual a small but very effective amount of ingredients recalling body odours is included. Typical ingredients out of the animal kingdom are musk and civet, which nowadays are usually replaced by musk-like aroma chemicals in larger quantities or specific blends based on such ingredients. The erogenous character is underlined by small amounts of fatty aldehydes and acids reminiscent of skin odours. Fresh citrus and leaf-like elements – together with spicy and fruity notes impart a more appealing character to the fragrance.

The principle structures and patterns of perfumes have not changed that dramatically throughout the history of perfumery. The difference between an ancient and a modern perfume lies in different raw materials, a different price range and a different way of compounding.

Until the second half of the nineteenth century the perfumer had at his disposal only products obtained by processing natural materials. Nevertheless, in the course of time refined processes were developed to isolate materials of a better quality and variety of scents. These processes, in the sequence of their appearance, include maceration of plant materials, water steam distillation and extraction using organic solvents. A real revolution started in the last quarter of the nineteenth century with the synthesis of aroma chemicals. The development of aroma chemicals can be divided into three periods, each of which inspired the perfumer to create specific fragrances. In the classical period from 1885–1950 the majority of aroma chemicals representing the different fragrance categories were synthesized.

In the industrial period, after World War and until approximately 1975, a new generation of inexpensive, stable and diffusive aroma chemicals were developed, fitting into the new mass market. In the third period – the period of trace components – extremely powerful so-called trace aroma chemicals were detected with the help of advanced analytic methods and afterwards synthesized; products which in many cases beside C, H and O also contain hetero atoms such as N and S.

The different aroma chemicals periods are reflected in corresponding perfume types. The first aroma chemicals of the classical period were mostly used in combination with a frame of rather expensive natural raw materials. Synthetic components in this case modified and modernized classical concepts. The perfumes stayed to be rather expensive and exclusive.

After World War II the role and the structure of a perfume started to change. Perfumes increasingly conquered the mass market. The price went down, and the perfume had to change its structure. More and more the perfumer created perfumes based on rather inexpensive synthetic aroma chemicals. At the same time the individuality of the character was more pronounced. The skeleton of the fragrance was constructed with aroma chemicals, whereas the natural ingredients introduced volume and harmony.

The trace aroma chemicals of the third period are used as characteristic elements in a new generation of perfumes. Modern fragrances in many cases have a rather simple structure using a combination of a few ingredients at high doses which never before had been used. In many cases these show a very good harmony in their development in a time frame. Due to the high dose of ingredients the modern period is also called the epoch of "overdose". The rather simple fundamental structure is now completed by adding trace aroma chemicals and other ingredients in smaller amounts.

Today perfumery is an applied art, which is designed for the market. This market now depends on the entire cultural condition of a society together with fashion trends and the general life-style. Different fragrance world markets are based on completely different backgrounds. In the United States mostly characteristic, powerful and diffusive perfumes are worn. In Japan, on the other hand, the perfume should be discreet and unobtrusive with the aim of being in harmony with the environment and society.

When creating a new perfume the perfumer has basically three different possibilities. The new idea can be based on a novel accord, an impression or a variation of an existing concept. New accords are presumably the most creative possibilities for novel perfumes. Accords in perfumery must be understood in a similar way as in music: a combination of a few ingredients leading to a new fragrance impression which is different from the sum of the odours of the components. The ratio of the ingredients even in a very simple accord are largely unpredictable. In many cases a new accord contains a novel, mostly synthetic, but sometimes also natural ingredient.

The second creative approach for a new perfume is the interpretation of an impression. This impression may be the scenery of a Mediterranean coastline or an Oriental bazaar. The third and most frequently used method to obtain novel fragrance concepts is the variation of existing perfume ideas. This can be done by changing a floral element (e.g. hyacinth for carnation) or a woody part against a sweet vanilla note. In spite of such rather small changes the performance of the new perfume might be quite different.

Despite the ever increasing restrictions limiting the use of many traditional ingredients, perfume will continue to be a part of our cultural and social worlds. Through his creativity, the perfumer will overcome these new challenges and create modern novel perfumes.

Cerebral Representation of Odour Perception

G. Kobal and B. Kettenmann

Introduction

The cerebral representation of odour perception in man is poorly understood compared to other sensory modalities such as hearing, vision and touch. This may result partly from the lack of appropriate instruments for specific stimulation of chemosensors, making investigations of these systems extremely difficult. Primary olfactory structures, namely the olfactory bulb, olfactory tract and piriform cortex, which have been studied in animal experiments, are also recognizable in humans (Price 1990). However, very little is known of neocortical regions that are involved in the processing of olfactory information. Findings in patients with brain lesions indicate that for the perception of odors the temporal lobe is of critical importance (Eichenbaum et al. 1983; Eskenazi 1986).

Recent progress in the field of neuronal imaging has enabled study of the functional topography of the olfactory system in greater detail. Results obtained by positron emission tomography (PET) show that in addition to a bilateral increase of cerebral blood flow (CBF) in the piriform cortex, the insular cortex and the right orbitofrontal cortex are also activated by odorous stimulation (Zatorre et al. 1992). Another experiment using functional magnetic resonance imaging (fMRI) has also shown a significant bilateral increase of CBF in the piriform cortex and the orbitofrontal cortex (Koizuka et al. 1994). A major disadvantage of these two imaging techniques is their low temporal resolution. By olfactory event related potentials (Finkenzeller 1966; Allison and Goff 1967; Kobal and Plattig 1978; Kobal 1981; Kobal and Hummel 1988; for review see Kobal and Hummel 1991) it has become possible noninvasively to record the activity of cortical neurons in fractions of a second. Recently, magnetic source imaging (MSI) has been used to identify brain areas activated after olfactory stimulation (Kettenmann et al. 1996).

The general goal of magnetoencephalography (MEG) is to localize magnetic fields measured at the surface of the scalp (Cohen 1972). These magnetic fields are generated by a number of cerebral neurons (electrically) active at the same time. Assuming that the human head is a spherical volume conductor

(Abraham-Fuchs al. 1988), and that electrical neuronal activity has the property of a current dipole possessing an electric field and a magnetic field, it is possible to calculate the location the orientation and the strength of the current sources creating the magnetic field measured at the surface of the sphere (Williamson and Kaufman 1981; Romani et al. 1982). In this model, not knowing the number of active dipoles, the magnetic field may be generated by one dipole or by several different ones (inverse problem; Helmholz 1853). Unfortunately, this is the situation in the active brain, and therefore a unique solution can not be obtained. Additionally, a radial dipole does not produce a magnetic field that can be measured with the usual order of the magnetometer. This dipole is silent and cannot be localized.

On the basis of a measured magnetic field a dipole position is estimated and followed by a nonlinear fit-strategy such as a Marquardt (1963) or Powell (1964) algorithm. With this procedure the location, strength and orientation of the theoretically determined dipole is iteratively changed in such a way that the magnetic field produced by this calculated dipole corresponds to the dipole measured by the magnetometer. The statistical procedure leading to the so-called equivalent current dipole is a least-squares solution. An extensive description of the data analysis applied can be found elsewhere (Scholz and Oppel 1992). Naturally the accuracy depends strongly on the signal to noise ratio (SNR) of the measured data and additionally increases with increasing depth of the dipole within the sphere. Also, the localization accuracy is better for a dipole centered below the measurement grid than below the outer part of the measurement grid. For the situation in the brain this error can be estimated only by simulations (Hari 1988; Janday 1987; Meijs 1988; Barth 1986).

By linking the magnetically defined equivalent current dipoles to the anatomical data of MRI (Stefan et al. 1990), it is now possible to visualize the location of activated areas in the subjects' brain and to check them for their anatomical and physiological plausibility.

In addition to these basic problems caused by physics, the reliability of the estimations is affected by external error sources, for example, magnetic noise cause by electronic devices or artifacts caused by the subjects themselves or the subjects' organs, such as heart activity (Abraham-Fuchs et al. 1988; Hansen et al. 1988; for review see Hämäläinen et al. 1993).

Employing a whole-head neuromagnetometer (Helsinki, Finland), Kettenmann et al. (1996) found bilateral activation in the superior temporal sulcus at approximately 700 ms using vanillin, phenylethyl alcohol and hydrogen sulfide. These three substances were chosen because they are specific odorants, i.e. do not activate the trigeminal nerve, and therefore more appropriate for studying the sense of smell than those used by Zatorre and Koizuka (Beidler and Tucker 1956; Silver et al. 1986; Kobal and Hummel 1991; Hummel and Kobal 1992; Doty et al. 1978).

The study presented here sought to confirm the results obtained with the whole-head magnetometer by employing a planar 37-channel sensor array (Erlangen, Krenikon), and additionally to identify the neuronal generators underlying the earlier components of the event-related potentials in the time interval between 200 and 700 ms after olfactory stimulation.

Material and Methods

Subjects

Ten healthy volunteers participated in the experiments (5 men and 5 women; 20–40 years of age, mean 28). They were carefully trained in avoiding eye blinking and other movement artifacts. Respiratory airflow in the nose that may affect the stimuli quantitatively was avoided by the subjects performing a special breathing technique (velopharyngeal closure, Kobal 1985).

The study was conducted in accordance with the revised version of the Helsinki/Hong Kong Declaration and was approved by the Ethics Committee of the University of Erlangen-Nuremberg.

Stimulation

For olfactory stimulation an apparatus was employed which delivered the stimulants without altering the mechanical or thermal conditions at the mucosa (Kobal 1985; Kobal and Hummel 1988). This monomodal olfactory stimulation was achieved by mixing pulses of the odorants in a constantly flowing air stream (total flow rate 140 ml/s) with controlled temperature and humidity (36.5 °C, 80 % relative humidity). Stimuli were applied nonsynchronously to breathing. Odor concentration was defined once in the beginning of the experiment by gas chromatography for vanillin. In case of H_2S predefined concentrations in pressure gas cylinders (22 ppm) were used. Before each sessions the olfactometer was calibrated, and the concentration was calculated by the flow rate of dilution.

The olfactometer was especially designed for this experiment. Twelve separately temperature controlled teflon tubings were fed through a grid with 3 × 3 cm wholes, incorporated in the wall of the shielded room. This did not alter the quality of shielding (measured by frequency distribution). All parts of the olfactometer consisted of nonmagnetic materials such as teflon, silicon, plexiglas, glass, gas and water. Even at a distance of 5 m between the outlet of the olfactometer and the solenoid valves the olfactometer can provide steep increase of odor pulses, which was verified by measuring CO_2 pulses with a thermistor (for more details see Kobal 1985). Subjects were seated comfortably in a magnetically shielded, ventilated chamber which could be monitored by means of a video system. White noise (approximately 60 dB SPL) applied to both ears was used to mask the switching clicks of the stimulator. The sound was transfered via air conduction through two hollow plastic tubings which were used as a connection between an acoustic stimulator outside the shielded room and the subjects' ears. Each subject participated in six experimental sessions on each of four experimental days (three experimental sessions for one nostril). In one experimental day either one of the two substances hydrogen sulfide (0.8 ppm) or vanillin (2.1 ppm) was tested with the sensor array positioned over one hemisphere. Sites of sensor location (left/right hemisphere MEG recording) and application of the two odorants was randomized across experimental days. Three sessions were performed for each nostril. During each of the three sessions 30 stimuli of the same substance were applied by way of teflon tubing (6 cm length, 2 mm inner diameter). To avoid habituation an interstimulus interval (isi) of 40 s and a stimulus duration of 200 ms was used so that there was no residual odorant left in the tubings. Additionally, the three sessions performed for one nostril were separated by breaks of 10 min. Subsequently data were averaged across these sessions if the head position of the subject had not changed (controlled by laser motion detector).

Olfactory Event Related Potentials

Olfactory event related potentials (OERP) were obtained from electrodes positioned at the vertex (Cz/A1). They were used as temporal markers during the analysis of the magnetic responses.

Olfactory Event Related Magnetic Fields

The olfactory event related magnetic fields (OERMF) were obtained by means of a biomagnetic system (Siemens, Krenikon) with a sensor array of 37 first-order gradiometers (baseline 7 cm) in a circular arrangement of 19 cm diameter (Hoenig et al. 1991). It was possible to obtain isocontour plots from the region of interest without repositioning. Electroencephalographical (EEG) and MEG data were recorded with a sampling rate of 500 Hz, a bandpass filter 0.1–70 Hz and filtered offline with a 30 Hz lowpass digital filter. The source analyses were based on signals averaged from artifact free records ($30 < n < 90$).

For data evaluation we used a map correlation 0.92, defined as:

$$\frac{\sum_{i=1}^{N} (xi - \bar{x})(yi - \bar{y})}{\sqrt{\sum_{i=1}^{N} (xi - \bar{x})^2 \sum_{i=1}^{N} (yi - \bar{y})^2}}$$

We used an interval length with a minimum of 0.006 s. The upper and lower limits for the strength of the reconstructed source was defined as $>0.007 < 0.03$ mA mm (deduced from electrophysiology).

Furthermore, an upper limit for the rate of change of the source strength was defined (factor < 10). The acceptable localization error was set to 20 mm as a maximum (defined as the area in which the equivalent current dipole has its possible location).

A magnetic field was called consistent if it lasted over a minimum time period of 10 ms. As a result the field patterns were individually and interindividually reproducible, equivalent current dipoles (ECDs) could be localized at nearly the same latency in about the same anatomical structure.

The time of best fit (TOBF) for one ECD estimated gives the time point were the isofield map of this special ECD shows its best "map correlation", which means that at this TOBF the measured map of the ECD has the best correlation with the theoretically calculated map, it has the smallest localization error and the best SNR. This does not mean that the neuronal source is only active at this time point. It can already start being active several milliseconds before and after this TOBF, but dependent on the actual situation it can be masked by additional neuronal activity from other sources.

The SNR of the data determines the accuracy in biomagnetic source reconstruction. In order to increase the SNR we used the averaging procedure (Abraham-Fuchs et al. 1990). A vertical electro-oculogram was used to detect signals coinciding with eye blinks or movements. Records contaminated with EOG deflections >200 μV were rejected. The noise level of the pretrigger period of the averaged session was estimated and used as a baseline. The noise level of all 64 measurements was in the range of 0.00003 pT^2 and 0.000488 pT^2, with a mean value of 0.000222 ± 0.000128 pT^2. The signals of the ECDs were in the range of eight to ten times higher than the calculated noise. No average across sessions was calculated.

MRI was used to provide accurate images of the brain's anatomy. For the alignment of the functional MEG information with this tomographic information a head coordinate system, defined by the nasion and the two preauricular points, was created for each subject. Contrast giving water pellets (0.3 mm diameter) were attached to the subjects skin during the MRI, and subsequently their locations were projected into the coordinate system of the MEG data. Individually shaped realistic conductor models which might provide better localization accuracy were not supported by the Krenikon software. To deduce the positioning of the subjects head with respect to the sensor array after head positioning the three landmarks were digitized with a 3-D digitizer (Isotrak, Polhemus Navigation Sciences, Colchester, VT, USA) and aligned with the coordinate system received from the MRI. This method of alignment presupposes that the subject is not moving during the measurement since dislocations can not be detected (controlled by a laser motion detector). To minimize the possibility of moving, the head was stabilized with a vacuum pillow.

Control measurements were carried out to exclude the possible contamination of the measured signals by tactile or auditory artifacts. Humidified blanks delivered to the nostrils did not result in activity in the MEG or in the EEG measurements.

Results

The signal quality of the evoked responses was sufficient for source localization in eight of the ten subjects. Consistent magnetic fields were identified in both hemispheres following the stimulation of each nostril. In 60% of the measurements reproducible dipolar field patterns were obtained 226–380 ms after stimulus onset, preceding or following the first major positive electric deflection of the event-related potential (P1). This equivalent current dipole was termed ECD I. In 44% of the measurements a reproducible dipolar distribution was obtained 306–486 ms after stimulus onset, corresponding to the ascending or descending slope of the N1 component, which was termed ECD II. In the left hemisphere this dipole was not identifiable in any of the subjects after stimulation with hydrogen sulfide. It was identifiable only in the right hemisphere in 36% of the measurements. The most stable dipolar field pattern appeared 518–730 ms after stimulus onset (in 66% of the measurements; ECD III) corresponding to the P2 component of the electrical response.

Figure 1 shows OERMFs recorded from one subject over the right hemisphere after stimulation of the right nostril with vanillin. In this case ECDs with best fits were obtained at 238 ms (ECD I), 308 ms (ECD II) and 524 ms (ECD III) after stimulus onset. The source orientations indicated a current flow towards central/parietal regions for ECD I and ECD III. For ECD II a current-flow pointed in the opposite direction, consistent with the polarity of the peaks of the OERPs.

In five subjects, and 14% of all measurements, all of the three ECDs could be identified during one session. In all other cases where ECD I was identified it was localized in the area between the superior temporal plane and the parainsular cortex. In seven out of eight patient a generator was localized in the left hemisphere after stimulation of the left nostril with vanillin. This was statistically significant (chi-square test: 4.5; df: 1; $p=0.034$). ECD II was localized in the anterior-central parts of the insula. In seven out of eight patient this generator was localized in the right hemisphere after stimulation of the right nostril with vanillin. This was also statistically significant (chi-square test: 4.5; df: 1; $p=0.0339$). ECD III was obtained in the superior temporal sulcus. In seven out of eight patient a statistical significance was obtained for this gene-

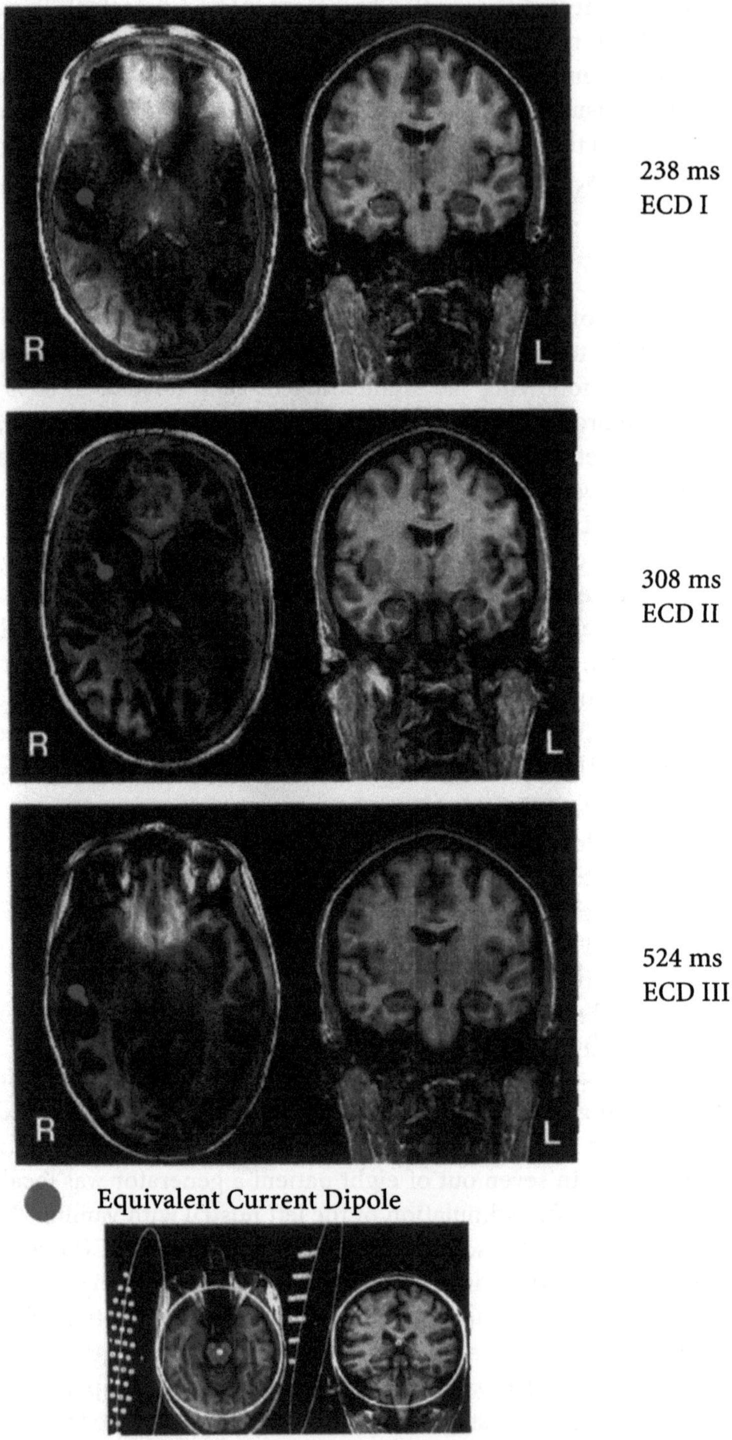
R
L
238 ms
ECD I
R
L
308 ms
ECD II
R
L
524 ms
ECD III
Equivalent Current Dipole

rator localized in the left hemisphere after stimulation of the left nostril with hydrogen sulfide (chi-square test: 4.5; df: 1; $p=0.0339$). An example of the localizations after stimulation with hydrogen sulfide is given in Fig. 2.

Intraindividually, spatial differences of localization sites for one type of ECD were less than 20 mm. Individually, the angle of orientation varied between 10° and 30° in all three dimensions. The dipole strength varied between 0.009 and 0.03 mA mm.

Discussion

Localization results of the OERFs demonstrated that odorants specifically activate neocortical areas, i.e., during the period of time when the ERP is obtained, areas between the superior temporal plane and the parainsular cortex, anterior-central parts of the insula and the superior temporal sulcus were active. These electro(magneto)physiological data confirm the hypothesis that there is a direct connection between primary olfactory areas and the insular cortex (Mesulam and Mufson 1982). Physiological and axonal tracer experiments in animals consistently demonstrated inputs from the primary olfactory cortical areas to the ventral agranular insular area (Clugnet and Price 1987; Carmichael et al. 1994).

The results of this study describing activity in the superior temporal sulcus (ECD III) also confirm findings of a previously published report using a whole-head neuromagnetometer (Kettenmann et al. 1996). These data indicate for the first time by different measurements, the activation of the superior temporal sulcus after olfactory stimulation. This finding is supported by the fact that there are axonal connections between the inferior orbitofrontal areas that receive input from specific olfactory structures, i.e. the primary olfactory cortex (Carmichael and Price 1995) and the superior temporal sulcus. With one exception both the dipole locations and the dipole orientations were reproducible for the responses after stimulation with both odorants. Hence, both odorants seem to activate similar cortical areas. The data also showed bilateral neocortical activation. This must be considered when discussing the hypothesis that olfactory input is primarily processed ipsilaterally to the stimulated nostril (Gordon and Sperry 1969; Youngentoub et al. 1982).

Fig. 1. Localization of neuronal activity after vanillin stimulation of the right nostril. Example of one subject. In this subject all three ECDs (ECD I–III) were obtained. Symbols, the active cortical regions in the axial and the coronal view (arrow size corresponds to the size of the dipole vector). Lower right, positioning of the sensor array and the model sphere used for calculation. The sensors are placed over the temporal lobe of the right hemisphere

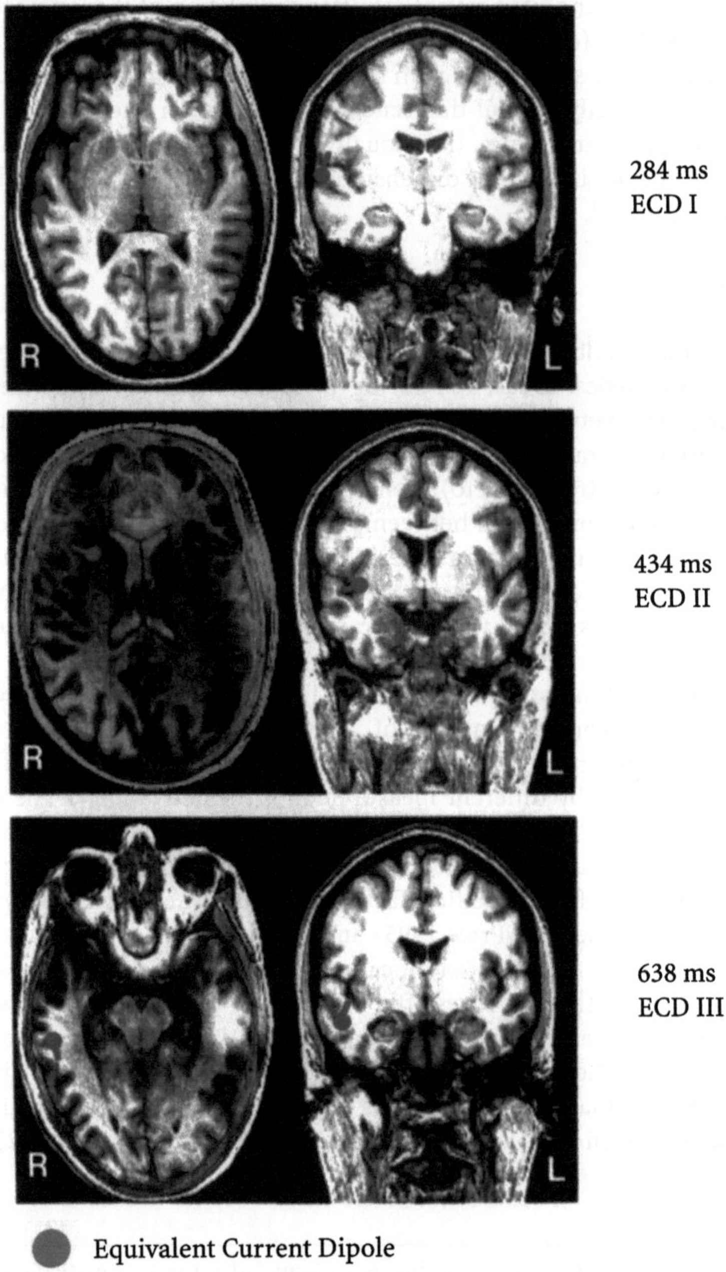

Fig. 2. Localization of neuronal activity after hydrogen sulfide stimulation of the right nostril. Example of one subject. In this subject all three ECDs (ECD I–III) were obtained. Symbols, the active cortical regions in the axial and the coronal view (arrow size corresponds to the size of the dipole vector)

Also in animal studies it has been demonstrated that there are bilateral connections between the anterior olfactory nucleus, the anterior part of the piriform cortex and neocortical areas. The fibers cross in the anterior commissure and are distributed equally in both hemispheres (Price 1990). However, there was one exception in the bilaterality of our results. We were not able to identify the ECD II in the left hemisphere after stimulation with hydrogen sulfide. This might indicate the coding of qualitative differences between hydrogen sulfide and vanillin. Of course, this hypothesis must be extensively tested using a larger scale of odorants. An earlier study demonstrated that amplitudes and latencies of OERPs elicited by vanillin and hydrogen sulfide are correlated with their hedonic properties (Kobal et al. 1992). Responses to hydrogen sulfide had significantly shorter latencies and smaller amplitudes after stimulation of the left nostril than to responses after stimulation of the right nostril. In contrast, latencies were longer when the left nostril was stimulated with vanillin and the amplitudes of the N1/P2 components were significantly larger than responses after stimulation of the other nostril. This finding was reproduced in another experiment where subjective estimates of the odorants showed that after stimulation of the left nostril, the more pleasant the perception of the odor was, the larger were the amplitudes and the longer were the latencies (Kobal et al. 1989).

In the light of the results of the present study this could mean that different cortical areas are activated after stimulation with odorants of different hedonic properties. There is also some evidence for lateralization of hedonic information from clinical studies. Pleasant emotions seem to be processed predominantly by the left hemisphere and unpleasant emotions by the right hemisphere (Davidson 1984; Dimond et al. 1976). The missing ECD II in the left insular cortex following hydrogen sulfide stimulation may justify the speculation that the observed differences in the responses to vanillin and hydrogen sulfide have their origin in the asymmetrical activation of the insular region. Of course, this does not yet explain why the differences in the OEP were observed only when left and right nostril stimulation was compared.

Another indication for lateralization was found by Hummel et al. (1995) investigating patient suffering from temporal lobe epilepsy. When olfactory stimuli were presented ipsilaterally to the epileptic focus, peak latencies of the OERP were prolonged in comparison to OERPs obtained after contralateral stimulation. Additionally, the topographical distribution of the P2 component changed in patients with right-sided foci. In these patients the amplitude of P2 was maximal at Cz, whereas in previous studies in normal subjects, maximal P2 amplitudes were always obtained at Pz (Hummel et al. 1992; Livermore et al. 1992).

The significance of olfaction in humans is stressed by the fact that olfactory dysfunctions can produce severe impairments in the quality of life. Infections (e.g. postviral anosmia), degeneration (e.g. hyposmia in Alzheimer's and Parkinson's disease) or a tumor affecting the olfactory bulb (Murphy 1987) belong to those diseases not yet sufficiently curable. In addition, the sense of smell plays a role in complex and controversial discussed disorders, such as idiopathic environmental intolerances (Hummel 1996). It is interesting to hypothesize that the underlying pathology results in changes of cortical functions. Possible dislocations and plastic changes might be easily studied using the technique of MSI.

In sum, for the first time, brain areas have been identified that generate some of the components of olfactory bioresponses (OERPs and OERFs), in humans. Deduced from our results we have strong evidence to believe that apart from the known primary olfactory areas these neocortical areas are of specific olfactory origin.

Acknowledgements. This research was supported by DFG grant Ko812/5-1. We thank Dr. Elisabeth Pauli, Department of Neurology, University of Erlangen-Nuremberg, for performing the statistical analysis of the data.

References

Abraham-Fuchs, Schneider S, Reichenberger H (1988) MCG Inverse solution: influence of coil size, grid size, number of coils and SNR. IEEE Trans Biom Eng BE-35:573-576

Abraham-Fuchs K, Härer W, Schneider S, Stefan H (1990) Pattern recognition in biomagnetic signals by spatio temporal correlation and application to the localization of propagating neuronal activity. Med Biol Eng Comput 28:398-406

Allison T, Goff WR (1967) Human cerebral evoked responses to odorous stimuli. Electroencephalogr Clin Neurophysiol 23:558-560

Barth DS, Sutherling W, Broffman J, Beatty J (1986) Magnetic localization of dipolar current source implanted in a sphere and a human cranium. Electroencephalogr Clin Neurophysiol 63:260-273

Beidler LM, Tucker D (1956) Olfactory and trigeminal nerve responses to odors. Fed Proc 15:14-21

Carmichael ST, Price J L (1995) Sensory and premotor connections of the orbital and medial prefrontal cortex. J Comp Neurol 363(4):642-664

Carmichael ST, Clugnet M-C, Price JL (1994) Central olfactory connections in the macaque monkey. J Comp Neurol 346:403-434

Clugnet M-C, Price JL (1987) Olfactory input to the prefrontal cortex in the rat. Ann NY Acad Sci 510:231-235

Cohen D (1972) Magnetoencephalography: detection of the brain's electrical activity with a superconducting magnetometer. Science 175:664-666

Davidson RJ (1984) Affect, cognition and hemispheric specialization. In: Izard CE, Kagan J, Zajonc R (eds) Physiological correlates of human behavior. London, Academic

Dimond SJ, Farrington L, Johnson P (1976) Differing emotional responses from right and left hemispheres. Nature 261:690-692

Doty RL, Brugger v WPE, Jurs PC, Orndorff MA, Snyder PJ, Lowry LD (1978) Intranasal trigeminal stimulation from odorous volatiles: psychometric responses from anosmics and normal humans. Physiol Behav 20:175-185

Eichenbaum H, Morton TH, Potter H, Corkin S (1983) Selective olfactory deficits in case HM. Brain 106:459-472

Eskenazi B (1986) Odor perception in temporal lobe epilepsy patients with and without temporal lobectomy. Neuropsychol 24:553-562

Finkenzeller P (1966) Gemittelte EEG-Potentiale bei olfaktorischer Reizung. Pflugers Arch 292:76-80

Gordon HW, Sperry RW (1969) Lateralization of olfactory perception in the surgically separated hemispheres of man. Neuropsychol 7:11-120

Hämäläinen M, Hari R, Ilmoniemi RJ, Knuutila J, Lounasmaa O (1993) Magnetoencephalography - theory, instrumentation, and applications to noninvasive studies of the working human brain. Rev Mod Phys 65:413-497

Hansen JS, Ko HW, Fisher RS, Litt B (1988) Practical limits on the biomagnetic inverse process determined from in vitro measurements in spherical conducting volumes. Phys Med Biol 33:105-111

Hari R, Joutsiniemi SL, Sarvas J (1988) Spatial resolution of neuromagnetic records: theoretical calculations in a spherical model. EEG Clin Neurophysiol 71:64-72

Helmholz H von (1853) Über einige Gesetze der Verteilung elektrischer Ströme in körperlichen Leitern, mit Anwendung auf die thierisch-elektrischen Versuche. Ann Phys Chem 89:211-233, 353-377

Hoenig HE, Daalmans GM, Bär L, Bömmel F, Paulus A, Uhl D, Weisse HJ, Schneider S, Seifert H, Reichenberger H, Abraham-Fuchs K (1991) Multichannel DC SQUID sensor array for biomagnetic applications. IEEE Trans Magn 27:2777-2785

Hummel T, Kobal G (1992) Differences in human evoked potentials related to olfactory or trigeminal chemosenory activation. Electroencephogr Clin Neurophysiol 84:84-89

Hummel T, Pauli E, Schüler P, Kettenmann B, Stefan H, Kobal G (1995) Chemosensory event-related potentials in patients with temporal lobe epilepsy. Epilepsia 26(1): 79-85

Hummel T, Roscher S, Jaumann MP, Kobal G (1996) Intranasal chemoreception in patients with multiple chemical sensitivities: a double-blind investigation. Reg Indus Health (submitted)

Janday BS, Swithenby SJ (1987) Analysis of magnetoencephalographic data using the homogeneous sphere model: empirical tests. Phys Med Biol 32(1):105-113

Kettenmann B, Jousmäki V, Portin K, Salmelin R, Kobal G, Hari R (1996) Odorants activate the human superior temporal sulcus. Neurosci Lett 203:1-3

Kobal G (1981) Elektrophysiologische Untersuchungen des menschlichen Geruchssinns. Thieme, Stuttgart

Kobal G (1985) Pain-related electrical potentials of the human nasal mucosa elicited by chemical stimulation. Pain 22:151-163

Kobal G, Plattig K-H (1978) Methodische Anmerkungen zur Gewinnung olfaktorischer EEG-Antworten des wachen Menschen (objective Olfaktometrie) Z EEG-EMG 9:135-145

Kobal G, Hummel T (1988) Olfaction: chemosensory evoked potentials in patients with olfactory disturbances. Rhinology 26 [Suppl]:1-18

Kobal G, Hummel T (1991) Olfactory evoked potentials in humans. In: Getchell TV, Doty RL, Bartoshuk LM, Snow JR, Jr (eds) Smell and taste in health and disease. Raven, New York, pp 255-275

Kobal G, Van Toller S, Hummel T (1989) Is there directional smelling? Experientia 45:130-132

Kobal G, Hummel T, Van Toller S (1992) Differences in human chemosensory evoked potentials to olfactory and somatosensory chemical stimuli presented to left and right nostrils. Chem Senses 17(3):233-244

Koizuka I, Yano H, Nagahara M, Seo R, Shimada K, Kubo T, Nogawa T (1994) Functional imaging of the human olfactory cortex by magnetic resonance imaging. ORL 56:273–275

Livermore A, Hummel T, Kobal G (1992) Chemosensory evoked potentials in the investigation of interactions between the olfactory and the somatosensory (trigeminal) system. Electroenceph. Clin Neurophysiol 83:201–210

Marquardt DW (1963) An algorithm for least-squares estimation of nonlinear parameters. J Soc Ind Appl Math 11:431–441

Meijs JW, ten Voorde BJ, Peters JM (1988) On the influence of various head models on EEGs and MEGs. In: Pfurtscheller G, Lopes da Silva FH (eds) Functional brain imaging. Springer, Berlin Heidelberg New York, pp 31–45

Mesulam M-M, Mufson EJ (1982) Insula of the old world monkey. I. Architectonics in the insulo-orbito-temporal component of the paralimbic brain. J Comp. Neurol 212:1–22

Murphy C (1987) Olfactory psychophysics. In: Neurobiology of taste and smell. Wiley, New York, pp 251–274

Price JL (1990) Olfactory system. In: The human nervous system. Academic, p 29

Powell MJD (1964) An efficient method for finding the minimum of a function of several variables without calculating derivatives. Computer J 7:155–162

Romani GL, Williamson SJ, Kaufman L (1982) Biomagnetic instrumentation. Rev Sci Instrum 53:1815–1845

Scholz B, Oppelt A (1992) Probability based dipole localization and individual localization error calculation in biomagnetism. Proc Ann IEEE Med Biol Soc 14:1766–1767

Silver WL, Mason JR, Marshall DA, Maruniak JA (1986) Rat trigeminal, olfactory and taste responses after capsaicin desensitization. Brain Res 333:45–54

Stefan H, Schneider S, Abraham K, Bauer J, Neubauer U, Röhrlein G, Huk WJ (1990) Magnetic source localization in focal epilepsy; first experiences with multichannel MEG correlated to MR brain imaging. Brain 113:1347–1359

Williamson SJ, Kaufman L (1981) Biomagnetism. J Magn. Magn. Mat. 22:129–201

Youngentoub SL, Kurtz DB, Leopold DA, Mozell MM, Hornung DE (1982) Olfactory sensitivity: is there laterality? Chem Senses 7:1–9

Zatorre RJ, Jones-Gotman M, Evans AC, Meyer E (1992) Functional localization and lateralization of human olfactory cortex. Nature 360:339–340

Part II
Beneficial Biological Effects

The Structure, Origin and Function of Human Axillary Odours

G. Preti, A. I. Spielman and J. J. Leyden

Introduction

Human body odours generally arise from the interaction of the resident microorganisms with skin gland and other secretions and are a function of the location on the body where the odor is being produced. The amounts of moisture and skin gland secretions as well as oxygen availability determine the type and number of flora present on different areas of the body. The mouth, axillae, genital region and feet support greater varieties and numbers of bacteria due to their occluded and moist environment; consequently these are also the primary odor-producing areas found on humans [1, 2].

Metabolic disorders such as diabetes or trimethylaminuria and microbiological infections in certain areas will give rise to abnormal and sporadic malodor production [3, 4]. Although our research has examined several odor-producing areas at different times [4–6], the research presented here will focus upon the odor produced in the axillary region and its putative function.

The identity of the volatile chemicals responsible for axillary odours (commonly referred to as "body odour") is of both commercial and biological importance. Commercially, more than 1.5 billion dollars a year are spent in the United States alone on products to eliminate, attenuate or mask the odours produced in the axillae. The axillae can support a large population of aerobic microflora because of moisture and secretions from eccrine, apocrine, apoeccrine and sebaceous glands. These microflora are responsible for axillary odour production. Several studies have demonstrated that diphtheroid bacteria are important odor producers, and apocrine gland secretions are the principle odour-producing substrate [7, 8].

Biologically, extracts of human axillary secretions from both males and females have been shown to alter the length and timing of the female menstrual cycle. The latter effect suggests that human axillary secretions contain physiologically active materials that function as primer pheromones capable of altering neuroendocrinology via chronic exposure.

The Characteristic Axillary Odours and Their Origin

Prior to our recent research, a number of investigations of axillary secretion constituents focused upon the interesting steroidal molecules found in the underarm area. Both radioimmunoassay techniques as well as combined gas chromatography/mass spectrometry (GC/MS) were employed to identify volatile, odoriferous steroids in the axillae [9, 10], particularly 5α-androst-16-en-3β-ol (androstenol) and 5α-androst-16-en-3-one (androstenone). These compounds have musky, urine-like odors which were thought by some authors to be suggestive of axillary odors [7, 9, 10]. However, our recent studies have presented both organoleptic and analytical evidence to demonstrate that the mixture of C_6-C_{11} branched, straight-chained and unsaturated acids present in axillary sweat, constitute the characteristic axillary odor [11–13]. In terms of relative abundance, these acids, in particular (*E*)-3-methyl-2-hexenoic acid (*E*-3M2H), are present in far greater quantity that the $C_{19}\Delta^{16}$-volatile steroids. In the combined male samples we analyzed, *E*-3M2H is the dominant component and present at far greater concentration than androstenone: ~357 ng/µl extract of *E*-3M2H versus ~0.5 ng/µl extract of androstenone [11]. In combined female samples, the straight-chain acids were present in greater relative abundance than *E*-3M2H; further, no androstenone was seen in female extracts. Androstenol was present, albeit in far lower concentration that E-3M2H or the other acids: ~150 ng/µl extract of *E*-3M2H versus ~3.5 ng/µl extract androstenol [13]. The *Z*-isomer of 3M2H is also present in each gender, however in different relative abundance: 10:1 (*E*: *Z*) in males and 16:1 (*E*: *Z*) in females.

Although *E*-3M2H is a major analytical component of the characteristic axillary odour in males, a number of components are necessary for the complete axillary "bouquet" (see Table 1). In addition, studies from both our laboratory [14] and another [15] have documented both the presence of a specific anosmia for both isomers of 3M2H and an olfactory threshold for the *E*-isomer that is of the same order of magnitude as that for androstenone [16]. Consequently, the strength and quality of the odour produced in the axillae appears to be related to the axillary bacterial populations and perhaps the concentrations of 3M2H present, but further, rigorous organoleptic studies must confirm this.

Studies performed and reviewed in the past several decades have demonstrated that the precursors to axillary odour reside in the apocrine glands [7–9, 17]. The characteristic axillary odours are a result of the interactions of odourless, aqueous soluble precursors present in apocrine secretions with the axillary microorganisms. We have examined ephinepherine-induced apocrine secretions and found that the water soluble components contain 3M2H and other constituents of the characteristic axillary odor bouquet bound, in some

Table 1. Volatiles constituting the characteristic axillary odour: compounds judged to be important contributors to the axillary odour by organoleptic evaluation of gas chromatographically separated axillary secretion extracts (adapted from [11] and [13])

Hexanoic acid	7-Octenoic acid
3-Methylhexanoic acid	4-Ethyloctanoic acid
4-Ethylpentanoic acid	Unsaturated C_9 acid[a]
(*Z*)-3-Methyl-2-hexenoic acid	Unsaturated C_{10} acid[b]
n-Heptanoic acid	4-Ethylnonanoic acid
2-Methylheptanoic acid	9-Decenoic acid
(*E*)-3-Methyl-2-hexenoic acid	10-Undecenoic acid
n-Octanoic acid	Phenylacetic acid[c]
4-Ethylheptanoic acid	

Female odours also included trace amounts of (*E*)-3-methyl-2-pentenoic and (*E*)-3-methyl-2-octenoic acid.
[a,b] Also seen in the characteristic female odours.
[c] Identified as its trimethylsilyl ester, see [11].

fashion, to non-volatile molecules [12]. These odorants can be released by base hydrolysis (5% NaOH) or by incubation with bacteria [12]. Separation and hydrolysis (by NaOH or enzymes) of the proteins found in apocrine secretions have demonstrated that 3M2H is carried to the skin surface bound to two proteins which we have designated as apocrine secretion odor binding proteins 1 and 2 (ASOB1 and 2). ASOB1 and ASOB2 have apparent molecular weights of 45 and 26 kDa, respectively, as measured by sodium dodecylsulfate-polyacrylamide gel electrophoresis (SDS-PAGE; [18]).

Antisera to each of these proteins were prepared using purified proteins pooled from several male donors. The antisera were employed to probe, by Western blotting, the proteins from a variety of body fluids (e.g., tears, forehead and areaolar sweat, submaxillary and parotid saliva, urine, ear wax, serum and nasal secretions). All fluids, except urine, contained an immunoreactive protein with the same electrophoretic migration pattern as ASOB1; areaolar sweat and ear wax were also positive for ASOB2 [18]. Three of these body fluids (tears, nasal secretions and whole saliva) were separated into aqueous and organic soluble fractions and hydrolyzed to demonstrate that 3M2H could be liberated from the aqueous soluble components, albeit at concentrations far lower (<60 – 300×) than when this procedure is performed on apocrine secretions [18]. These results suggest a widespread distribution of an ASOB1-like protein and perhaps its bound odors in a variety of body fluids.

Female apocrine secretion proteins have also been electrophoretically separated and probed with antisera to ASOB1 and 2. The electrophoretic pattern of proteins and Western blotting was qualitatively similar to that for male apocrine secretion proteins [19].

ASOB1 and 2 were localized in biopsied axillary tissue from males and females [19]. Specific immunoreactivity was detected at antisera dilutions of 1:4000, localized only in the apocrine glands. Eccrine and sebaceous glands showed no specific reactivity. No difference was noticed between the immunoreactive pattern for ASOB1 and 2. Male samples demonstrated higher immunoreactivity in the lumen of apocrine glands while females showed more immunoreactivity in the acinar structures [19].

Both the actual molecular weight and structure of ASOB2 purified by preparative SDS-PAGE have been determined using enzymatic digestions, separation of the resulting peptides (by high-performance liquid chromatography) and structure determination by matrix assisted laser desorption ionization time-of-flight mass spectrometry (MALDI-TOF-MS). These results determined that the primary amino acid sequence of ASOB2 is identical to that of apolipoprotein D (apoD) [20]. This, as well as *in situ* hybridization using an anti-sense oligonucleotide probe for apoD mRNA, demonstrates that the site of expression for the apocrine secretion apoD is the apocrine gland. We also found that the glycosylation pattern of apoD from apocrine secretion differs markedly from that found for apoD in serum [20]. This demonstrates that apocrine apoD undergoes different post-translational modification than serum apoD.

ApoD is a member of the $\alpha_2\mu$-microglobulin superfamily of proteins (also known as lipocalins) [21]. The physiological role of plasma apoD is not known. Although several putative ligands have been suggested by in vitro studies and theoretical considerations [22], our studies identify, for the first time, an in vivo ligand for apoD as it appears in apocrine secretion. We also determined that there is a 2:1 molar ratio of 3M2H to apocrine apoD. The significance of apoD being a member of the protein superfamily of lipocalins is further discussed below.

ASOB1 is also a glycoprotein produced within the apocrine glands; however its identity is not completely known at this time. As noted above, antisera to ASOB1 cross-reacts with 45 kDa proteins found in a variety of other body fluids, suggesting a broad distribution of a protein with similar antigenic sites. Consequently, our studies are focusing upon the identity of ASOB1 and other proteins in the apocrine secretion and their role in odor production, as well as the levels of characteristic axillary odours in individual male and female donors.

Do Axillary Components Function as Chemical Signals?

The possibility that human odors may function as chemical signals or "pheromones" has come under considerable discussion in both the scientific and popular press. Pheromones were first defined and researched in numerous insect species. Chemical signals in insects are responsible for specific behaviors, some of which involve genetic programming. These well-characterized behaviors include attraction and copulation, and are mediated by chemical signals defined as releaser pheromones [23]. While some odor-mediated releaser effects have been documented in non-human mammals (i.e., pigs; [24]), the more frequently documented effects of mammalian chemical signals has been endocrine alterations that may result in changes to estrous cycle length and timing [25], acceleration of puberty [26] induction of ovulation [27] and pregnancy block in recently mated females [28]. While many of these effects have been documented in rodents, similar effects have been reported in domestic animals [29, 30] and Old World primates [31]. The term, primer pheromone, is applied to chemical signals, such as these, that act to alter reproductive physiology via the hypothalamic-pituitary-gonadal axis.

Although humans have rich sources of odour which can generate volatile chemical signals and an olfactory sensory system to receive them, our responses to odour are mediated by past experience, context and numerous other sensory inputs. Consequently, one would not expect to see releaser pheromone effects in humans, and none have been rigorously documented. However, several studies have suggested that interpersonal relations among women as well as among men and women may affect the menstrual cycle by altering reproductive endocrinology. These relationships include the well-accepted menstrual synchrony effect first documented in all female living groups [32] and later replicated by others in co-educational facilities [33, 34]. Male stimuli also appear to alter menstrual cycle length and regularity [35].

Russell et al. [36] were the first to present evidence that menstrual synchrony may be mediated by axillary secretion components. Other studies have confirmed and extended these results [35, 37]. Consequently, axillary secretions appear to contain constituents that act as primer pheromones that are capable of altering neuroendocrine pathways. The identity of the active ingredient(s) is not currently known. However, our results suggest that if the odours that characterize the axilla are responsible for the alteration of menstrual cycles, then the chemistry involved is similar to that found in other mammalian pheromone systems where proteins carry volatile, physiologically active molecules excreted from the body. In addition, apocrine apoD is a member of the lipocalin family of carrier proteins [21]. This further strengthens the remarkable similarity between human axillary secretions and non-human mammalian odor sources where lipocalins have been shown to carry chemical signals used in pheromonal communication [38, 39].

References

1. Leyden JJ, Nordstrom KM, McGinley KJ (1991) Cutaneous microbiology. In: Goldsmith LA (ed) Physiology, biochemistry and molecular biology of the skin. Oxford University Press, New York, pp. 1403–1424
2. Labows JN, Preti G (1992) Human semiochemicals. In: Van Toller SN, Dodd GH (eds) Fragrance: the psychology and biology of perfume. Elsevier Applied Science, London, pp 69–90
3. Shelley ED, Shelley WB (1984) The fish odor syndrome: trimethylaminuria. JAMA 251:253–255
4. Preti G, Clark L, Cowart BJ, Feldman RS Lowry LD, Weber E, Young IM (1992) Non-oral etiologies of oral malodor and altered chemosensation. J Periodontol 63:790–796
5. Preti G, Lawley HJ, Hormann CA, Cowart BJ, Feldman RS, Lowry LD, Young IM (1995) Non-oral and oral aspects of oral malodor. In: Rosenberg M (ed) Bad breath: research perspectives. Ramot, Tel-Aviv, pp 149–173
6. Huggins GR, Preti G (1981) Vaginal odors and secretions. Clin Obstet Gynecol 24:355–377
7. Leyden JJ, McGinley KJ, Hoelzle K, Labows JN, Kligman AM (1981) The microbiology of the human axillae and its relation to axillary odors. J Invest Dermatol 77:413–416
8. Labows, JB, McGinley, KJ, Kligman, AM (1982) Perspectives on axillary odor. J Soc Cosmet Chem 34:193–202
9. Rennie PJ, Gower DB, Holland KT (1991) In-vitro and in-vivo studies of human axillary odour and the cutaneous microflora. Brit J Dermatol 124:596–602
10. Gower DB, Ruparelia BA (1993) Olfaction in humans with special reference to odorous 16-androstenes: their occurrence, perception and possible social psychological and sexual impact. J Endocrinol 137:167–187
11. Zeng XN, Leyden JJ, Lawley HJ, Sawano K, Nohara I, Preti G (1991) Analysis of characteristic odors from human male axillae. J Chem Ecol 17:1469–1492
12. Zeng XN, Leyden JJ, Brand JG, Spielman AI, McGinley K, Preti G (1992) An investigation of human apocrine gland secretion for axillary odor precursors. J Chem Ecol 18:1039–1055
13. Zeng XN, Leyden JJ, Spielman AI, Preti G (1996) Analysis of characteristic human female odors: qualitative comparison to males. J Chem Ecol 22:237–257
14. Wysocki CJ, Zeng XN, Preti G (1993) Specific anosmia and olfactory sensitivity to 3-methyl-2-hexenoic acid: a major component of human axillary odor. Chem Senses 18: 652–653 (abstr)
15. Baydar AE, Petrzilka M, Schott MP (1992) Perception of characteristic axillary odors. Perfum Flavor 17:2–9
16. Wysocki, CJ, Beauchamp GK (1991) Individual odor differences in human olfaction. In: Wysocki CJ, Kare MR (eds) Chemical senses: genetics of perception and communications, vol. 3, Marcel Dekker, New York, pp 353–373
17. Labows JN (1988) Odor detection, generation and etiology in the axillae. In: Felgen C, Laden K (eds) Antiperspirants and deodorants. Marcel-Dekker, New York, pp 321–343
18. Spielman AI, Zeng XN, Leyden JJ, Preti G (1995) Proteinaceous precursors of human axillary odor: isolation of two novel odor binding proteins. Experientia 51:40–47
19. Spielman AI, Harmony JAK, Stuart WD, Leyden JJ, Sunavala G, Turner G, Vowels BR, Lam WC, Yang S, Preti G (1997) Identification and immunohistochemical localization of protein precursors to human axillary odor in apocrine glands and secretions. Arch Dermatol (in press)
20. Zeng C, Spielman AI, Vowels BR, Leyden JJ, Biemann K, Preti G. A human axillary odorant is carried by apolipoprotein D. Proc Natl Acad Sci (USA) 93:6626–6630

21. Flower DR (1994) The lipocalin protein family: a role in cell regulation. FEBS Letters 354:7–11
22. Milne RW, Rassart E, Marcel YL (1993) Molecular biology of apolipoprotein D. Curr Opin Lipidol 4:100–106
23. Albone ES (1984) Mammalian semiochemistry: the investigation of chemical signals between mammals. Wiley, New York, pp 2–5
24. Reed HCB, Melrose DR, Patterson RLS (1974) Androgen steroids as an aid to detection of oestrus in pig artificial insemination. Brit Vet J 130:61–67
25. McClintock MK (1984) Estrous synchrony: modulation of ovarian cycle length by female pheromones. Physiol Behav 32:701–705
26. Vandenberg JG (1969) Male odor accelerates female sexual maturation in mice. Endocrinol 84:658–660
27. Gray GD, Davis HN, Zerylnick M, Dewsbury DA (1974) Oestrus and induced ovulation in montane voles. J Reprod Fert 38:193–196
28. Bruce HM (1959) An exteroceptive block to pregnancy in the mouse. Nature 184: 105
29. Izard MK, Vandenberg JG (1982) Priming pheromones from oestrous cows increase synchronization of oestrous in daily heifers after PGF-2 injection. J Reprod Fert 66:189–196
30. Signoret JP (1991) Sexual pheromones in the domestic sheep: importance and limits in the regulation of reproductive physiology. J Steroid Biochem Molec Biol 39:639–645
31. Stoddart DM (1990) The scented ape. Melbourne, Cambridge University Press, pp 207–245
32. McClintock MK (1971) Menstrual synchrony and suppression. Nature 229:244–245
33. Graham CA, McGrew WC (1980) Menstrual synchrony in female undergraduates living on a co-educational campus. Psychoneuroendocrinol 5:245–252
34. Quadagno DM, Shubeita HE, Deck J, Francoeur D (1981) Influence of male social contacts, exercise and all female living conditions on the menstrual cycle. Psychoneuroendocrinol 6:239–244
35. Preti G, Cutler WB, Krieger AM, Huggins GR, Garcia CR, Lawley HJ (1986) Human axillary secretions influence women's menstrual cycles: the role of donor extract from women. Horm Behav 20:474–482
36. Russell MJ, Switz GM, Thompson K (1980) Olfactory influences on the human menstrual cycle. Pharmac Biochem Behav 13:737–738
37. Cutler WB, Preti G, Krieger AM, Huggins GR, Garcia CR, Lawley HJ (1986) Human axillary secretions influence women's menstrual cycles: the role of donor extract from men. Horm Behav 20:463–476
38. Singer AG, Macrides F (1990) Aphrodisin: pheromone or transducer? Chem Senses 15:199–203
39. Robertson DHL, Benyon RL, Evershed RP (1993) Extraction characterization and binding analysis of two pheromonally active ligands associated with major urinary protein of house mouse (Mus musculus). J Chem Ecol 19:1405–1416

Communication by Odour – The Influence of Body Odour on the Attractiveness of Men

R. E. Maiworm and W. U. Langthaler

Introduction

Human olfactory communication is an important factor in many aspects of life. Mothers can distinguish their infants from those of others by smell alone (Schleid 1980). It is possible to recognize kin on the basis of body odour (Porter, Balogh, Cernoch, and Franchi 1986). Furthermore, couples can recognize one another by their scent. Male odours are perceived as stronger and less pleasant, while female odours are perceived as less intense and more pleasant (cf. Hold and Schleid 1977).

Certain constituents of underarm secretions, such as odoriferous steroids, are now being discussed as putative human pheromones. It is suggested that they may have an erotic effect. Androstenone and androstenol have been examined most often. After puberty, androstenone is produced in the underarm secretion of males in greater quantities than among women. For example, it has an effect on the choice of seat in a waiting room (Kirk-Smith and Booth 1978). Androstenol seems to have a significant effect on self-perception (Benton and Wastell 1989). Androsterone, another steroid, found on the surface of underarm hair (Thoth and Faredin 1983), has as yet not been studied, except as a test-control substance in conjunction with androstenol (Gustavson, Dawson, and Bonnet 1986). It has yet to be seen whether androsterone has an effect on human behaviour. In a series of experiments, androsterone, androsterol and androstenone were examined in regards to varying perceptions of men by women. Two of these experiments are examined here in greater depth.

Method

Procedure

The experiments was designed so that all variables remained identical except for the test substances, androstenone, androstenol and androsterone, in order to test the varying perception of men by women under the influence of the test substances.

Standardized full-body photographs were taken of all the test subjects. They assumed a standardized pose, in which one hand was in the right pocket, foot marks on the floor guided positioning, and marks were used to indicate angle and orientation of the face. In a separate study, the attractiveness of each test person had been assessed by 118 students. Five photographs were selected that span the range of the attractiveness scores as given by the student evaluations.

The double-blind study was administered by two female facilitators who knew nothing about the test groups or of the substances (e.g. putative pheromones). The subjects were tested individually and were treated identically, apart from the stimuli administered. Subjects were given a standardized written description of the experiment in which they were given to understand that they were taking part "in an experiment regarding the effects of the best known ingredients of perfumes". After the mood scale (the EWL, *Eigenschafts-Woerter Liste*; Jahnke and Debus 1978) was administered, one of the three test stimuli was applied to the upper lip of the subjects. The mood scales were completed before and after the rating of the photographs. The subjects had 5 min to read the questionnaire, which consisted of the rating scales for the assessment of the men. Each photographed man was rated on 20 bipolar, seven-point, adjective rating scales developed in previous studies (e.g. ranging from "sensitive" to "insensitive" along the scale: 3-2-1-0-1-2-3) (Maiworm and Langthaler 1992). They had one questionnaire for each man. The photographs were randomly presented and subjects subsequently rated them, one at a time, so that it was not possible to make comparisons between them. Each questionnaire was returned after it was completed. A standardized interview was conducted by a trained female facilitator after the experiment which covered questions about the phase of the subjects' menstrual cycle, oral contraception and sexual partners. At the end of the session the olfactory test for specific ansomia was carried out.

Results

In the first experiment (experiment 1), 1 mg 5α-androst – 16 en 3-ol and 1 mg. 3-hydroxy-5-androstan 17-one were placed in solution with ethanol. As a test control (placebo) ethanol alone was used. The 95 women taking part in the experiment were randomly divided into three groups. Androsterone effected perception in that men were perceived to be better, warmer, and friendlier, tending to be tougher, but less sexy (MANOVA with Bonferroni adjustment for multiple testing). Using androstenol, subjects perceived men to be less sexy and tended also to find them less erotic (Fig. 1).

In gauging the effect of these odiferous substances, other factors must be considered. The average attractiveness of a man is decisive in determining

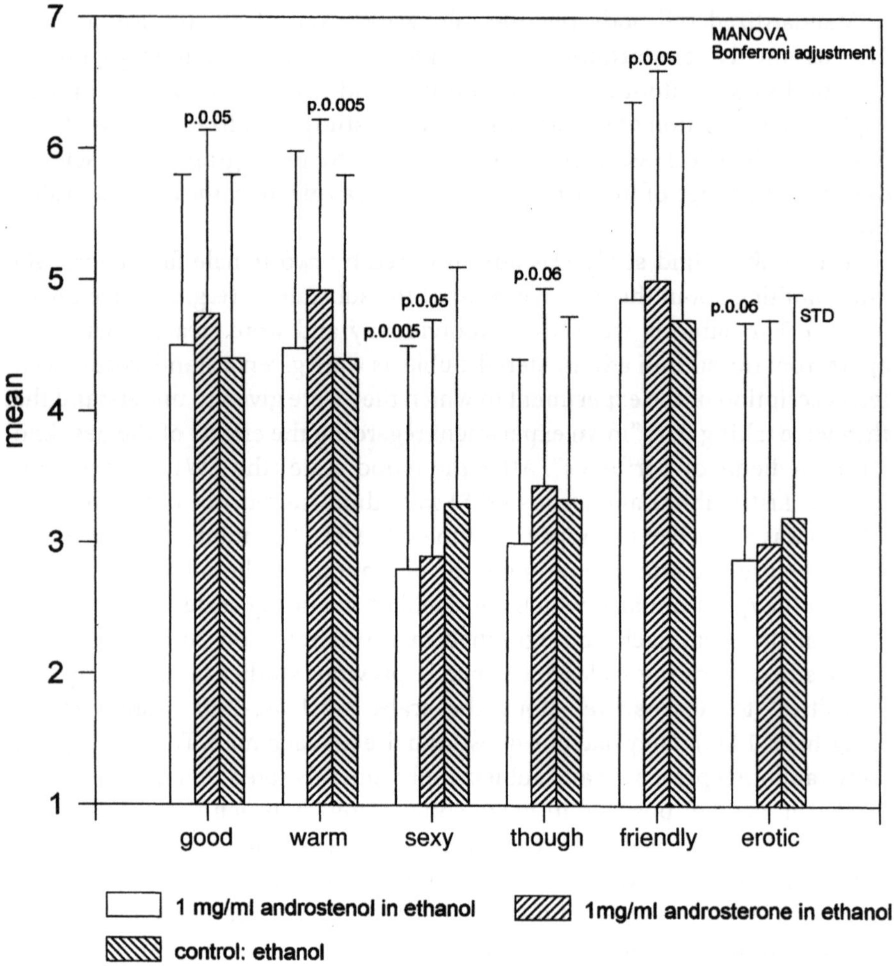

Fig. 1. Effects of androstenol and androsterone on the assessment of men: comparison to control

what effect androstenol and androsterone will have. Perceptions of both unattractive and highly attractive men were left relatively unaffected by these substances, while significant effects may be demonstrated with average men (see also Maiworm and Langthaler 1992). When adrosterone was administered, men of average attractiveness were perceived to be more sensitive, warmer, more intelligent, better, friendlier, nicer, more loveable, and more likeable (Fig. 2). Using androstenol they were perceived to be warmer, more intelligent, better, more loveable, more sympathetic, more expressive, more physically attractive, and more likeable than the results garnered from control results.

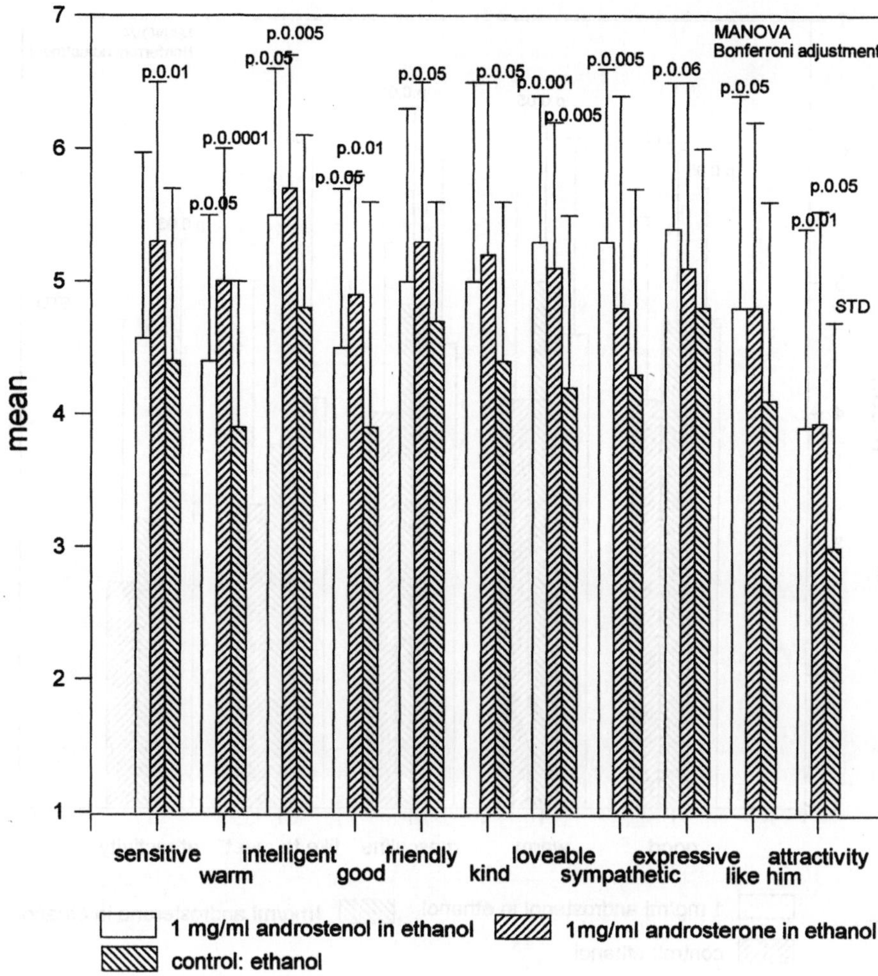

Fig. 2. Effects of androstenol and androsterone: average attractive man

The subject's position in terms of menstrual cycle is also important. During the middle of the menstrual cycle (days 10–19), no significant changes resulting from the test substances were noted. However, if a woman is in the first portion of her menstrual cycle (days 1–9) and androstenol is administered, men are perceived to be better, there is a tendency to find them more attractive, and the desire to meet them rises significantly. If androsterone is administered, men are perceived to be better, warmer and more masculine (Fig. 3).

In the last part of the cycle (days 20–29) women under the influence of androstenol perceive men as friendly and open, but as less attractive, less sexy,

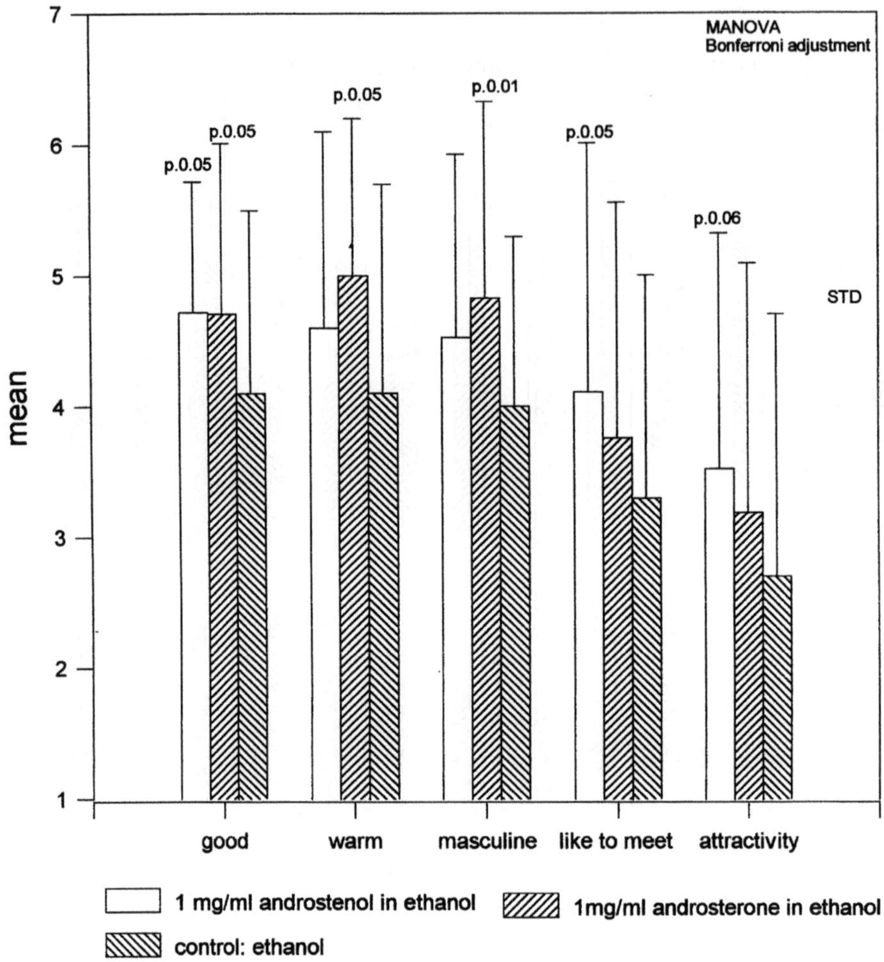

Fig. 3. Effects of androstenol and androsterone: first part of the menstrual cycle (days 1–9)

less erotic, and less arousing. Under androsterone they are perceived to be sensitive and emotional, but less sexy and attractive (Fig. 4).

Experiment 2

In the second experiment 0.5 mg. 5α-androst-16 en-3α-one was used in solution with white, pure, odourless vaseline oil and in solution with 99% pure ethanol. As test controls the solvents were used in their natural state. Eighty-six women took part in the experiment.

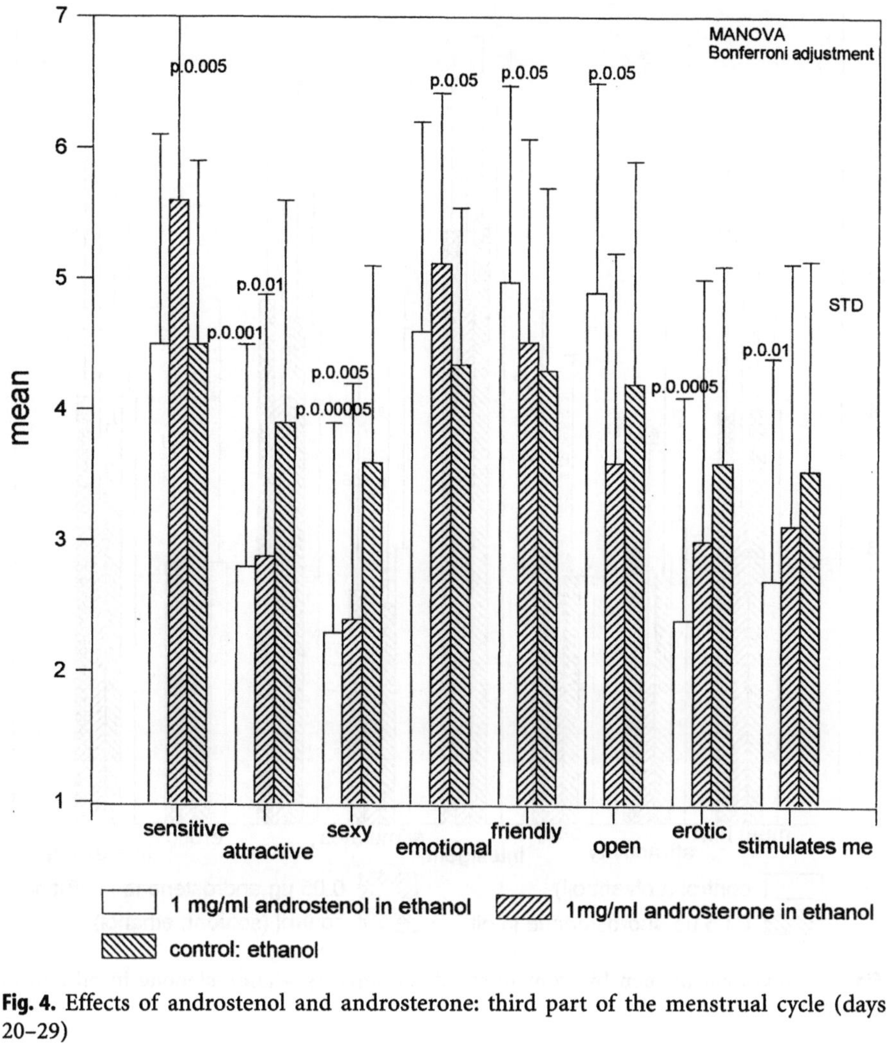

Fig. 4. Effects of androstenol and androsterone: third part of the menstrual cycle (days 20–29)

Using androstenone in ethanol, men received noticeably more negative marks. They were perceived as less attractive, less sexy, less intelligent, less trustworthy, less erotic, less interesting, less arousing, and the desire to meet them was also significantly reduced (Fig. 5). The results of androstenone in oil were not significantly different from the results of plain oil alone.

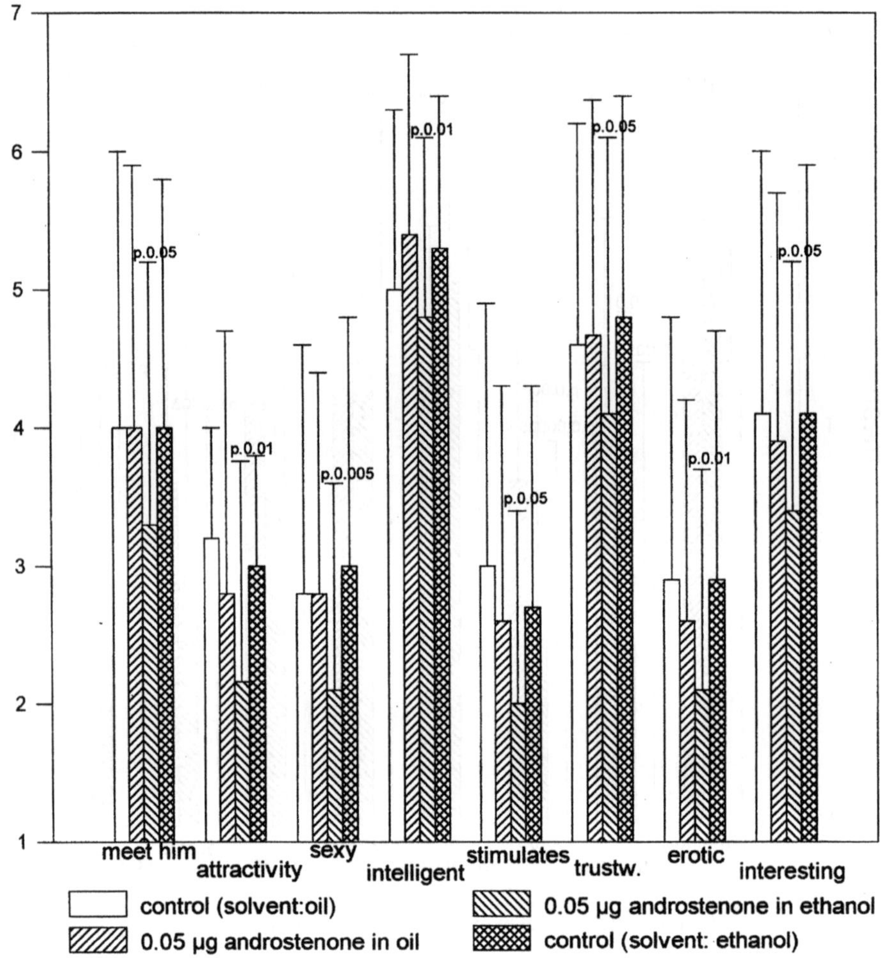

Fig. 5. Assessment of men by women: effects of solvents – androstenone in oil and in ethanol

Discussion

Experiment 1 clearly shows the effect of androsterone on the perception of men. The men received more positive ratings on a variety of scales. These significant effects are related to the erotic-sexual sphere but notably the men were gauged as less sexy and there was a tendency to find them less erotic. Given these test results, it appears to be problematic to use androsterone as a test control substance in conjunction with androstenol, as described in the experiments of Gustavson et al.

The effect of odoriferous secretions of human underarms appears to be influenced by various factors. Analogous to the model used for animals, the effect of chemical signals, especially pheromones, is usually influenced by the reproductive status of the signal recipient as well as that of the sender. In experiment 1, it may be seen that at different periods in the menstrual cycle androsterone and androstenol had different effects. Contrary to expectations, these substances showed no effect during the middle period of the menstrual cycle, in which ovulation is possible. Rather, these effects are greatest during the first period of the menstrual cycle. At the same time, both pleasant and less pleasant effects may be observed in the final period of the cycle. The unpleasant effects are related to the ero-sexual sphere. In respect to other attributes, such as friendliness, emotionality, and sensitivity, more pronounced responses may be noted.

In all studies concerned with the effects of androstenone, ethanol was used as the solvent. In experiment 2 it may be clearly seen that men are more harshly perceived when androstenone is used in conjunction with ethanol. This negative response to androstenone may result from the type of solution chosen. Odours in combination with one another smell very different than when experienced alone (Laing 1991). The unique smell of ethanol immediately after application could be responsible for the negative values found in conjunction with androstenone. These results call into question the use of ethanol as a solvent and probably the use of other odours as well in these sorts of tests.

References

Gustavson AR, Dawson ME, and Bonnet DG (1987) Androstenol, a putative human pheromone, affects human (homo sapiens) male choice performance. Brief communications. J Comp Psychol 101 (2): 120–122

Hold B and Schleid M (1977) The importance of human odour in non-verbal communication. Z Tierpsychol 423: 225–238

Jahnke W and Debus G (1978) Die Eigenschaftswörterliste. EWL. Hogrefe, Göttingen

Kirk-Smith MD and Booth DA (1980) Effects of androstenone on choice of location in other's presence. In: Van Der Starre H (ed) Olfaction and Taste 7. IRL, London, pp 397–400

Laing DG (1991) Characteristics of the human sense of smell when processing odor mixtures. Chem Senses 16: 257–269

Maiworm RE and Langthaler WU (1992) Influence of androstenol and androsterone on the evaluation of men of varying attractiveness levels. In: Müller-Schwarze D and Doty RL (eds) Chemical signals in vertebrates VI. Plenum, New York, pp 575–579

Porter RH, Balogh RD, Cernoch JM, and Franchi C (1986) Recognition of kin through characteristic body odors. Chem Senses 11: 389–395

Schleidt M (1980) Personal odor and nonverbal communication. Ethol Sociobiol 1: 225–229

Toth I and Faredin L (1983) Steroids excreted by human skin. Acta Med Hung 40: 139–145

Orientation of Insects in a Multitrophic System: The Role of Fragrances

P. CHRISTIANSEN-WENIGER, N. SIRI and S.G. MICHA

Introduction

Living organisms in terrestrial as well as aquatic environments are able to communicate by odours (Shorey 1976; Ritter 1979; Agosta 1992). Insects are "masters of fragrances" and many species depend on volatile chemicals for orientation and communication (Lewis 1984). Such volatile signals are defined as semiochemicals (Nordlund 1981) and the network of intraspecifically (pheromones) and interspecifically (allelochemicals) active substances represent a semiochemical web, which might offer possibilities for interference in order to control pests (Vinson 1986).

A complex of volatile-mediated interactions is demonstrated in the multitrophic system: plant – aphid – primary parasitoid – hyperparasitoid. Aphids, which damage plants mainly by the consumption of assimilates and transmission of viral diseases, have numerous predatory and parasitic enemies. Aphid parasitoids (primary parasitoids) such as *Aphidius* spp. or *Aphelinus* spp. oviposit into the aphid and their progeny develops inside the living host until the food source is completely exploited. Pupation of most primary-parasitoid species takes place within the so called aphid mummy. Parasitic enemies of these primary parasitoids are termed hyperparasitoids. They attack their hosts within the living aphid (e.g. *Alloxysta* spp.) or within the aphid mummy (e.g. *Dendrocerus* spp. or *Asaphes* spp.). Insects differ in their degree of specialization and are divided into monophagous, oligophagous or polyphagous species according to the number of host species they exploit. Besides the parasitic exploitation of a host, some parasitoids (*Aphelinus* spp. and *Asaphes* spp.) show predatory behaviour by feeding on the host as adult insect (host feeding).

Allelochemicals which mediate interactions between these four trophic levels can be classified according to benefit (Nordlund 1981): release of a "kairomone" benefits only the receiver, whereas the emitter benefits from the action of an "allomone". When both the emitter and the receiver benefit from an odour, it functions as "synomone". The use of volatile signals by aphids, primary parasitoids and hyperparasitoids, and the role of experience in relation to odour response is discussed in the present article.

Orientation of Aphids

The colonization of host plants mainly depends on the foraging behaviour of winged (alate) aphid morphs. Visual cues play an important role in their orientation (Kennedy and Ludlow 1974; Hardie et al. 1989; Nottingham et al. 1991a), but olfactory cues are also involved (Chapman et al. 1981; Nottingham et al. 1991b; Isaacs et al. 1993; Nottingham and Hardie 1993; Pettersson et al. 1994). Hence, aphids are able to distinguish between odours from host and nonhost plants, using the former as kairomones and the latter as allomones. Tests in a Y-tube olfactometer, where insects were offered the choice between two different odours, revealed that alate *Sitobion avenae* (F.) preferred host plants infested by conspecifics to aphid-free plants (Micha 1995). It remains uncertain whether the attraction was caused by odours from the infested plant, by a synergistic effect of plant and aphid volatiles, or by odours from settled aphids, acting as an aggregation pheromone (Kay 1976; Petterson et al. 1995). The same aphid species avoided artificially injured host plants (Micha 1995), indicating the release of an allomone from damaged plant tissue (MM Blight and JA Pickett, cited by Hardie et al. 1994a). Pettersson et al. (1996) found aphid repellent properties in cereal plants which grew next to aphid-infested plants. They suggest a defence reaction (antixenosis) induced in plants as a response to herbivore attack in the neighbourhood, which supports the idea of a communication between stressed plants.

Aphids do communicate between each other by odours. Attacked aphids are known to release a cornicle secretion, which contains a volatile alarm pheromone, analysed as the terpenoid, (E)-β-farnesene (Bowers et al. 1972; Edwards et al. 1973). This pheromone elicits defence, running or dropping behaviour of neighbouring aphids. Sex pheromones are emitted only in autumn, when holocyclic aphid species produce sexual morphs in order to enable genetic recombination. These pheromones, which are single compounds or mixtures of monoterpenoids (nepetalactone and nepetalactol, Dawson et al. 1990; Pickett et al. 1992), are released by female aphids (oviparae) to attract conspecific males. Attraction of males was enhanced by the mixture of sex pheromone and host-plant components, indicating a synergistic effect of the different volatiles (Campbell et al. 1990; Hardie et al. 1994b).

Aphid detection of semiochemicals associated with the higher trophic level (primary parasitoids) is not yet proven. Alate *S. avenae* could not detect traces of their parasitic enemies (*Aphidius uzbekistanicus* Luzhetzki) on a glass surface (Micha 1995).

Orientation of Primary Parasitoids

Primary parasitoids are efficient aphid antagonists; this is afforded partly by their remarkable host-finding ability (Chambers et al. 1986; Höller 1988; Stilmant 1994). The parasitoids thereby rely on semiochemicals which derive from plants and aphids.

The relationship between primary parasitoids and plants is mutualistic: primary parasitoids are detrimental to the pest population and plants provide host-finding cues to primary parasitoids. It is therefore not surprising that *A. uzbekistanicus* was attracted in a Y-tube olfactometer to volatiles from aphid-infested host plants (Micha and Wyss 1995). These kairomones were still present, when the aphids were removed from the plant before the experiment. Aphid-free parts of infested plants were tested similarly. In order to exclude any contamination by aphids (e.g. honeydew), a week old aphid colony was bound to a basal leaf part via a clip cage (Way 1973). The positive response of *A. uzbekistanicus* towards odours from the aphid-free apical leaf area of the same leaf proved the production of attractants by the plant. However, the induced synomone production remained in infested leaves and synomone production was not induced systemically within the plant. Plant injury by aphid probing might not lead to the release of semiochemicals as indicated by an absent reaction of *A. uzbekistanicus* towards injured plant leaves (Micha 1995).

Other tests in a Y-tube olfactometer showed a strong attraction of *A. uzbekistanicus* towards the aphid alarm pheromone, (E)-β-farnesene (Micha and Wyss, in press). (E)-β-farnesene is apparently a host-finding kairomone for primary parasitoids, and probably acts over shorter distances as responses were limited to relatively high doses of this chemical. The alarm pheromone, which is produced by a large number of aphid species, is an unspecific volatile. It is therefore not a reliable kairomone to mono- or oligophagous primary-parasitoid species and other more host-specific kairomones could be expected.

Synthetic aphid sex pheromone compoments attracted *Praon* spp. in the field (Hardie et al. 1991, 1994c; Powell et al. 1993). Catches of other primary parasitoid species, however, were very low or absent. Honeydew, the sugary excretion of aphids, provides food for adult parasitoids and is known to function as a contact kairomone for primary parasitoids (Budenberg et al. 1992). However, the substance, which has few volatile elements (Micha 1995), showed poor results in a Y-tube olfactometer

Primary parasitoids are capable of detecting the presence of their enemies, the hyperparasitoids. Odours from *Alloxysta victrix* (Westwood) elicited dispersal behaviour of *A. uzbekistanicus* females (Höller et al. 1994). 6-Methyl-5-hepten-2-one (MHO) was the main component of this semiochemical, which otherwise functions as spacing and sex pheromone of *A. victrix* (Micha et al. 1993).

Orientation of Hyperparasitoids

Volatile signals for host-finding cues of hyperparasitoids are provided by three lower trophic levels (plants, aphids and primary parasitoids). However, only aphids profit from the attraction of hyperparasitoids as they are antagonists of primary parasitoids.

A. victrix and *Dendrocerus carpenteri* (Curtis) were much more attracted by volatiles from infested plants than by odours from plants or aphids alone (Siri 1993). Allelochemicals from aphids and plants may have acted synergistically, or odours produced after aphid infestation (see above) may have been detected by the test insects. The same volatile signals may be used by both primary parasitoids and hyperparasitoids. Single compounds of leaf extracts were tested with *A. victrix*, revealing a high attractive effect of linalool and a strong repellent effect of 1-octen-3-ol (Siri 1993).

The aphid alarm pheromone, (E)-β-farnesene, which was used as kairomone by primary parasitoids (see above), also attracted *A. victrix*, thus acting as a synomone (Siri 1993). The alarm pheromone or odours from infested plants are very general features of aphid colonies and hyperparasitoids, once in a colony, must detect other, more reliable signals in order to find their specific hosts. *D. carpenteri* and *Asaphes vulgaris* Walker were thereby attracted to odours from the shell of an aphid mummy of its primary-parasitoid host, *A. uzbekistanicus* (Christiansen-Weniger 1992; Siri 1993). The insects were more attracted over a short range (35-mm petri dish) than over the longer distance in a Y-tube olfactometer (at least 120 mm).

As host suitability varies, so does the attractiveness of hosts. *Aphelinus varipes* (Förster) is a primary parasitoid, which is rarely attacked in the field (Höller 1989). Methanol extracts of its aphid mummy or parts of it elicited virtually no attraction of the hyperparasitoid, *A. vulgaris* (Christiansen-Weniger 1994a). Moreover, similar extracts repelled *A. vulgaris* from attacking a more suitable host, *Aphidius ervi* Haliday (Christiansen-Weniger 1992). The strongest repulsion was caused by the extracted late larval hindgut, which showed secretory activity in the colon (Christiansen-Weniger 1994b). The findings suggest the production of a protective allomone.

The Role of Learning in the Host-Finding Behaviour of Primary Parasitoids and Hyperparasitoids

The ability to learn host-finding cues characterizes many hymenopteran parasitoids (Vet et al. 1990; Turlings et al. 1993). The insects are thereby able to associate a new volatile signal with a host, provided that the new signal is experienced together with the target (host).

A. uzbekistanicus required a period of learning in order to show a positive response towards volatile signals of infested plants (Micha and Wyss 1995). Learning was most effective when the parasitoids had access to infested plants for at least one hour with a subsequent break of at least 16 h. Experiences with plants or aphids alone showed no effect. In other words, a period of experience improved the original faint attraction of naive aphid parasitoids to infested host plants (Sheehan and Shelton 1989; Grasswitz and Paine 1993).

Hyperparasitoids also appear to rely on learning behaviour. Choice tests before and after contact to previously unknown stimuli uncovered the relevance of host feeding in the host-acceptance behaviour of *A. vulgaris* (Christiansen-Weniger 1991). Host acceptance was modified after the insects had the opportunity to feed and oviposit for three days on a new host in a no-choice situation. Oviposition under the exclusion of host feeding had no effect (Christiansen-Weniger 1992). *A. vulgaris* might be able to switch between different host species at any period of its life cycle, which indicates one reason for the high degree of polyphagy of this species.

References

Agosta WC (1992) Chemical communication: the language of pheromones. Scientific American Library, New York

Bowers WS, Nault LR, Webb RE, Dutky SR (1972) Aphid alarm pheromone: isolation, identification, synthesis. Science 177:1121–1122

Budenberg WJ, Powell W, Clark SJ (1992) The influence of aphids and honeydew on the leaving rate of searching aphid parasitoids from wheat plants. Entomol Exp Appl 63:259–264

Campbell CAM, Dawson GW, Griffiths DC, Pettersson J, Pickett JA, Wadhams LJ, Woodcock CM (1990) Sex attractant pheromone of damson-hop aphid Phorodon humuli (Homoptera, Aphididae) J Chem Ecol 16:3455–3465

Chambers RJ, Sunderland KD, Stacey DL, Wyatt IJ (1986) Control of cereal aphids in winter wheat by natural enemies: aphid-specific predators, parasitoids and pathogenic fungi. Ann Appl Biol 198:219–231

Chapman RF, Bernays EA, Simpson SJ (1981) Attraction and repulsion of the aphid, Cavariella aegopodii, by plant odors. J Chem Ecol 7:881–888

Christiansen-Weniger P (1991) Some aspects of host selection by two aphid hyperparasitoids: Asaphes vulgaris Wlk, Asaphes suspensus (Nees) (Hymenoptera: Pteromalidae) Bull IOBS/WPRS 14:94–101

Christiansen-Weniger P (1992) Wirt-Parasitoid-Beziehung zwischen Blattlausprimärparasitoiden und den Blattlaushyperparasitoiden Asaphes vulgaris Wlk. und Asaphes suspensus (Nees) (Hymenoptera: Pteromalidae). Thesis, University of Kiel, Germany

Christiansen-Weniger P (1994a) Studies on semiochemicals affecting the host acceptance behaviour of Asaphes vulgaris Wlk (Hymenoptera: Pteromalidae) Norw J Agr Sc Supplement 16:277–282

Christiansen-Weniger P (1994b) Morphological observations on the preimaginal stages of Aphelinus varipes (Hym, Aphelinidae) and the effects of this parasitoid on the aphid Rhopalosiphum padi (Hom, Aphididae) Entomophaga 39:267-274

Dawson GW, Griffiths DC, Merritt LA, Mudd A, Pickett JA, Wadhams LJ, Woodcock CM (1990) Aphid semiochemicals-a review, and recent advances on the sex pheromone. J Chem Ecol 16:3019-3030

Edwards LJ, Siddall JB, Dunham LL, Uden P, Kislow CJ (1973) Trans-farnesene, alarm pheromone of the green peach aphid, Myzus persicae (Sulzer) Nature 241:126-127

Grasswitz TR, Paine TD (1993) Influence of physiological state and experience on the responsiveness of Lysiphlebus testaceipes (Cresson) (Hymenoptera, Aphidiidae) to aphid honeydew and to host plants. J Insect Beh 6:511-528

Hardie J, Poppy GM, David CT (1989) Visual responses of flying aphids and their chemical modification. Physiol Entomol 14:41-51

Hardie J, Nottingham SF, Powell W, Wadhams LJ (1991) Synthetic aphid sex pheromone lures female parasitoids. Entomol Exp Appl 61:7-99

Hardie J, Isaacs R, Pickett JA, Wadhams LJ, Woodcock CM (1994a) Methyl salicylate and (-)-(1R, 5S)-myrtenal are plant-derived repellents for black be an aphid, Aphis fabae Scop (Homoptera: Aphididae) J Chem Ecol 20:2847-2855

Hardie J, Storer JR, Nottingham, SF, Peace L, Harrington R, Merritt LA, Wadhams LJ, Wood DK (1994b) The interaction of sex pheromone and plant volatiles for field attraction of male bird-cherry aphid, Rhopalosiphum padi. Brighton Crop Protection Conference, Pests and Diseases 3:1223-1230

Hardie J, Hick AJ, Höller C, Mann J, Merritt LA, Nottingham SF, Powell W, Wadhams LJ, Witthinrich J, Wright AF (1994c) The responses of Praon spp. parasitoids to aphid sex pheromone components in the field. Entomol Exp Appl 71:95-99

Höller C (1988) Effizienzanalyse der Parasitoiden an Getreideblattläusen. Thesis, University of Kiel, Germany

Höller C (1989) Aphelinus varipes (Förster) (Hymenoptera, Aphelinidae), a promising parasitoid of cereal aphids. Bull IOBC/WPRS 12:43-53

Höller C, Micha SG, Schulz S, Francke W, Pickett JA (1994) Enemy-induced dispersal in a parasitic wasp. Experientia 50:182-185

Isaacs R, Hardie J, Hick AJ, Pye BJ, Smart LE, Wadhams LJ, Woodcock CM (1993) Behavioural responses of Aphis fabae to isothiocyanates in the laboratory and field. Pestic Sc 39:349-355

Kay RH (1976) Behavioural components of pheromonal aggregation in Aphis fabae Scopoli. Physiol Entomol 1:249-254

Kennedy JS, Ludlow AR (1974) Co-ordination of two kinds of flight activity in an aphid. J Exp Biol 61:173-196

Lewis T (ed) (1984) Insect communication. 12th symposium of the Royal Entomological Society of London. Academic, London

Micha SG (1995) Die Bedeutung von Semiochemikalien im tritrophischen System aus Hafer (Avena sativa), Große Getreideblattlaus (Sitobion avenae) und Blattlausparasitoid (Aphidius uzbekistanicus). Thesis, University of Kiel, Germany

Micha SG, Wyss U (1995) Bedeutung von Pflanzenduftstoffen bei der Wirtssuche von Aphidius uzbekistanicus (Hymenoptera, Aphidiidae), eines Parasitoiden der Großen Getreideblattlaus (Sitobion avenae). Gesunde Pflanzen 47:300-307

Micha SG, Wyss U (1997) Aphid alarm pheromone (E)-β-farnesene: a host finding kairomone for the aphid primary parasitoid Aphidius uzbekistanicus (Hymenoptera: Aphidiinae) Chemoecology 7:132-139

Micha SG, Stammel J, Höller C (1993) 6-Methyl-5-heptene-2-one, a putative sex and spacing pheromone of the aphid hyperparasitoid, Alloxysta victrix (Hymenoptera: Alloxystidae) Eur J Entomol 90:439-442

Nordlund DA (1981) Semiochemicals: a review of the terminology. In: Nordlund DA, Jones RL, Lewis WJ (eds) Semiochemicals, their role in pest control Wiley, New York, pp 13–28
Nottingham SF, Hardie J (1993) Flight behaviour of the black bean aphid, Aphis fabae, and the cabbage aphid, Brevicoryne brassicae, in host and non-host plant odour. Physiol Entomol 18:389–394
Nottingham SF, Hardie J, Tatchell GM (1991a) Flight behaviour of the bird cherry aphid, Rhopalosiphum padi. Physiol Entomol 16:223–229
Nottingham SF, Hardie J, Dawson GW, Hick AJ, Pickett JA, Wadhams LJ, Woodcock CM (1991b) Behavioural and electophysiological responses of aphids to host and nonhost plant volatiles. J Chem Ecol 17:1231–1242
Pettersson J, Pickett JA, Pye BJ, Quiroz A, Smart LE, Wadhams LJ, Woodcock CM (1994) Winter host component reduces colonization by bird-cherry-oat aphid, Rhopalosiphum padi (L.) (Homoptera, Aphididae), and other aphids in cereal fields. J Chem Ecol 20:2565–2574
Pettersson J, Quiroz A, Stephansson D, Niemeyer HM (1995) Odour communication of Rhopalosiphum padi on grasses. Entomol Exp Appl 76:325–328
Pettersson J, Quiroz A, Fahad AE (1996) Aphid antixenosis mediated by volatiles in cereals. Acta Agric Scand B 46:135–140
Pickett JA, Wadhams LJ, Woodcock CM, Hardie J (1992) The chemical ecology of aphids. Ann Rev Entomol 37:67–90
Powell W, Hardie J, Hick AJ, Höller C, Mann J, Merritt L, Nottingham SF, Wadhams LJ, Witthinrich J, Wright AF (1993) Responses of the parasitoid Praon volucre (Hymenoptera: Braconidae) to aphid sex pheromone lures in cereal fields in autumn: Implications for parasitoid manipulation. Eur J Entomol 90:435–438
Ritter FJ (ed) (1979) Chemical ecology: odour communication in animals. Elsevier, Amsterdam
Sheehan W, Shelton AM (1989) The role of experience in plant foraging by the aphid parasitoid Diaretiella rapae (Hymenoptera: Aphidiidae) J Insect Behav 2:743–759
Shorey HH (1976) Animal communication by pheromones. Academic, New York
Siri N (1993) Analysis of host finding behaviour of two aphid hyperparasitoids (Hymenoptera: Alloxystidae, Megaspilidae). Thesis, University of Kiel, Germany
Stilmant D (1994) Differential impact of three Sitobion avenae parasitoids. Norw J Agr Sc Supplement 16:89–99
Turlings TCJ, Wäckers FL, Vet LEM, Lewis WJ, Tumlinson JH (1993) Learning of host-finding cues by hymenopterous parasitoids. In: Papaj DR, Lewis AC (eds) Insect learning. Ecological and evolutionary perspectives. Chapman and Hall, New York, pp 51–78
Vet LEM, Lewis WJ, Papaj DR, van Lenteren JC (1990) A variable-response model for parasitoids foraging behaviour. J Insect Behav 3:471–490
Vinson BS (1986) The role of behavioral chemicals for biological control In: Franz JM (ed) Biological plant and health protection. Fischer, Stuttgart, pp 74–87
Way MJ (1973) Population structure in aphid colonies. Entomol Soc NZ Bull 2:76–84

Chemical Signals During Raids by the Robber Bee *Lestrimelitta limao* on Other Stingless Bee Nests (Hymenoptera, Apidae, Meliponinae)

R. RADTKE

Introduction

Workers of the neotropical robber bee species *Lestrimelitta limao* do not visit flowers to collect pollen and nectar. Instead, they raid nests of other stingless bees (Meliponinae) in organized groups of up to 1000 individuals. During a raid they collect honey, pollen and nest construction material. The significance of species-specific volatiles for the organization of raids by *L. limao* was originally postulated by Moure et al. (1958) and later by Nogueira-Neto (1970). Using biotests, I attempted to characterize those volatiles which release those behavioural reactions in the robber bees observed during naturally occurring raids.

Materials and Methods

Studies on the behaviour of the stingless bees and biotests were executed at the Biological Research Station of the University of Tübingen at the PUC University in Porto Alegre, RS, Brazil. The bees were kept in observation hives in the laboratory and in the meliponarium of the institute.

The volatile samples were pentane extracts of heads, thoraces and abdomens of worker bees. GC/MS analysis of these samples and the synthesis of the volatiles used in the biotests were performed by members of Prof. Francke's group at the Institute of Organic Chemistry and Biochemistry, University of Hamburg. In the biotests single volatiles and mixtures were presented for 1 min, 1 cm in front of the nest entrance tube, and for 3 min inside the nest. The amount of the tested substances corresponded to 1–20 bee equivalents.

The behaviour of worker bees during the consecutive phases of a raid was studied under natural conditions and in biotests by direct observation and by analysis of video documentation. The typical behavioural elements of the individual phases were identified and described. The aim of the experimental part of this work was to identify those chemical substances in the volatile bouquet of the robber bees which elicit each of the behavioural elements typical for the individual phases of a raid. GC/MS analysis allowed the individual compounds of the bouquets of the robber bees to be identified. The reactions of the bees were analyzed and compared with behaviour observed under control conditions.

Results

By GC/MS analysis, 61 individual substances were identified in the volatile bouquet of *L. limao*. The bouquet is composed of hydrocarbons, alcohols, carbonic acids, aldehydes, terpenes and esters. One terpene, citral, represented 57.2% of the volatiles, the highest relative amount of any substance.

Robber bee scouts often spent several days searching before they found a host nest to rob. They circled the host nest several times at close range and sometimes landed near to its entrance hole. They never marked the host nest with volatiles. The scout bees did not elicit defense behaviour when they made contact with guard bees of the host nest. They also did not leave scent marks on the ground when returning from a newly discovered host nest to their home nest.

After having returned to her home nest, a successful scout robber bee recruited nest mates by bumping into them while beating her wings. Under natural conditions, recruits started to move rapidly towards the entrance tube where they assembled. Bumped bees turned to bump other nest mates so that this behaviour spread rapidly in the nest. In biotests strong wing beating and bumping could be elicited by applying 6-methyl-5-hepten-2-one, a mixture of ethyl esters or acetates (Table 1).

Following in-hive recruitment, recruited bees spent 2–15 min in a highly agitated state in the entrance tube. The "runway assembly phase" always preceded mass take-off. Before and during mass take-off, up to 15 bees could be observed to engage in a distinct flight pattern in front of the entrance tube. They faced the nest and flew in vertical loops, repeatedly approaching to and retreating from the entrance. It was not possible to find a chemical releaser for this flight behaviour. Mass take-off by in-hive recruits, however, could be triggered by presenting citral or several ethyl esters to the assembly of agitated bees in the entrance tube.

Raiding parties flew at a cruising height of up to 10 m even across water to reach a host nest. Using biotests, it was not possible to lure raiding parties away from their direct flight path to the host nest by any volatile. Therefore suggestions that bees in raiding parties flew in a scent plume released by the guiding scout bee could not be confirmed.

At the nest entrance of host nests of *Tetragonisca angustula* and *Plebeia wittmanni*, 6-methyl-5-hepten-2-one and citral elicited the defence behaviour of guard bees of the host nest.

Table 1. Behaviour sequence of workers of *L. limao* during raids on host nests, and the components of the volatile bouquet of the robber bees which release the typical behaviour of the bees of each phase of a raid.

	Observed behaviour	Behaviour-releasing substances
1	A scout bee recruits hive mates inside its own nest by body contacts	6-methyl-5-hepten-2-one Mixture of ethyl esters, head extract Mixture of acetates
	↓	
2	Robber bees run excitedly out of their nest interior into the entrance tube	No chemical releasers found
	↓	
3	Robber bees fly out of their nest entrance tube	Citral Ethyl octadecenoate Ethyl octadecadienoate Ethyl octadecatrienoate
	↓	
4	The scout bee guides the recruited robber bees to a host nest along a scent trail or in a scent plume	Guidance along a scent trail could be excluded but guidance in a scent plume of volatiles could not be confirmed
	↓	
5	The robber bees attack a host nest; the host guard bees try to defend their nest	6-methyl-5-hepten-2-one Citral
	↓	
6	End of the raid	Citral

After 2–3 days of continuously raiding a host nest, the robber bees stopped raiding and left it. During this leaving phase, robber bees released a strong lemon-like odour, possibly citral. In two cases, a raid could be stopped when citral was introduced inside a nest of *Plebeia*.

Discussion

The main behavioural elements of the robber bee during raids can be experimentally released with the chemical signals identified in biotests. Whenever a behavioural element was released, the reaction of the bees was restricted to that single element of the whole sequence (Table 1). However, no chemical signal has so far been identified that triggers the transition to the next behavioural element in a raid.

Certain volatiles such as 6-methyl-5-hepten-2-one and citral elicit different reactions at different locations in the nest and during different phases of a raid. The reactions are typical and specific for each of the distinct phases of a raid. The reactions of the bees also depend on the context in which a chemical signal is released or perceived, and on the disposition of the bees themselves. Citral, for example, functions as a repellent to *L. limao* in biotests when applied during the time between two raids. The bees retreat from the site of application. If, however, the bees have gone through the initial stages of in-hive recruitment, citral elicits mass take-off from the nest entrance tube. When offered in their own nest, citral elicits wing beating and nondirected locomotion. If, however, citral is presented at the end of a raid in a nest of *P. wittmanni*, for instance, the robber bees assemble and leave the host nest (Radtke 1994).

Volatiles thus have multiple signalling effects. Their biological activity is determined by the context in which they are perceived and by the disposition of the receivers.

References

Moure JS, Nogueira-Neto P, Kerr WE (1958) Evolutionary problems among the Meliponinae. Proceedings of the Tenth International Congress on Entomology, vol 2, pp 481–493

Nogueira-Neto P (1970) Behavior problems related to the pillages made by some parasitic stingless bees (Meliponinae, Apidae). Essays in Memory of T. C. Schnairla, pp 416–434

Radtke R (1994) Die kleptoparasitische neotropische Biene *Lestrimelitta limao*: Verhalten und chemische Kommunikation bei Raubzügen auf Nester anderer Stachelloser Bienen. Thesis, University of Tübingen

Part III
Adverse Effects in Humans

Molecular Aspects of Fragrance Sensitisation

J. P. Lepoittevin and V. Mutterer

Introduction

From time immemorial, perfumes have been part of human culture and approximately 3000 "fragrance" molecules are currently used in the perfume industry [1]. These fragrance molecules are not, in general, used in isolation, but are combined to create a characteristic perfume; a single perfume contains from 10 to 300 different molecules [2], which, nowadays, are often synthetic and completely characterised. Fragrance molecules are found in a large number of manufactured products, but the main source of exposure is still, without doubt, perfumes and cosmetics. It is estimated that 95% of the female population and at least 75% of the male population come into daily contact with cosmetic products [3] and it is, therefore, not surprising that perfumes represent a major source of sensitisation. The frequency of sensitisation to perfumes is estimated as 1%–2% in the general population [4] and almost 8% in contact eczema patients [5].

A major advance in the field of epicutaneous testing has been the development and widespread use of standardised and completely characterised products. Mixtures or impurities make the interpretation of results very difficult and have been the cause of many substances being classified as sensitising agents, when the allergen was, in fact, a degradation product or impurity [6, 7]. The testing of a mixture of compounds is thus an important source of error. Chemical substances, especially allergens, are not inert entities, but are liable to undergo modification and/or interact with their surroundings, forming new compounds [8]. This principle, which applies to a pure product, is even more important in the case of mixtures, containing several molecules, the compatibility of which is often poor or even unknown. Such modifications and interactions can lead to increased (synergistic) or decreased (antagonistic) reactivity.

By definition, perfumes are mixtures of molecules, and all problems inherent in the use of molecular mixtures, whether during the sensitisation or challenge phases, apply to these products. Perfume sensitisation must not, therefore, be considered as an interaction of the skin with a single molecule, but with a complex mix, with all the attendant problems this implies.

General Remarks On Mixes

Not all mixes are the same; two main categories can be distinguished [9]: those consisting of a mixture of molecules that are chemically and structurally unrelated and those containing molecules with similar structures.

Heterogeneous Mixes

It is the first category, the "heterogeneous mixes", which poses the most problems for the chemist, since the presence, in the mixture, of several molecules, which differ widely in size and reactivity, can result in many interactions during skin penetration, biodistribution of molecules between the various cutaneous compartments, metabolism or interaction with antigen presenting cells.

Homogeneous Mixes

The second category of mixes, the "homogeneous mixes," consists of a mixture of molecules that are very similar in structure and reactivity. The factors controlling molecular recognition during the elicitation phase of the allergic response are highly dependent on the chemical group and the spatial geometry of the molecule. In order to detect sensitisation to a certain group, it is therefore sometimes necessary to combine several molecules in which it is present, but with different geometries. In this case, all the molecules possess the same chemical reactivity, are metabolised in the same way and have analogous physico-chemical properties.

Perfumes

Perfumes fall into the first and more complex category, the heterogeneous mixes. The presence of dozens, or even hundreds, of different molecules makes all types of interaction between molecules possible; the main sources of interaction encountered during sensitisation and/or challenge are described below.

Principle Causes of Interactions Seen in Heterogeneous Mixes

During sensitisation and challenge, molecules must first penetrate into the epidermis, where they undergo biodistribution and are eventually metabolised, forming reactive haptens, which then react with nucleophilic residues in proteins to form antigens [10].

Skin Penetration

Factors which control the penetration of organic molecules across the stratum corneum are of prime importance. Skin penetration is mainly a function of lipophilicity [11], represented by the partition coefficient, P, for an octanol/water mixture; the greater the value of log P (and hence the lipophilicity of the molecule), the greater the permeability. The second factor to take into account is the volume of the molecule; this can be modelled using various parameters, such as molecular weight (MW) [12] or molecular volume (MV) [13].

The penetration constant, Kp, (in cm/h) can, for example, be expressed either as a function of log P and MW:

$$\log Kp = a \log P + b\,MW + c \tag{1}$$

or as a function of the water solubility expressed as a function of log P and the melting point (MP):

$$\log Sa = a \log P + b\,(MP - 25) + c \tag{2}$$

For lipophilic substances, skin permeability increases in a quasi-linear fashion with an increase in log P until log P reaches a value of about 3, at which point it plateaus, then decreases in the form of a parabola fitting the equation:

$$\log Kp = a \log P - b\,(\log P)^2 \tag{3}$$

For a given value of log P, smaller molecules penetrate most easily.

The presence, in the perfume, of molecules of widely different physicochemical properties, lipophilicity (log P), MW or MV inevitably results in differences in rates of penetration. The effects of one molecule on the penetration rate of another must also be taken into account, e.g. the presence of certain lipophilic or amphiphilic molecules results in increased skin penetration.

Metabolic Conversion of Pro-Haptens Into Haptens

The rate of metabolism of pro-haptens into haptens by the various epidermal enzyme systems is another very important point [14]. For a given enzyme system, this will depend on the concentration of not only the pro-hapten (reaction substrate), but also of the hapten (reaction product). In the case of a mixture of pro-haptens, e.g. a mixture of allylic alcohols, there will be competition between the different molecules for the reactive site of the enzyme and their metabolism will be affected. In the case of a reversible system, the presence of a large amount of reaction product can lead to the slowing, or even reversal, of the reaction. Finally, the presence of several different molecules, all substrates for the same enzyme system, can result in the phenomenon of enzyme induction, with increased enzyme biosynthesis and a resultant increase in enzyme activity.

Generation of Antigenic Sites

Antigenic sites are generated on proteins when haptens react with nucleophilic residues on the different amino acids. The degree of modification of a protein by any given molecule is mainly determined by [15]:

1. The kinetic rate constant (k) for the hapten-protein reaction.
2. The residence time of the molecule in the epidermis, a function of log P (octanol/water).
3. The dose (D) of product reaching the reaction site.

The degree of alkylation, or relative alkylation index (RAI), can be expressed as:

$$\mathrm{RAI} = a \log k + b \log P + c \log D \qquad (4)$$

When several molecules of different types are simultaneously present in the epidermis, there will be competition for the finite number of nucleophilic sites on the proteins and antigenic competition leads to an under-expression of the least reactive haptens and thus to a modified sensitisation spectrum.

The Fragrance Mix

One good example of a heterogeneous mix that mimics a perfume is the fragrance mix [16], a well-known mixture which has been tested over many years and which contains seven components of very varied nature (Fig. 1) and reactivity. Compared with certain preparations, which contain more than 300 different molecules, it is a very simple "perfume," but it can be used to illustrate the different aspects of, and problems inherent in, molecular mixtures.

General Remarks

The fragrance mix contains three large terpene families:

1. Three cinnamic derivatives.
2. Two eugenol derivatives (eugenol and isoeugenol).
3. Two linear monoterpenes.

These three families of molecules differ greatly, not only in their structure, but also in their method of sensitisation. The mix is completed by an extract of oak moss, which itself contains a large number of products.

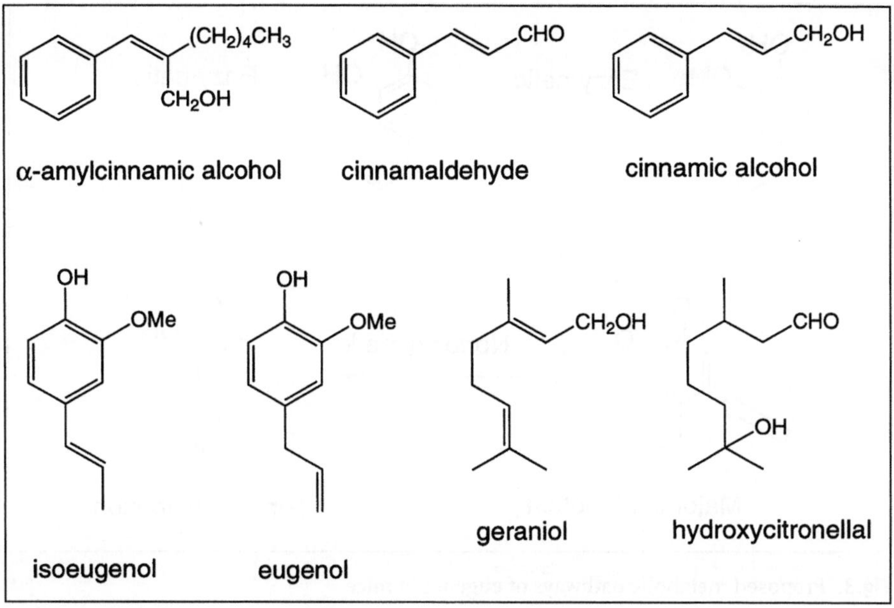

Fig. 1. Chemical structures of the fragrance mix constituents

Cinnamic Derivatives

The mix contains three such derivatives with different sensitisation profiles, as cinnamic aldehyde and α-amylcinnamic aldehyde can be considered as haptens, whereas cinnamic alcohol is a pro-hapten, partially metabolised to cinnamic aldehyde. The joint presence of cinnamic alcohol and cinnamic aldehyde can result in a enzyme reaction in equilibrium (Fig. 2), which is displaced as a function of the respective amounts of the two molecules.

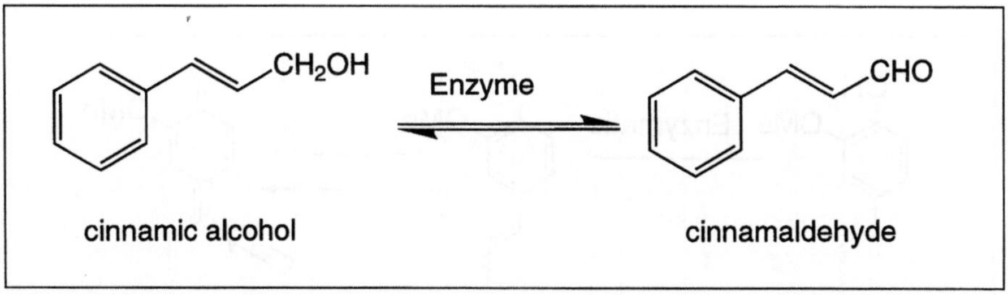

Fig. 2. Metabolic equilibrium between two related molecules – cinnamic alcohol and cinnamaldehyde

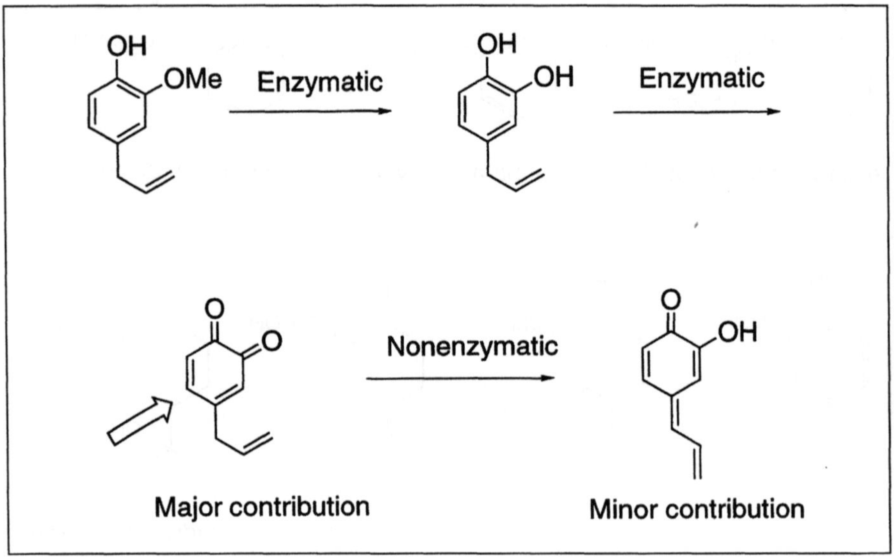

Fig. 3. Proposed metabolic pathways of eugenol in mice

Eugenol Derivatives

The fragrance mix contains eugenol and isoeugenol, which, like cinnamic alcohol, must undergo a metabolic oxidation step (in this case, a more complex one) to form the reactive hapten. Recent studies on the mechanism of activation of eugenol derivatives seem to indicate that these two molecules follow different metabolic pathways, explaining the observed difference in reactivity and the low degree of allergic cross-reaction between them [17]. The weaker sensitising agent, eugenol, seems to require an initial demethylation step, forming a catechol, which is then oxidised to the highly reactive ortho-quinone (Fig. 3), while isoeugenol is itself sufficiently reactive to be directly oxidised to the equally highly reactive paraquinone methide (Fig. 4).

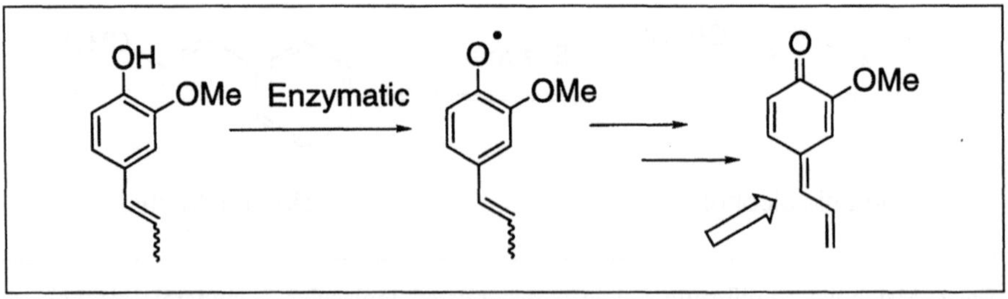

Fig. 4. Proposed metabolic pathways of isoeugenol in mice

Linear Monoterpene Derivatives

Two such derivatives, geraniol, a pro-hapten which must be oxidised to the aldehyde, and hydroxycitronnellal, an aldehyde hapten, are present in the fragrance mix. Again, the problem of the joint presence of an alcohol and aldehyde of related structure arises, together with the possibility of altered enzymatic metabolism.

Observations on Mix Reactivity

All the types of interaction described above are encountered in this mix, a mixture of haptens and pro-haptens with different structures and properties. Because of these interactions, the mix must be considered as a whole, rather than simply as the sum of its components, a point clearly made by the experience of many clinicians, when testing the fragrance mix, that a positive response to the mix is not always accompanied by a positive result to one, or more, of the constituents tested in isolation.

This frequent observation clearly shows that the eliciting potential of the mix is greater than the sum of the eliciting potentials of its constituents and that the mixture results in a marked synergistic effect. It is highly probable that this observation, made during challenge, applies equally well to the sensitisation stage.

This observation, carried out on a relatively simple and well characterised mixture, gives an indication of the extent of the possible reactions (both positive and negative) that can occur in more complex mixtures, produced on the basis of organoleptic requirements without, in any way, taking into account the compatibility of the constituent.

Conclusion

Sensitisation to even a simple mixture of molecules with very different physico-chemical properties results in many interactions during skin penetration, metabolism and epitope formation by reaction with the nucleophilic residues of proteins. In certain cases, such interactions can, without doubt, result in a decrease in sensitising potential, but most probably result, in many cases, in an increase in sensitisation potential. These effects are, as yet, poorly quantified, but deserve all our attention, since the prevention policy currently in use in the perfume industry, of considering the allergising potential of isolated molecules, is clearly limited, and the increasing number of cases of sensitisation to perfumes should prompt us to look at the perfume as a whole.

References

1. Nater JP, De Groot AC (1985) Unwanted effects of cosmetics and drugs used in dermatology. Elsevier, Amsterdam
2. Fisher AA (1980) Perfume dermatitis. Part 1. General considerations and testing procedures. Cutis 26:458–460
3. Nielsen NH, Menné T (1993) Sensibilisation de contact aux constituants des cosmétiques dans une population Danoise non sélectionnée. La Glostrup allergy study, Danemark. Ann Dermatol Venereol 120:33–36
4. Nielsen NH, Menné T (1992) Allergic contact sensitisation in an unselected Danish population. The Glostrup study, Denmark. Acta Derm Venereol (Stockh) 72:456–460
5. Wilkinson JD, Andersen K, Camarasa J et al. (1989) Preliminary results on the effectiveness of two forms of fragrance mix as screening agents for fragrance sensitivity. In Frosch PJ, Dooms-Goossens A, Lachapelle JM, Rycroft RJG, Scheper EJ (eds) Current topics in contact dermatitis. Springer, Berlin Heidelberg New York, pp 127–131
6. Karlberg AT, Bohlinder K, Boman A, Hacksell U, Hermansson, Jacobsson S, Nilsson JLG (1988) Identification of 15-hydroperoxyabietic acid as a contact allergen to Portuguese colophony. J Pharm Pharmacol 40:42–47
7. Dooms-Goossens A, Bruze M, Buysse L, Fregert S, Gruvberger B, Stals H (1995) Contact allergy to allylglycidylether presents an impurity in 3-glycidyloxypropyltrimethoxysilane, a fixing additive in silicone and polyurethane resins. Contact Dermatitis 33:17–19
8. Dupuis G, Benezra C (1982) Allergic contact dermatitis to simple chemicals. Marcel Dekker, New York
9. Les "MIX": Du fondamental à la clinique. Le point de vue du chimiste. In: Progrés en dermato-allergologie, vol 1. GERDA éditeur. Médiscript, Viterne, France, pp 185–192
10. Basketter DA, Dooms-Goossens A, Karlberg AT, Lepoittevin JP (1995) The chemistry of contact allergy: why is a molecule allergenic? Contact Dermatitis 32:65–73
11. Flynn GL (1990) Physicochemical determinants of skin absorption. In Gerrity TR, Henry CJ (eds) Principles of route-to-route extrapolation of risk assessment. Elsevier, Amsterdam, pp 93–127
12. Potts RO, Guy R (1992) Predicting skin permeability. Pharm Res 9:663–669
13. Barratt MD (1995) Quantitative structure activity relationships for skin permeability. Toxicol In Vitro 9:27–37
14. Hotchkiss SAM (1992) Skin as a xenobiotic metabolizing organ. In Gibson SS (ed) Progress in drug metabolism. Taylor & Francis, London, pp 217–262
15. Roberts DW, Williams DL (1982) The derivation of quantitative correlations between skin sensitization and physicochemical parameters for alkylating agents and their application to experimental data for sultones. J Theor Biol 99:807–825
16. Andersen KE, Burrows D, White IR (1995) Allergens from the standard series. In Rycroft RJG, Menné T, Frosch PJ (eds) Textbook of contact dermatitis, Springer, Berlin Heidelberg New York, pp 416–458
17. Bertrand F, Basketter DA, Roberts DW, Lepoittevin JP (1996) Skin sensitisation to eugenol and isoeugenol in mice: possible metabolic pathways involving ortho-quinone and quinone methide intermediates. Chem Res Toxicol 10:335–343

Identification of Fragrance Sensitizers by QSAR

J. J. Hostýnek, P. S. Magee and H. I. Maibach

Background

Fragrance materials consistently place among the most common causes of allergic contact dermatitis (ACD), and are the leading cause of ACD in cosmetics in particular [1]. The term cosmetics encompasses a broad spectrum of products of potentially daily use. Skin contact with stay-on products can extend up to 12 h or more; they often are applied repeatedly making constant reexposure and thus the cumulative effect of potential sensitizers unavoidable. Among these, perfumes and colognes in particular consist entirely of highly complex mixtures of fragrance chemicals in appropriate solvent systems, with concentrations ranging from 5% to 40% in the finished formulation. It is also a remarkable feature of those chemicals that their molecular size and lipophilicity combine to make most of them good skin penetrants [2], a prerequisite for immune system activation. Reliable numbers for the frequency of fragrance allergy are hard to come by. Nevertheless, occasionally published data indicate that the prevalence of allergic disease is rising in many countries [3], and so is the evidence that for an important part of cutaneous cosmetic intolerance the cause lies in their fragrances. In a European study for instance, the overall incidence of allergy to fragrance materials among dermatology patients was 7.8% [4], and has been estimated to run as high as 18% in a survey of a normal, asymptomatic cohort of women [5].

It is understandable from such figures that reliable tests allowing prospective recognition of allergens among the myriad chemicals used in fragrance composition rate high priority for the cosmetics industry, as well as for public health officials and medical practitioners. Sensitization is the hazard that the fragrance and cosmetics industries are most intent on avoiding, and the condition that dermatologists are most intent on curing. It is thus a legal requirement in the European Union now that new substances be tested for their potential to cause skin sensitization [6]. Current interest runs high among toxicologists and the general public as well in replacing established animal tests with alternatives that reduce, or even replace the use of animals. Quantitative structure activity relationship (QSAR) is one such method which objectively describes the interaction between chemicals and biological systems [7], and is now increasingly used in the prediction of a variety of toxicological endpoints, ACD among them. As no fully validated in vitro model to assess ACD potential is available or likely to be developed in the foreseeable future, empirically derived, mechanistically based QSAR models thus hold the potential for becoming valid alternatives to extensive animal testing, particularly if they can be confirmed as robust predictors of allergy.

Such a biologically based, comprehensive QSAR model combining both structural alerts with barrier diffusion criteria has been developed through systematic analysis of known contact allergens, which identifies both functional features that make a chemical an allergen, as well as the physicochemical properties which determine penetration of a compound through the stratum corneum [8]. The model has performed well in validation studies [9] which included matching its performance with the *vivo* test by the murine local lymph node assay [10].

Purpose

Given the preeminent position of fragrance chemicals as potential allergens in products of everyday use, it seemed appropriate to test the predictive performance of our QSAR model when it is applied to a selection of such compounds. As skin sensitization is becoming a commonly assessed toxicological endpoint, verification of model performance was made easy by the preexisting historical data base of experience obtained live with the human model over years of dermatological and allergological observation. Predictions by the QSAR model validated against human experience were also going to be matched with the performance of the expert system DEREK on the same set of compounds. DEREK (Deductive Estimation of Risk from Existing Knowledge) is a rulebase consisting of over 50 structural alerts developed in the United Kingdom [11], and is entirely based on the results of over 300 chemicals screened for allergenicity in the guinea pig maximization test. The diverse nature of clinical data used for validation of the two prophetic systems, man vs. guinea pig, also appeared to offer an opportunity for matching prophetic performance of our QSAR model with the most widely used traditional skin sensitization test, the guinea pig maximization test of Magnusson and Kligman [12].

Materials and Methods

Criteria for Compound Selection

The safety of the myriad fragrance chemicals used in compounding is monitored by the International Fragrance Research Association (IFRA). When necessary, IFRA issues recommendations on the use of these materials, including restrictions on use levels and advisories not to use substances at all when indicated by safety concerns. Thus, to date the use of nearly 100 fragrance raw materials has been either restricted or prohibited, in greatest part due to their allergenic properties [13]. As selecting compounds of well established sensitizing properties was important for our validation project, 33 ACD active compounds were selected among the fragrance raw materials restricted or prohibited by IFRA due to their potential for sensitization [13]. An additional 3 ACD actives were selected among chemicals identified as contact allergens: geraniol [14], benzyl salicylate [14] and lilial [15]. The 14 inactive aroma chemicals (NON) were confirmed as nonallergens through a Medline search for the years 1966–1995 and RIFM Fragrance Raw Materials Monographs, again reflecting the result of maximization tests in humans, published in Food and Chemical Toxicology (formerly Food and Cosmetic Toxicology [16]).

Prerequisite for all compounds selected for the study (Table 1) was their listing in the standard reference book on perfumery chemicals by S. Arctander [17].

Table 1. Performance of the QSAR model and an expert system (DEREK) in predicting ACD activity of 50 fragrance compounds

Compound	CAS	ACD/NO[c]	QSAR[d]	DEREK[d]
Dihydrocoumarin[b]	119-84-6	1	1	1
Hydroxycitronellal[a]	107-75-5	1	0	1
Isoeugenol[a]	97-54-1	1	1	1
Cinnamaldehyde[b]	104-55-2	1	1	1
trans-2-Hexenal diethylacetal[b]	67746-30-9	1	1	1
Citral[b]	5392-40-5	1	1	1
Cyclamen alcohol[b]	4756-19-8	1	1	0
p-*tert*-Butyl phenol[b]	98-54-4	1	1	1
Methyl crotonate[b]	623-43-8	1	1	1
Pseudomethyl ionones[b]	26651-96-7	1	1	1
Cinnamic alcohol[a]	104-54-1	1	1	0
Limonene (dipentene)	138-86-3	0	1	1
4-Methoxyacetophenone	100-06-1	0	1	0
3,5,5-Trimethylhexyl acetate	58430-94-7	0	1	1
Hexylsalicylate	6259-76-3	0	1	1

Table 1 (continued)

Compound	CAS	ACD/NO[c]	QSAR[d]	DEREK[d]
Benzylsalicylate	118-58-1	1	0	0
2-Phenylethyl alcohol	60-12-8	0	1	1
Phenylacetaldehyde[b]	122-78-1	1	1	1
Musk ketone	81-14-1	0	1	0
Musk xylene	81-15-2	0	1	1
trans-2-Heptenal[b]	18829-55-5	1	1	1
Diethyl maleate[b]	75554-12-3	1	1	1
Lilial	80-54-6	1	1	1
Fixolide	1506-02-1	0	1	0
Benzyl dimethylcarbinol	100-86-7	0	1	1
2-*n*-Pentylidene cyclohexanone[b]	25677-40-1	1	1	1
Methyl salicylate	119-36-8	0	1	1
Isoamyl salicylate	87-20-7	0	1	1
Methyl *N*-methylanthranilate	85-91-6	0	1	0
1-(4-Methoxyphenyl)-1-penten-3-one[b]	104-27-8	1	1	1
trans-2-Hexenal dimethyl acetal[b]	18318-83-7	1	1	1
Geraniol	106-24-1	1	1	0
7-Methoxycoumarin[b]	513-59-9	1	1	1
Amylcyclopentenone[a]	25564-22-1	1	1	1
3-Propylidenephthalide[a]	17369-59-4	1	1	1
6-Methylheptadienone[a]	1604-28-0	1	1	1
4-Methyl-3,5-hydrocinnamaldehyde[a]	99-72-9	1	1	1
Folione[a]	111-12-6	1	1	0
Allylheptyne carboxylate[a]	73157-43-4	1	1	0
1-Octene-3-yl acetate[a]	2442-10-6	1	0	0
6-Isopropyl-2-decalol[b]	34131-99-2	1	0	0
3-Methyl-2(3)-nonene nitrile[a]	53153-66-5	1	0	1
Hexahydrocoumarin[b]	700-82-3	1	1	1
Versalide	88-29-9	0	1	0
Perillaldehyde[a]	2111-75-3	0	1	1
Hydroabietyl alcohol[b]	70775-80-3	1	0	0
Dimethyl citraconate[b]	617-54-9	1	1	1
Anisylidene acetone[b]	943-88-4	1	1	1
Pentyl cyclopentanone propanone	40942-73-2	0	1	0
Benzylidene acetone[b]	122-57-6	1	1	0

[a] Restricted use in fragrances by IFRA.
[b] Prohibited use, or restricted to use with quenching in fragrances by IFRA.
[c] Rating as allergen (1) or inactive (0) in human use.
[d] Correct (1) or incorrect (0) classification by QSAR or DEREK.

Table 2. QSAR Model descriptors and coefficients ($n = 70$; $r^2 = 0.750$; $s = 0.275$; $F = 15.81$)

Descriptor	Coefficient	*t* value
Molar refraction MR	0.0116	2.49
Lipophilicity factor PL	-0.161	-3.38
Hydrogen bond acceptors HBA	0.0498	2.88
Hydrogen bond donor groups HBD	-0.129	-2.91
Aliphatic esters ICOOR	-0.284	-3.55
Michael reactants ICONJ	0.570	6.47
Reactive halides IX	0.160	4.73
Aromatic alcohols IArOH	0.596	6.18
Aromatic amines $IArNH_2$	0.503	4.82
Primary alcohols IOH	0.207	2.51
Reactive nucleophiles and electrophiles IUNIQ	0.512	4.12
Intercept	0.118	

The Statistical Discriminant Model

A discriminant model, referred to as QSAR for brevity, based on 72 carefully selected ACD and NON active compounds was developed and used successfully in diverse studies [8, 10]. It is based on a combination of transport/binding descriptors and dichotomous (0/1) descriptors reflecting protein reactivity. A full description of the model and its development is featured in our primary reference [8]. As experience is gathered in subsequent studies, it is reflected in stepwise improvement of the model, and accordingly in its performance. The version used here represents the latest such improvement; the descriptors used are presented in Table 2 and characterized as follows.

Molar refraction (MR) is the basically polarizable molecular volume, modeling London forces in nonspecific binding; PL (lipophilic contribution of logP) models lipophilic interactions of a compound with proteins and membranes; HBA, a simple count of the electron pairs on N and O, models the concentration potential of hydrogen-bond acceptor groups; HBD, a simple count of the N-H and O-H groups, models the concentration potential of hydrogen-bond donor groups; ICOOR codes 1/0 for simple aliphatic esters and models esterase degradation; ICONJ codes 1/0 for conjugated olefins activated by groups that cause Michael addition of SH and NH_2 protein end-groups; IX codes 1/0 for reactive aliphatic or aromatic halides; IArOH codes 1/0 for phenols easily metabolized to reactive quinones; $IArNH_2$ codes 1/0 for anilines easily metabolized to reactive quinones; IOH codes 1/0 for primary alcohols easily oxidized to reactive aldehydes; IUNIQ codes 1/0 for strong nucleophiles and for unusually reactive electrophiles that occasionally require coding as alerts. Previous studies of diverse molecular structures have shown the discriminating power of the equation to fall in the range of 79%–88% correct classification, predicting nonallergens somewhat more efficiently than allergens [8]. In SAR studies, classifications with Yest values falling in the range 0.4–0.6 are usually considered indeterminate. In this study, however, as a comparison was intended with the DEREK system which simply classifies compounds as YES/NO from an input molecular structure, for the sake of consistency an allergen was defined as any compound with a Yest score >0.5, and as a nonallergen with a score <0.5.

Results

As shown in Table 3, of the 50 fragrance chemicals the discriminant model (QSAR) correctly predicts 44, with 88% concordance. All of the 6 incorrect QSAR predictions, identified in Table 1 with "0", are false-negatives rated as allergens from human experience. Thus, the QSAR model again performs better in the identification of nonallergens, with specificity (predicted negatives/true negatives) of 100%, than on allergens, where sensitivity of the QSAR model (predicted positives/true positives) is 83%.

The performance of DEREK, also tabulated in Table 3, gives correct predictions for 34 (68% concordance). Individual scores are listed in Table 1, giving higher sensitivity or prediction of allergens (26/36 = 72%) than specificity, i.e., prediction of nonallergens (8/14 = 57%).

Table 3. Predictive accuracy of QSAR model and DEREK expert system

	QSAR		DEREK	
	n	%	*n*	%
Concordance	44/50	88	34/50	68
Sensitivity	30/36	83	26/36	72
Specificity	14/14	100	8/14	57

Discussion

The false-negative classification of six allergens shows certain shortcomings still exist in our QSAR model which require correction. The ACD compounds classified as inactives are hydroxycitronellal, benzylsalicylate, 1-octen-3-yl acetate, 6-isopropyl-2-decalol, 3-methyl-2(3)-nonene nitrile and hydroabietyl alcohol. The Yest value for hydroxycitronellal is borderline-negative, and by statistical convention would fall in the indeterminate range. Evidently coding for an active aldehyde group alone falls short for correct classification. Benzylsalicylate becomes active upon hydrolysis to the prohapten benzyl alcohol in the skin, and at present the model falls short of coding for 2-step metabolism. Hydroabietyl alcohol fails to predict correctly due to its high lipophilicity value, which correlates negatively for skin penetration ability, a point that is due for correction in subsequent modeling. 3-Methyl-2(3)-nonene nitrile is a mixture of olefins, one of which (2-nonene nitrile) is potentially protein reactive. Coding is subjective, however, as acrylonitriles that are alkyl disubstituted in the beta-position are not normally Michael-reactive. The model fails because we declined to code ICONJ = 1 for this substructure. The remaining two compounds: 1-octen-3-yl acetate and 6-isopropyl-2-decalol appear devoid of alerts that would lead to ACD activity, and are stigmatized by IFRA for reasons that elude structural rationale.

The divergence in predictive power exhibited between the QSAR model and DEREK in this comparative exercise (Table 3) is readily explained by the diversity of the two systems. One hallmark of the QSAR model is the significance attributed to size and polarity as factors determining the ability of structures to penetrate the stratum corneum. A second element, albeit insufficiently elaborated at this stage, is coding for pro-haptens in the QSAR model, particularly as it concerns multistage metabolism in the epidermis. Note that, according to the developers of DEREK, these are criteria scheduled for further development of the DEREK expert system also, as new rulebases are continually added there in the endeavor to arrive at better qualitative predictions [11]. Most importantly, however, the difference in performance is due to the difference in databases used in the development of the two prophetic algorithms, and in the particular nature of the test set chosen in the present instance. The QSAR model predicts penetration and sensitization events likely to occur in the human skin upon open epicutaneous exposure, an event reflecting an actual real-life scenario, and is tested against data obtained entirely from human experience. DEREK, on the other hand, entirely rests on guinea pig maximization test (GPMT) data, a model designed to maximize the sensitivity of the animal to allergen action. A worst-case scenario is created in that test, especially when the animal is treated with Freund's Complete Adjuvant, resulting in a lowered skin irritation threshold, and is likely to exhibit an "angry back" or "excited skin syndrome" [18]. In following that test protocol, the effect of the stratum corneum barrier is defeated by definition, in the induction as well as the elicitation phase [19]. In addition, false-positive reading of patch test reactions are possible when following that protocol if animals are not adequately rechallenged at lengthy intervals to distinguish specific from nonspecific irritant reactions [20]. This apparent tendency by DEREK to overstate sensitization potential becomes especially evident in the difference between specificity and sensitivity obtained from the two methods of analysis. While performance of the QSAR is 100% in the classification of nonallergens, there DEREK's accuracy appears to be the least, reflecting the main characteristic of the test method it is based on. DEREK correctly identifies the ability of chemical substructures to react with native protein groups, defined as alerts, but does not fully account for the probability of their reaching the viable tissues in the skin yet. DEREK identifies the sensitizers; QSAR predicts whether they sensitize man.

Summary

Performance of two prophetic systems: the QSAR model and DEREK, was matched in classifying 50 fragrance chemicals commonly used in perfumery composition for their contact sensitization potential. While the QSAR model proves to be a robust predictor of allergenicity in man, yielding 88% concordance, in its present form DEREK appears primarily geared towards systematic identification of protein-reactive structural elements.

References

1. Fisher AA (1995) Fisher's contact dermatitis. Rietschel RL, Fowler, JF Jr (eds) Williams & Wilkins, Baltimore, pp 448–456
2. Hostýnek JJ (1995) Predicting absorption of fragrance chemicals through human skin. J Soc Cosmet Chem 46:221–229
3. Smit HA, Coenraads PJ (1993) Epidemiology of contact dermatitis. In: Burr ML (ed) Epidemiology of contact dermatitis. Karger, Basel, pp 29–48
4. Wilkinson JD, Andersen K, Camarasa J (1989) Preliminary results on the effectiveness of two forms of fragrance mix as screening agents for fragrance sensitivity. In: Frosch PJ, Dooms-Goossens A, Lachapelle J-M, Rycroft EJ, Scheper EJ (eds) Current topics in contact dermatitis. Springer, Berlin Heidelberg New York, pp 127–131
5. Guin JD, Berry VK (1980) Perfume sensitivity in adult females. J Am Acad Dermatol 3:299–302
6. EC (1993) Council directive, 7th Amendment to Directive 67/548/EEC. Official Journal of the European Communities 35:L154
7. Hansch C, Leo A (1995) Exploring QSAR – fundamentals and applications in chemistry and biology, vol 1. American Chemical Society, Washington, DC
8. Magee PS, Hostýnek JJ, Maibach HI (1994) A classification model for allergic contact dermatitis. Quant Struct Act Relat 13:22–33
9. Magee PS, Hostýnek JJ Maibach HI (1994) Modeling allergic contact dermatitis. In: Rougier A, Goldberg AM, Maibach HI (eds) In vitro skin toxicology. Liebert, New York, pp 281–291
10. Hostýnek JJ, Lauerma AI, Magee PS, Bloom E, Maibach HI (1995) A local lymph-node assay validation study of a structure-activity relationship model for contact allergens. Arch Dermatol Res 287:567–571
11. Ridings JE, Barratt MD, Cary R, Earnshaw CG, Eggington CE, Ellis MK, Judson PN, Langowski JJ, Marchant CA, Payne MP, Watson WP, Yih TD (1996) Computer prediction of possible toxic action from chemical structure: an update on the DEREK system. Toxicology 106:267–279

12. Magnusson B, Kligman AM (1969) The identification of contact allergens by animal assay. The guinea pig maximization test. J Invest Dermatol 52:568
13. Ford RA (1991) The toxicology and safety of fragrances. In: Müller PM, Lamparsky, D (eds) Perfumes: art, science, technology. Elsevier Applied Science, London, pp 441-463
14. Scheinman PL (1996) Allergic contact dermatitis to fragrances: a review. Am J Contact Dermatitis 7:65-76
15. Frosch PJ, Pilz B, Andersen KE, Burrows D, Camarasa JG, Dooms-Goossens A, Ducombs G, Fuchs T, Hannuksela M, Lachapelle J-M, Lahti A, Maibach HI et al. (1995) Patch testing with fragrances: results of a multicenter study of the European Environmental and Contact Dermatitis Research Group with 48 frequently used consituents of perfumes. Contact Dermatitis 33:333-342
16. Opdyke DLJ (1979) Monographs on fragrance raw materials. Pergamon, Oxford
17. Arctander S (1960) Perfume and flavor materials of natural origin. Arctander, Montclair
18. Nethercott JR, Lawrence M (1983) The effect of the guinea pig maximization protocol on the irritant response to deodorized kerosene-the excited skin syndrome. Contact Dermatitis 9:439-443
19. Klecak G (1996) Test methods for allergic contact dermatitis in animals. In: Marzulli F, Maibach HI (eds) Dermatotoxicology. Hemisphere, New York, pp 437-460
20. Kligman AM, Basketter DA (1995) A critical commentary and updating of the guinea pig maximization test. Contact Dermatitis 32:129-134

Fragrances as a Cause of Contact Dermatitis in Cosmetics: Clinical Aspects and Epidemiological Data

A.C. de Groot and P.J. Frosch

Introduction

Perfumes are so much a part of our culture that we take them for granted, but if they were suddenly taken from us, society would suffer immeasurably. We do pay a price for their service, and part of that concerns dermatological and other medical reactions.

Contact with Fragrances and Fragranced Products

The use of fragrances is ubiquitous and not limited to cosmetic products used primarily for their scent such as perfumes, eaux de cologne, eaux de toilette, deodorant and aftershave [1]. Virtually all cosmetics and toiletries contain fragrance materials; even "unscented" or "fragrance-free" products may contain a "masking" perfume. Flavours used in oral hygiene products – toothpaste, mouthwash, and dental floss – are fragrance chemicals. Scented household products include detergents, cleaners, softeners, deodorizing sprays, polishes, solvents and waxes. In industry, cutting fluids, electroplating fluids, paints, rubber, plastics, insecticides, herbicides and additives used in air conditioning water may all be scented. Eugenol is widely used by dentists. Paper and paper products – including diapers, facial tissues, moist toilet paper and sanitary napkins – may cause a reaction. Fabrics and clothes may contain fragrance materials, especially after they are laundered or treated with a fabric softener. Topical drugs often contain perfumes, and ventilating systems may spread fragrances. The distinction between fragrances and spices is often indistinct. Many synthetic fragrances are used as spices and flavours. Natural fragrances such as cinnamon, clove, vanilla and cardamom are added to foods, soft drinks, lozenges, chewing gum, candies, ice cream and tobacco.

Perfumes are widely used. Of 811 female clients of beauticians 91% report using perfume/cologne and 82% deodorant [2]. Of 35 490 persons asked in the United States 61% used deodorant and 34% colognes [3]. Other fragrance-containing products not primarily intended for their smell, such as soap, shampoo and toothpaste are used by almost everybody. Thus it can be stated that virtually everyone is in daily contact with fragrance materials.

Modes of Contact

Contact with fragrances may be from direct product application to the skin or mucous membranes (toothpaste, mouth fresheners, feminine hygiene sprays, perfumed eyedrops), by occasional contact with an allergen-contaminated product such as towels and pillows, contact with products used by partners, friends or coworkers ("consort" or "connubial" contact dermatitis [4]), airborne contact [5], and systemic exposure by inhalation and ingestion (fragrances, flavours and spices in foods and drinks, cough syrup).

Sites of Contact with Fragrances

Any part of the body may be in contact with fragranced cosmetics: *scalp:* shampoo, hair lacquer, hair gel; *face:* skin care products, aftershave, perfumed tissue handkerchiefs, airborne from perfumes on clothing; the *eyelids:* eye cosmetics; the *lips:* lipstick, toothpaste; the *neck:* aftershave, perfume; the *trunk:* body lotion; the *axillae:* deodorant and antiperspirant; the *arms and legs:* body lotion; the *perianal area:* fragranced (moistened) toilet tissue; the *vulvar area:* feminine hygiene sprays, sanitary napkins, topical drugs; the *hands:* moisturizing creams, soap; and the *feet:* scented antiperspirants.

Epidemiology of Adverse Reactions to Fragrances in Cosmetics and Toiletries

Adverse reactions to fragrances/fragranced cosmetics appear to be far from rare. Guin and Berry [6] conducted a questionnaire study in 90 student nurses; 29 (32%) gave a history of cutaneous fragrance intolerance. When patch tested with the "fragrance mix" (a composition of 8 commonly used fragrances to identify subjects with fragrance allergy), 15/90 (18%) gave a positive reaction. Of these 15, 12 (80%) had indeed a positive history of fragrance sensitivity. Of the nurses with a negative patch test reaction, only 21% considered themselves to be fragrance sensitive [6]. De Groot et al. [7] interviewed 1609 adult subjects and 196 (12%) reported reactions to various kinds of cosmetics and toiletries in the preceding 5 years. Sixty-nine of these (35% of the reactors and 4.3% of the total population) attributed their reactions to products primarily used for their smell (45 deodorants, 16 aftershaves and 8 perfumes).

The Medical Product Agency introduced a cosmetic control system in Sweden in 1989. Between 1989 and 1994, 191 reports of cosmetic side effects were evaluated. The majority of adverse effects involved only the skin, and 90% were eczematous reactions. Seventy percent of the cases of dermatitis

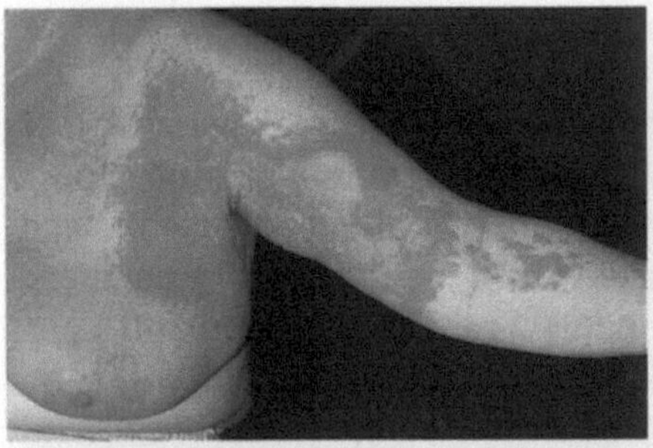
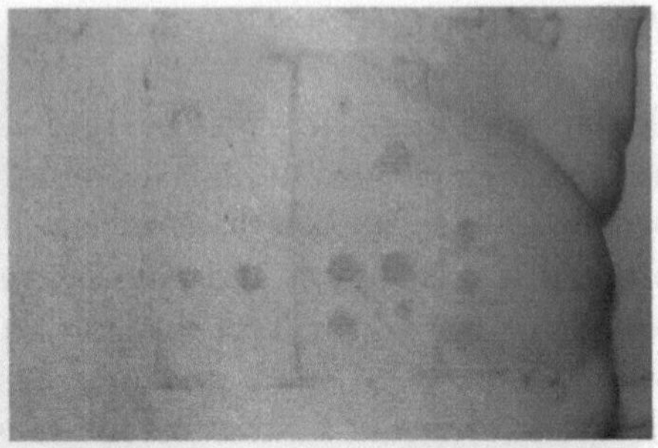
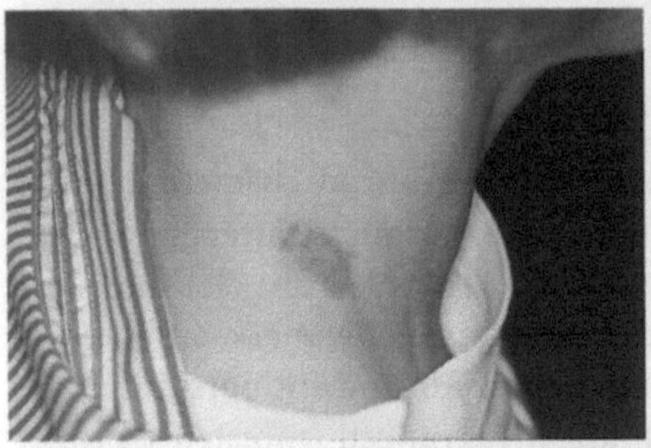
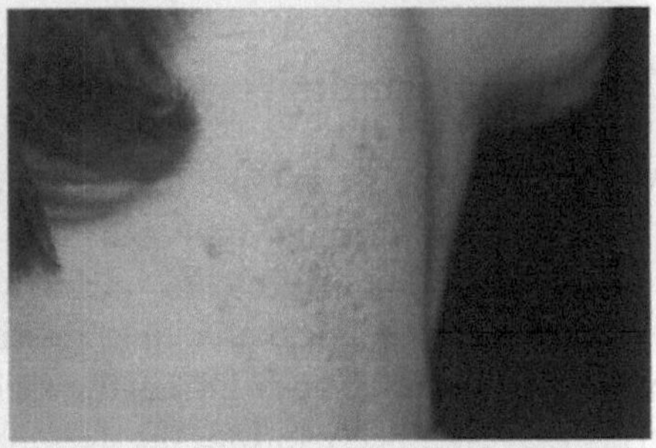
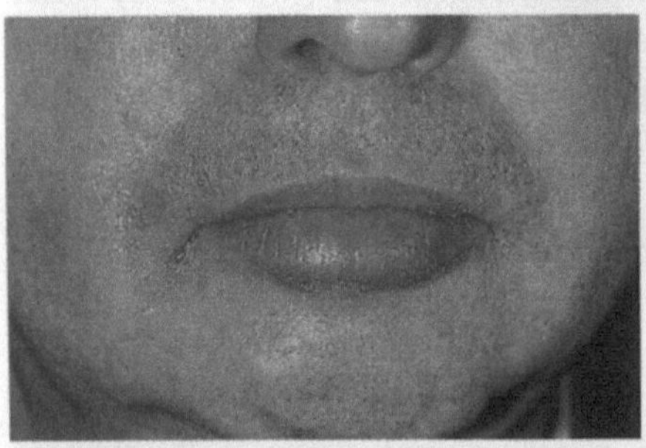
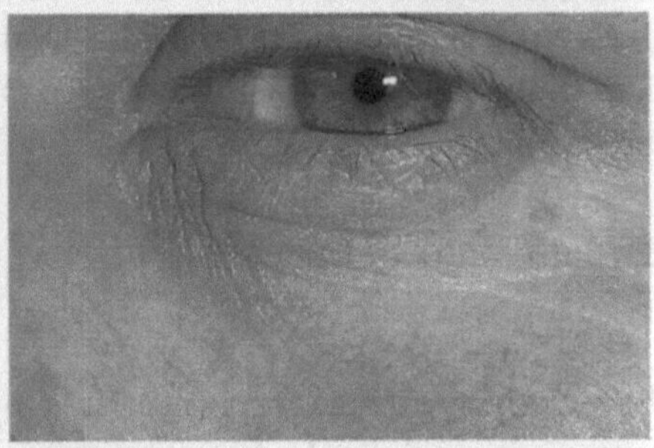
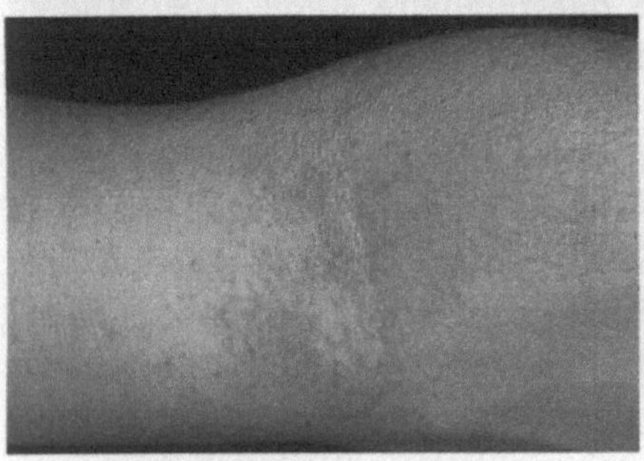
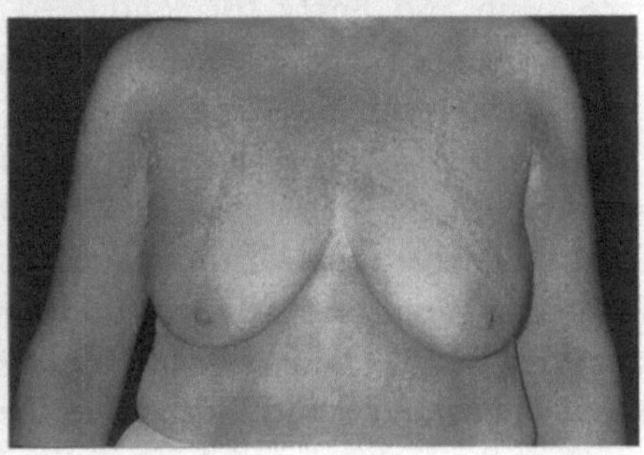

Fig. 1. Severe axillary dermatitis with erythema multiforme-like lesions due to a deodorant

Fig. 2. Multiple sensitivities to fragrances as detected by patch testing (patient from Fig. 1)

Fig. 3. Well-defined patch of allergic contact dermatitis due to the habit of applying the perfume to the same spot on the neck

Fig. 4. Lichenoid contact dermatitis due to a perfume spray

were classified as allergic. Patch testing with cosmetic ingredients revealed fragrances to be the leading cause (22/79 positive reactions [8]).

Considering the extensive use of balsams, fragrances, spices, and flavour additives to food, the frequency of contact allergy to these groups of materials is relatively small. In absolute numbers, however, fragrance allergy is common. The prevalence in dermatitis patients seen by dermatologists is high; in most countries the fragrance mix is among the "top five" allergens, usually number two after nickel sulphate, and yields between 6%–11% positive reactions. Indeed, fragrances are common causes of allergic contact dermatitis. At least 35% of all allergic reactions to cosmetics are due to perfume ingredients [9]. In studies investigating contact allergy to cosmetic products, perfumes account for 4% – 18% of all reactions, and deodorants/antiperspirants cause 5% – 17% of all cases of allergic contact dermatitis [10]. This may actually be an underestimation of the real importance of fragrance sensitivity. People rarely consult a dermatologist with a rash caused by perfume, toilet water, cologne, or deodorant. When this occurs, the culprit is usually obvious, and they simply stop using the fragrance on their skin. Even in the general population, fragrance sensitivity is not rare. In Denmark 567 unselected individuals aged 15 – 69 were tested with the fragrance mix (TRUE test system), and 6 (1.1%) had a positive reaction [11]. The frequency in men (1.1%) was identical to that in women (1.0%). In men, shaving with a razor is said to increase the risk of becoming sensitized by fragrances by a factor of three, possibly by creating small cuts in the skin facilitating penetration of applied perfume substances derived from soaps, shaving foams and aftershave lotions [12].

Types of Adverse Reactions to Fragrances

Allergic contact dermatitis is the adverse reaction most commonly seen by dermatologists. Other side effects include irritant dermatitis, photocontact dermatitis, immediate contact reactions (contact urticaria), and pigmented cosmetic dermatitis.

Allergic Contact Dermatitis: Clinical Picture (Figs. 1 – 8)

In spite of the daily contact of virtually everybody with fragrances, and despite the high frequency of positive patch test reactions to the fragrance mix in pa-

Fig. 5. Severe long-standing allergic cheilitis due to carvone contained in a toothpaste
Fig. 6. Discrete patchy periorbital dermatitis caused by the perfume in an "antiwrinkle cream"
Fig. 7. Repeated open application test in the antecubital space was positive (patient from Fig. 6)
Fig. 8. Severe widespread allergic contact dermatitis (caused by the perfume in a bath oil)

tients routinely tested for suspected contact dermatitis, literature on the clinical picture of perfume dermatitis is rather scant. In not a single study routinely testing the fragrance mix has the clinical picture of patients with positive reactions to the mix been investigated and compared with contact dermatitis patients not sensitized to fragrances. It can be expected, however, that the neck, the skin behind the ear and the axillae are often implicated, being exposed to products with high concentrations of fragrances (perfume, deodorant). Also, the sensitive skin of the face and the eyelids should be particularly susceptible to developing allergic contact dermatitis to fragrances in skin care products, decorative cosmetics and cleansing preparations, and from airborne contact [5]. Micro-traumata from shaving facilitates (photo) contact allergy to aftershave fragrances [12]. Indeed, among the 167 patients with suspect fragrance allergy investigated by Larsen et al. [13] the face was most frequently affected (40%).

Meynadier et al. [14] investigated 28 patients with fragrance sensitivity. Twelve were sensitized to perfumes or perfumed products, five to perfumes in topical drugs, seven to both; in four, the relevance was uncertain. One patient had pruritus sine materia on the eyelids from fragrance sprayed on her clothes. Several had allergic contact dermatitis on the face and coeur. Most of these were erythematous; in some cases the eruption resembled nummular eczema, seborrhoeic dermatitis, sycosis barbae, or lupus erythematosus. More acute lesions with papules, vesicles and oozing are sometimes observed. Lesions in the skin folds may be mistaken for atopic dermatitis. Dermatitis due to perfumes or toilet water tends to be "streaky". Facial psoriasis may be induced/aggravated by allergic contact dermatitis from fragrances.

Hand eczema is common in fragrance sensitive patients. Santucci et al. identified 54 patients sensitive to the fragrance mix. The hands were most frequently affected (41%), followed by the face (25%), diffuse (17%), axillae (9%) and legs (4%) [15]. Malten et al. also found the hands to be the most frequently affected in patients with suspected allergic cosmetic fragrance dermatitis [16]. Indeed, patients with hand eczema have an odds ratio of 2.6 of being sensitized to the fragrance mix compared to patients without hand dermatitis [17]. This may be explained by contact with fragranced cosmetics and toiletries (soap, shampoo, hand cream), perfumed topical drugs, perfumed household products, flavouring materials used in the kitchen, and vegetable foods. Dyshidrotic eruptions are ascribed to ingestion of spices. We think that fragrances are rarely the sole cause of hand eczema, including occupational cases. Usually patients first have irritant dermatitis or atopic dermatitis, which is later complicated by contact allergy to products used for treatment (fragranced topical drugs) or prevention (hand creams and lotions) of hand dermatitis, or to other perfumed products in the household, hobby, or work environment. Atopic dermatitis located at other body sites, perianal dermatitis, and vulvar dermatitis may also be complicated by fragrance allergy.

Irritant Dermatitis

Few well-documented cases of irritant dermatitis from fragrance materials are found in the literature. A large number of persons developed rashes after the introduction of a lemon-scented detergent in a hospital. The temperature-dependent, primary irritant reaction from the lemon perfume was due to the chemical citral. The problem was solved by washing the dishes in colder or luke-warm water rather than hot water [18]. Meynadier et al. [14] state that irritant reactions occur frequently and are caused especially by products with high concentrations of perfume, notably deodorants and antiperspirants. However, these authors provide no clinical data or literature references to substantiate their claims. Of course, deodorants and antiperspirants are an important cause of irritation, favoured by the humid climate in, and anatomical occlusion of the axillae. However, this may well be caused by the alcohol content or other ingredients rather than by the fragrance materials.

Photocontact Dermatitis

Compared to contact allergic reactions, photocontact dermatitis from fragrances is unusual. Only musk ambrette, a fragrance fixative used both in the food and cosmetics industry, has caused a considerable number of photocontact allergy reactions since its first description in 1979 [19]. It is (or was formerly) present in colognes, toiletries and perfumes, especially for men, and in fragrant oil used by Muslims before prayers. Pigmented photoallergic contact dermatitis, airborne pigmented contact dermatitis and lichenoid photocontact dermatitis have all been described. Persistent light reactions are not rare, sometimes leading to erythroderma. Photocross-reactions have been observed to musk moskene and musk xylene. Photodermatitis may be acquired by "connubial" or "consort" exposure.

The photoallergenic and phototoxic properties of coumarin derivatives, notably 6-methylcoumarin, are well known [20]. Coumarin itself, which is widely present in fragrances, does not appear to induce clinical photosensitization. 6-Methylcoumarin is no longer used in the cosmetics industry.

Occasionally, positive photopatch tests have been observed to the fragrance mix, and some phototoxic reactions were noted. Reactions to oak moss and its ingredients lichen acids are usually of the contact allergic type, but photosensitivity may occur to oak moss, atranorin and evernic acid.

In patients with persistent light reactions in chronic actinic dermatitis, a greater incidence of contact sensitivity reactions to certain fragrance materials than in patients with polymorphic light eruption and in patients with nonlight contact dermatitis was found [21], suggesting that in some subjects with persistent light reaction a significant factor is likely to be exposure to substances such as fragrance materials which have the ability to produce dermatitis, not only from contact allergic sensitivity but also through photocontact reactions involving either phototoxic or photoallergic mechanisms [21]. Recently 21% of 89 patients with chronic actinic dermatitis were found to be allergic to fragrances and 6% had photocontact allergy to musk ambrette, which seems to confirm the association [22]. Even more of these patients (36%) were found to be allergic to the sesquiterpene lactone mix, containing allergenic constituents of Compositae plants. Some fragrance materials may cross-react with Compositae, and indeed have sesquiterpene lactones been suggested as "screening agents" for fragrance sensitivity.

Immediate Contact Reactions (Contact Urticaria)

Contact urticaria to fragrances is usually nonallergic (nonimmune immediate contact reactions [23]), caused by a nonallergic histamine-liberating effect. Well known causes are balsam of Peru, cinnamic aldehyde [23], cinnamic acid, cinnamyl cinnamate, benzyl benzoate and benzyl alcohol. Immediate contact reactions can also affect the respiratory tract, as some individuals suffering from chronic respiratory problems experience worsening or precipitation of their symptoms on exposure to some fragrance materials [6].

Pigmented Cosmetic Dermatitis

In Japan in the 1960s and 1970s many women with bizarre hyperpigmentations of the face were observed. Before the relationship with cosmetics was discovered, such patients were diagnosed as suffering from Riehl's melanosis or "melanosis feminae faciei". The skin manifestations of (what was later called) pigmented cosmetic dermatitis consisted of diffuse or patchy brown hyperpigmentation on the cheeks and/or forehead; sometimes the entire face was affected. Occasionally, erythematous macules or papules, suggesting a mild contact dermatitis, were observed. Itching was sometimes present. In 1964 contact allergy to cosmetics was first suspected to be the cause of melanosis feminae faciei; yet it would take nearly 10 years before the term "pigmented cosmetic dermatitis" was coined by Nakayama et al. [24]. Systematic investigation of patients suffering from pigmented cosmetic dermatitis with patch testing and photopatch testing cosmetic ingredients confirmed that many patients with "melanosis feminae faciei" had contact allergy to cosmetics. It was found that the major sensitizers in cosmetics were coal tar dyes (used in decorative cosmetics) and fragrances. Common causative fragrance materials included jasmine absolute, ylang-ylang oil, cananga oil, sandalwood oil, benzyl salicylate, benzyl alcohol, methoxycitronellal (a derivative of hydroxycitronellal), β-santalol, geraniol, geranium oil, and patchouli oil. Photocontact allergy was less important in the development of pigmented cosmetic dermatitis.

On the basis of their clinical and patch testing experience, Nakayama et al. developed the "allergen controlled system" for the production of safer cosmetics, and major cosmetic companies in Japan began to stop using various sensitizers in their products in 1977. Since 1978 the number of patients suffering from pigmented cosmetic dermatitis has decreased remarkably.

Pigmented cosmetic dermatitis was and is hardly observed in Western countries, as the persistent secondary hyperpigmentation to contact dermatitis, which causes the clinical picture, is common in Mongoloids but is not observed in Caucasians. Nowadays, cases of pigmented cosmetic dermatitis from fragrances are reported infrequently.

Berloque Dermatitis. Berloque dermatitis is characterized by pigmentation, classically in a droplet or pendant-like configuration, usually over the sides of the neck in adult females. This cosmetic reaction used to be very frequent, and was caused by a phototoxic reaction to 5-methoxypsoralen (bergapten) in bergamot oil present in perfumes, resulting in hyperpigmentation with or without preceding erythema. This incidence of berloque dermatitis already declined in the 1960s, by the reduction of the concentration of natural bergamot oil in perfumes and the use of bergamot oil free of bergapten. Nevertheless, cases were still reported in 1981 [25].

Other Adverse Reactions

Depigmented airborne contact dermatitis from santalol and musk ambrette released from burning incense has been observed [26]. A pemphigoid-like allergic reactions was thought to be caused by cinnamic aldehyde [27]. Contact dermatitis from the application of spray cologne to the chest and the abdomen in a female patient resulted in the development of erythema multiforme with progression to toxic epidermal necrolysis and ultimately her death [28]. Erythema multiforme-like allergic contact dermatitis was also caused by a deodorant.

Fragrances can induce or worsen respiratory problems [29]. Guin and Berry interviewed 90 student nurses. In 4 asthma was thought to be aggravated or precipitated by exposure to fragrances, 25 developed rhinitis, and 5 ascribed (worsening of) episodes of urticaria to contact with fragrances [6]. Shortness of breath and sneezing from inhalation of fragrances was also found in a similar interview study [7]. Persons with respiratory allergy commonly experience aggravation around cosmetic counters, candle shops and perfumes worn by other people, for example, in church. This is thought to be due to a direct release of histamine rather than an allergic mechanism, caused by fragrance ingredients known to cause nonimmunological immediate contact reactions [6].

References

1. Fischer T (1995) Perfumed products. In: Guin JD (ed) Practical contact dermatitis. McGraw-Hill, New York, pp 355–371
2. De Groot AC, Beverdam E, Tjong Ayong C, Coenraads PJ, Nater JP (1988) The role of contact allergy in the spectrum of adverse effects caused by cosmetics and toiletries. Contact Dermatitis 19:195–201
3. Westat Inc (1975) An investigation of consumers' perceptions of adverse reactions to cosmetic products. National Technical Information Service, US Department of Commerce, Washington
4. Morren MA, Rodrigues R, Dooms-Goossens A et al. (1992) Connubial contact dermatitis: a review. Eur J Dermatol 2:219–223
5. Dooms-Goossens A, Deleu H (1991) Airborne contact dermatitis: an update. Contact Dermatitis 25:211–217
6. Guin JD, Berry VK (1980) Perfume sensitivity in adults females. A study of contact sensitivity to a perfume mix in two groups of student nurses. J Am Acad Dermatol 3:299–302
7. De Groot AC, Nater JP, van der Lende R, Rijcken B (1987) Adverse effects of cosmetics: a retrospective study in the general population. Int J Cosmet Sci 9:255–259
8. Berne B, Boström Å, Grahnén AF, Tammela M (1996) Adverse effects of cosmetics and toiletries reported to the Swedish Medical Product Agency 1989–1994. Contact Dermatitis 34:359–362
9. Dooms-Goossens A, Kerre S, Drieghe J, Bossuyt L, Degreef H (1992) Cosmetic productts and their allergens. Eur J Dermatol 2:465–468
10. De Groot AC, Weyland JW, Nater JP (1994) Unwanted effects of cosmetics and drugs used in dermatology, 3rd edn. Elsevier, Amsterdam, pp 442–451
11. Nielsen NH, Menné T (1992) Allergic contact sensitization in an unselected Danish population. Acta Derm Venereol (Stockh) 72:456–460
12. Edman B (1994) The influence of shaving method on perfume allergy. Contact Dermatitis 31:291–292
13. Larsen W, Nakayama H, Lindberg M et al. (1996) Fragrance contact dermatitis. A worldwide multicenter investigation. I. Am J Contact Dermatitis 7:77–83
14. Meynadier JM, Meynadier J, Peyron JL, Peyron L (1986) Formes cliniques des manifestations cutanées d'allergie aux parfums. Ann Dermatol Venereol 113:31–39
15. Santucci B, Cristaudo A, Cannistraci C, Picardo M (1987) Contact dermatitis to fragrances. Contact Dermatitis 16:93–95
16. Malten KE, van Ketel WG, Nater JP, Liem DH (1984) Reactions in selected patients to 22 fragrance materials. Contact Dermatitis 11:1–10
17. Christophersen J, Menné T, Tanghøi P et al. (1989) Clinical patch test data evaluated by multivariate analysis. Contact Dermatitis 21:291–299
18. Rothenborg HW, Menné T, Sjølin K-E (1977) Temperature dependent primary irritant dermatitis from lemon perfume. Contact Dermatitis 3:37–48
19. Cronin E (1984) Photosensitivity to musk ambrette. Contact Dermatitis 11:88–92

20. Kaidbey KH, Kligman AM (1981) Photosensitization to coumarin derivatives. Arch Dermatol 117:258–265
21. Addo HA, Ferguson J, Johnson BE, Frain-Bell W (1982) The relationship between exposure to fragrance materials and persistent light reactions in the photosensitivity dermatitis. Br J Dermatol 107:261–274
22. Menagé H du P, Ross JS, Norris PG, Hawk JLM, White IR (1995) Contact and photocontact sensitization in chronic actinic dermatitis; sesquiterpene lactone mix is an important allergen. Br J Dermatol 132:543–547
23. Safford RJ, Basketter DA, Allenby CF, Goodwin BFJ (1990) Immediate contact reactions to chemicals in the fragrance mix and a study of the quenching action of eugenol. Br J Dermatol 123:595–606
24. Nakayama H, Matsuo S, Hayakawa K et al. (1984) Pigmented cosmetic dermatitis. Int J Dermatol 23:299–305
25. Zaynoun ST, Aftimas BA, Tenekjian KK, Kurban AK (1981) Berloque dermatitis – a continuing cosmetic problem. Contact Dermatitis 7:111–116
26. Hayakawa R, Matsunaga K, Arima Y (1987) Depigmented contact dermatitis due to incense. Contact Dermatitis 16:272–274
27. Goh CL, Ng SK (1988) Bullous contact allergy from cinnamon. Dermatosen 36: 186–187
28. Thompson JA Jr, Wansker BA (1981) A case of contact dermatitis, erythema multiforme, and toxic epidermal necrolysis. J Am Acad Dermatol 5:666–669
29. Schleuter DP (1978) Airway response to hair spray in normal subjects and subjects with hyperreactive airways. Chest 75:544–547

How Do We Test for Fragrance Allergy?

W. G. Larsen

Fragrances can cause a number of local and systemic reactions. The following are the most common:

- Contact dermatitis – allergic and irritant
- Phototoxicity – allergic and toxic
- Systemic contact dermatitis and toxicity
- Urticaria – immunological and nonimmunological
- Asthma and rhinoconjunctivitis
- Pigmentation and depigmentation

Contact Dermatitis

The most common reactions seen by dermatologists to fragrance materials is allergic contact dermatitis [1, 2], and this review focuses on testing for contact dermatitis. During the 1980s numerous cases were reported of photodermatitis due to musk ambrette [3] and 6-methyl coumarin [4]. The reactions to musk ambrette were photocontact dermatitis primarily in men due to aftershave lotions. There was a limited outbreak of 6-methyl coumarin photosensitivity due to increased concentrations of 6-methyl coumarin in a certain fragranced sunscreen. Both of these chemicals were removed from the market so reactions are rarely seen The International Fragrance Association [5] has recommended that musk ambrette not be used on any preparation that touches the human skin. Years ago there were perfumes that contained oil of Bergamot which caused phototoxic reaction due to the psoralen. Today psoralen-free oil of Bergamot is used. The fragrance materials that cause phototoxic contact dermatitis are the following[5]:

- 5-Acetyl-1,1,2,3,3,6-hexamethylindane
- Angelica root oil (*Angelica archangelic* L.)
- Bergamot oil expressed (*Citrus aurantium* L. *bergamia* Wright et Arn.)
- Cumin oil (*Cumin cyminum* L.)
- Fig leaf absolute (*Ficus carica*)
- Lemon oil cold presses (*Citrus limon* L. Burm. F.)

- Lime oil, expressed (*Citrus aurantifolia* Swingle)
- Methyl *N*-methylanthranilate
- Orange peel oil, bitter (*Citrus aurantium* L.)
- Rue oil (*Ruta graveolens* L.)
- Tagetes absolute (*Tagetes patula* L.)
- Tagetes minute absolute (*Tagetes minuta* or *T. glandulifera*)
- Tagetes oil (*Tagetes erecta* L.; *T. glandulifera* Schrank)
- Verbena oil (*Lippia citriodora* Kunth)

Detection of Fragrance Dermatitis

During the 1960s and 1970s Balsam of Peru was a marker for fragrance dermatitis. In the late 1970s a fragrance mixture (FM) was introduced as a screening preparation. The FM consists of the following eight [8] chemicals:

- Cinnamic alcohol
- Cinnamic aldehyde
- Isoeugenol
- Eugenol
- Hydroxycitronellal
- Geraniol
- α-Amyl cinnamic aldehyde
- Oak moss absolute

Originally the fragrance mixture consisted of these eight [8] chemicals at a concentration of 2% each in petrolatum. This proved to be irritating so the concentration was reduced to 1% of each component for a total of 8% in petrolatum. This 8% fragrance mixture (8% FM) proved effective in detecting approximately 70% to 80% of fragrance allergic reactions [6, 7]. In most screening series it ranks second to nickel in percentage of positive reactions. Recently the emulsifier sorbitan sesquioleate has been added to enhance the effectiveness of the mixture.

A New Fragrance Mixture

There have been numerous studies to try to improve the screening ability of the 8% FM. In 1989 Wilkinson and coworkers tested over 2400 consecutive patch test patients to the standard 8% FM and a new one at 9.5% [8]. This new 9.5% FM was similar to the standard fragrance mixture except that dihydrocoumarin and citral were substituted for the oak moss and amyl cinnamaldehyde. The overall incidence of allergy to fragrance materials as measured by these two mixtures was 7.8% for the 8% FM and 6.7% for the new 9.5% FM. Both dihydrocoumarin and citral gave significant number of positive reactions. However, the workers did not pursue the use of this new fragrance mixture since citral and dihydrocoumarin are no longer commonly used in perfumes.

Testing with Fragrance Materials Based on Quantity Used in the United States

Recently Frosch and members of the European Environmental Contact Dermatitis Research Group tested 48 frequently used fragrance chemicals in an effort to determine the frequency of reactivity in dermatological patients with contact dermatitis [9]. The 48 fragrance materials were chosen based on the frequency of use of these materials in three types of 400 commercial products on the United States market. These three products were perfumes, household products and soaps. For most fragrance materials a concentration of 1% – 5% was used. Petrolatum was the best vehicle compared to isopropyl myristate and diethylphthalate.

All patients were tested to the standard series used in Europe which included the 8% FM and its eight [8] constituents. A total of 1323 patients were tested in the 11 centers. The 8% FM was positive in 8.3% if the patients and allergic reactions to the constituents were most frequent to oak moss, isoeugenol, eugenol, cinnamic aldehyde and geraniol. Of the 48 new fragrance materials 41 tested were negative. Allergic reactions were observed only ten times to seven materials of the new fragrance materials. The positive reactions were to Iso E Super™ (1,1,6,7-tetramethyl-6-acetyl decalene isomers) (n=2), Lyral (4-(4-hydroxy-4-methylpentyl)-3-cyclohexenel-1-carboxaldehyde) (n=3), Cyclacet (3,4-dihydroxycyclopentadien-2/3-yl acetate) (n=1), dimethylbenzyl carvinyl acetate (DMBCA) (n=1), Vertofix™ (Acetylcedrene) (n=1), Citronellal (n=1), and amyl salicylate (n=1). The clinical relevance of the positive reactions to any of the seven fragrance materials was not proved in a single case. Thus they concluded that the top fragrance materials commonly used in various products caused few reactions in dermatological patients and these appeared to be clinically irrelevant with the possible exception of Lyral. However, this data should be interpreted in light of the relatively small number of patients tested (only 100 in most centers).

Fragrance Mixture and Sorbitan Sesquioleate

In fragrance mixture positive patients it has been observed that testing to the eight constituents of the mixture is negative in a substantial number of cases. In 1991 Enders studied this discrepancy and found that by adding sorbitan sesquioleate (SSO) to each individual component the reactivity to individual components was greatly enhanced.

In 1992 Frosch [10] and members of the Europe Environmental Contact Dermatitis Research Group studied this phenomenon in a larger patient base consisting of 709 consecutive patients. They found that when testing the constituents without SSO, 41.5% showed an allergic reaction versus 54.7% with the SSO.

Three-Year Study of Fragrance Materials

In 1992 a 3-year world wide multicenter (United States, Europe, Japan) investigation was launched to expand the information on fragrance sensitization [11]. The purpose was to determine the prevalence of responses to selected fragrance materials in patients with known allergy and to further evaluate the risk factors and association with such responses. In 1992, 167 subjects were evaluated in seven centers worldwide with the 8% FM, the eight ingredients in the fragrance mixture, six other well-known fragrance allergens, balsam of Peru and 15 less well studied fragrance materials (Table 1). By design one-half of these patients were fragrance sensitive by history only and the other half were fragrance sensitive by past positive patch tests to fragrance materials. Eighty-five percent of the patients were female. The face and hands were the most common sites of clinical involvement. Of these patients 47.3% reacted to

Table 1. Responses to fragrance ingredients ($n = 167$)

Ingredient	Responses (%)	Ingredient	Responses (%)
Fragrance mix 8	47.3	α-Amyl-cinnamic aldehyde 5	3.0
Balsam of Peru 25 (N-125)	27.2	Benzyl salicylate 2	3.0
Ylang-ylang oil 10	17.4	Patchouli oil (C V Kaimun Medan) 10	3.0
Cinnamic aldehyde 1	14.4	Helional (IFF) 5	2.4
Hydroxycitronellal 4	13.8	Cedramber 5	1.8
Isoeugenol 4	13.8	Anisyl alcohol 5	1.8
Hydroxycitronellal 7	13.8	Benzyl alcohol 5	1.2
Oak moss absolute 5	13.2	Violet leaves absolute 2	1.2
Eugenol 5	7.8	Lilial 5	1.2
Narcissus absolute 2	6.6	Coumarin 5	1.2
Cinnamic alcohol 5, lanolin	6.6	Lanolin (purified) as is	1.2
Sandela (Givaudan) 5	6.6	Floropal 5	1.2
Sandalwood oil 10	6.6	Musk ambrette 5	1.2
Majantol (Drom) 5	5.4	Ligustral (Schiff's base) 5	0.6
Benzyl salicylate 5	4.8	Helional (Schiff's base) 5	0.6
Galbanum resin 2	4.8	Cashmeran 5	0.6
Geraniol 5	3.0	Petrolatum as is	0.6
Sandalore (Givaudan) 5	3.0	Sorbitan sesquioleate 20	0.6

Table 2. Differences in response in patients of different races: percentage allergic

Test substance	Caucasians ($n=117$)	Asians ($n=48$)	p
Fragrance Mix 8%	52.8	25.5	<0.01
Isoeugenol	15.8	4.2	0.04
Oakmoss absolute	14.2	2.1	0.03
Benzyl salicylate	1.7	10.6	0.01

the fragrance mixture. There were fewer positive responses elicited to the 8% FM, isoeugenol and oak moss absolute in Asians when compared to Caucasians. In contrast Asians were more likely to exhibit a response to benzyl salicylate (Table 2). The response to the 8% FM in the United States and Europe were similar. Oak moss absolute produced more responses in Europe than in the United States or Japan.

Frequent reactions were seen to the 8% FM, balsam of Peru, ylang-ylang oil, narcissus absolute and sandalwood oil. Reactions to the 8% FM were concordant with 290 of a total of 328 positive responded to the individual test materials (i.e. 88.4% of all positives). Sensitivity of ylang-ylang oil, Narcissus and sandalwood oil as a possible second group of screening test substances to be formulated as a mixture was evaluated. Testing with these three naturals would pick up 19 positives that would have been missed with the 8% FM alone, yield an attributable improvement in positive response frequency of 6%. Thus, by using both mixtures, a detection rate of 309 positives, or 94.2% of the responses obtained by testing with all the individual fragrance in gredients. Balsam of Peru was tested on only 148 of the study patients (not tested in Japan). Balsam of Peru elicited six positive responses that were missed by the two mixtures. Thus balsam of Peru improved the proportion of positive responses to individual ingredients that were predicted to 315 or 96%. The data thus suggests that using a second fragrance mixture consisting of the natural materials ylang-ylang oil, narcissus and sandalwood oil might be useful in extending the usefulness of the 8% FM. The second study in 1993 showed a significant number of reactions to Jasmine absolute 10% in petrolatum and spearmint oil 5% in petrolatum. The final study in 1994 showed a significant number of reactions to clove bud oil 10% in petrolatum. This year an international study comparing the 8% FM with a newly designed natural fragrance mixture was started.

This new fragrance mixture consists of five nature fragrance materials in petrolatum:

- Ylang-Ylang oil 2%
- Narcissus absolute 2%
- Sandalwood oil 2%

Table 3. Synthetic jasmine with components of the 8% FM

Benzyl acetate	31.90%	Anethol USP	0.50%
Benzyl alcohol	11.76%	Cycloprop	0.80%
Phenyl ethyl alcohol	12.69%	Nonalactone	0.50%
Linalool	11.10%	Methyl anthranilate	1.00%
Gamma decalactone	2.28%	Cinnamic alcohol	1.00%
Para cresyl methyl ether	0.13%	Cinnamic aldehyde	1.00%
Benzyl salicylate	4.52%	Eugenol	1.00%
Hexyl cinnamic aldehyde	6.34%	Isoeugenol	1.00%
Hydroxycitronellal	1.00%	Geraniol	1.00%
Butyl cinnamic aldehyde	3.88%	Oakmoss absolute Yugo. (Charabot)	1.00%
Methyl dihydro jasmonate	3.00%		
Indol	0.80%	Jasmine absolute Egyptian (Charabot)	1.00%
Ethyl benzoate	0.80%		

- Jasmine absolute 2%
- Spearmint oil 2%

The composition of the natural mixture is based on the results obtained in the three year international study. The natural fragrance mixture is being used to determine whether it extended the screening ability of the original 8% FM. The disadvantage of natural materials is that these substances are not chemically defined and may vary from batch to batch depending on where and when the natural materials are processed. Balsam of Peru is also being tested as is a newly designed synthetic jasmine. This synthetic jasmine also contains the ingredients of the 8% FM (Table 3).

The Future

Fragrance are constantly changing in the marketplace as new synthetic materials are developed. Therefore, epidemiological studies are important to determine which fragrance materials are causing allergic reactions. Some patients are found to be allergic to a perfume but have negative reactions to the fragrance mixture and balsam of Peru. These patients are of great interest since they presumably have an allergen which has not been well defined. These patients should be tested to all of the components of the perfume in order to determine the specific allergen. By doing this we will find new allergens and can consider them in future fragrance screening series. Most perfume companies are cooperative and provide individual constituents of the perfumes for patch testing. Normally four fractions of the perfume are provided. When a positive reaction is encountered, that particular fraction is further broken down into all of the individual components. This procedure was recently reported by Handly and Burrows [12] who had two patients who broke out to a perfume in two separate deodorant preparations. These workers tested the components of the perfume and found that the patients were allergic to lyral and acetyl cedrene. This case is a great interest since only three cases of lyral sensitivity have previously been reported and no cases of acetyl cedrene have been recognized. Thus they discovered a new fragrance material, acetyl cedrene, which may be of value in epidemiological studies.

At the present time, the 8% FM and balsam of Peru in a screening series is essential since they detect approximately 80% of fragrance sensitivity. Adding a synthetic jasmine to the screening series is also useful [13].

References

1. Adams RM, Maibach HI (1985) A five year study of cosmetic reactions. J Am Acad Dermatol 13:1062–1069
2. Larsen WG (1985) Perfume dermatitis. J Am Acad Dermatol 12:1–9
3. Raugi GJ, Storrs FJ, Larsen WG (1979) Photoallergic contact dermatitis to men's perfumes. Contact Dermatitis 5:251–260
4. Jackson RT, Nesbitt LT Jr, DeLeo VA (1980) 6-Methylcoumarin photocontact dermatitis. J Am Acad Dermatol 2:124–127
5. Ford R (1991) The toxicology and safety of fragrances. In: Muller PM, Lamparsky D (eds) Perfumes: art, science, technology. Elsevier, New York, pp 441–463
6. Calnan CD, Cronin E, Rycroft R (1980) Allergy to perfume ingredients. Contact Dermatitis 6:500–501
7. Johansen JD, Menne T (1985) The fragrance mix and its constituents: a 14-year material. Contact Dermatitis 32:18–23
8. Wilkinson JD Andersen K, Camarasa J, Ducombs F, Frosch P, Lahti A, Menne T, Rycroft RJG, White I (1989) Preliminary results on the effectiveness of two forms of fragrance mix as screening agents for fragrance sensitivity. Current Topics in Contact Dermatitis, Springer Heidelberg, pp 127–131
9. Frosch PJ, Pilz B, Andersen KE, Burrows D, Camarasa JG, Dooms-Goossens A, Ducombs G, Fuch T, Maibach HI, Menne T, Rycoft RJG, Shaw S, Wahlberg JE, White IR, Wilkinson JD (1995) Patch testing with fragrances: results of a multicenter study of the European Environmental and Contact Dermatitis Research Group with 48 frequently used constituents of perfumes. Contact Dermatitis 33:333–342
10. Frosch PJ, Pilz B, Burrows D, Camarasa JG, Lachapelle JM, Lahti A, Menne T, Wilkinson JD (1995) Testing fragrance mix. Is the addition of sorbitan sesquioleate to the constituents useful? Contact Dermatitis 32:266–272
11. Larsen WG, Nakayama H, Fischer T, Elsner P, Burrows D, Jordan W, Shaw S, Wilkinson J, Marks J, Sugawara M, Nethercott J (1996) Fragrance contact dermatitis: a worldwide multicenter investigation. Am J Contact Derm 7:77–83
12. Hadley J, Burrows D (1994) Allergic contact dermatitis from the synthetic fragrances lyral and acetyl cedrene in separate underarm deodorant preparations. Contact Dermatitis 31:288–290
13. Larsen WG (1977) Perfume dermatitis: a study of 20 patients. Arch Dermatology 113:623

Fragrance Hypersensitivity and Its Control

Hideo Nakayama

Fragrances have been used by mankind more than 3000 years, judging from the perfume container discovered in an ancient ruin in India and from a fresco showing ladies enjoying perfume in Egypt. They will surely also be used in the future since they are a kind of art, and at the same time are a part of our daily necessities such as cosmetics, toiletries and food. Some fragrances, however, have been demonstrated to be allergenic, and responsible for causing cosmetic dermatitis. Therefore discovering these "trouble making" fragrances was the first stage. Replacing them with alternative fragrances was then necessary at the second stage. This combination project has been carried out in Japan since 1970. This is a short report on the history of the project.

Project to Discover Common Cosmetic Sensitizers

In the 1960s many Japanese women suffered severe cosmetic dermatitis. There are two clinical types: the first is ordinary allergic contact dermatitis with symptoms of erythema, swelling, itching, papules and fine scaling. Histopathological findings spongiosis of the epidermis and perivasular lymphocytic and monocytic infiltration of the upper dermis, a typical feature of type IV hypersensitivity. The second type is a bizarre reticular or diffuse brown or black hyperpigmentation of the face, which could not be cured by any treatment before 1972, when a treatment by the name of "allergen control" started (Fig. 1).

Biopsy revealed that the causation of this persistent hyperpigmentation was pigmentary incontinence, an accumulation of melanin released from the cytolysis of basal and suprabasal prickle layer cells by the attack of lymphocytes. As this pigmentary disorder of the face was so disastrous and was suspected to result from contact hypersensitivity, because of the presence of cytolysis associated with lymphocyte invasion, a project was started to discover the unknown contact allergens in cosmetics in 1970 [2].

A total of 477 cosmetic components, including fragrances, pigments, base materials and preservatives, were patch tested for 2 days to detect their irritancy on a few volunteers as the first trial. Then 287 selected components were

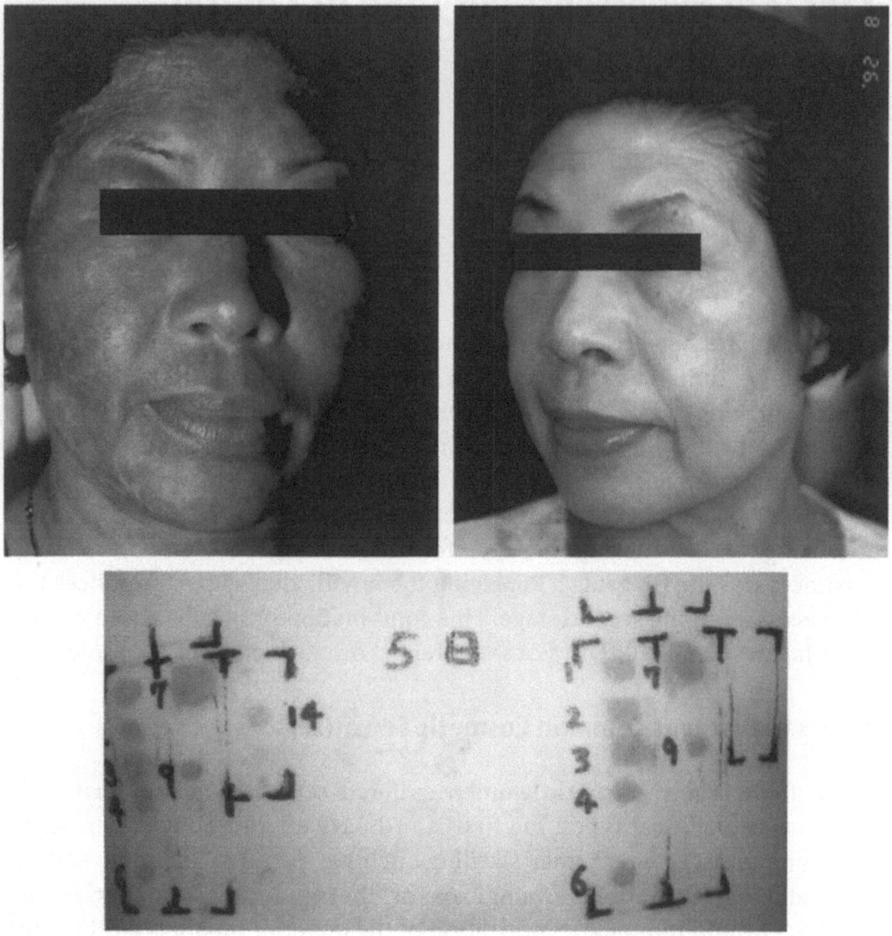

a c

b

Fig. 1 a–c. A 50-year-old woman suffering from severe pigmented cosmetic dermatitis of the face. **a** The dark brown diffuse pigmentation could not be cured by any antisymptomatic treatment. **b** A patch test showed that she was strongly sensitized to a variety of fragrances such as jasmine, canaga oil, ylang-ylang oil, geraniol, eugenol, hydroxycitronellal, balsam of Peru, and lavender oil, which were patch-tested at nonirritating concentrations. *Left*, there was no exacerbation of photopatch testing with UV-A, irradiated at 5.85 j/cm^2. Pigments showed negative results. Allergen control, i.e., the use of only allergen-free soaps (solid Minon) and cosmetics (As ceine) prevented further recurrence of the dermatitis, and she was cured completely after 2 years of use. **c** Relapse did not occur as she avoided contamination of ordinary cosmetics and soaps for 15 years

patch tested on 30–40 healthy volunteers to confirm the highest concentrations without causing irritation as the second trial. These concentrations were chosen because a previous test reported by a dermatologist and a fragrance company failed to discover cosmetic allergens when these components were patch tested at 0.1%–0.5% concentrations, revealing that such concentrations must have been too low to detect the causative contact allergens. Primary sensitizers, such as methyl heptine carbonate and costus root oil, were discovered at this second trial, and it was decided not to test these further on the patients [2].

In the third trial the cosmetic components which showed negative results on the 30–40 healthy volunteers were rearranged into ten groups, and patch tested on dermatitis patients. This was 6 years before the invention of the Finn-Chambers; therefore these patch test materials were patch-tested using a classical vinyl patch test plasters carrying round cotton pads of 8 mm in diameter (Miniplaster, Torii Pharmaceutical, Japan). The fragrance materials were patched for 2 days and were removed on the morning of the 2nd day so that the reading of the 2nd day (approximately 48 h) could be made a few to several hours after the removal of the patch test. The reading was made on the 2nd, 3rd and 7th days of the patch test. The patients were classified into pigmented cosmetic dermatitis, cosmetic dermatitis without pigmentation and dermatoses other than cosmetic dermatitis. The statistical significance using the *F* test was calculated between two groups, a cosmetic dermatitis group, including pigmented and nonpigmented cosmetic dermatitis, and controls, including dermatoses other than cosmetic dermatitis and healthy volunteers. Those cosmetic components which showed significant high *F* values were regarded as cosmetic allergens on the condition that the positive patch test reactions were allergic in nature, and reproducible [3]. Those which showed almost no positive reactions at such high concentrations of 5%–10%, showing *F* test values from 0 to 5, were regarded as cosmetic components which did not sensitize, even though they had been used in quantity by the industry. An example of the reactivity is shown in Table 1.

A number of common cosmetic sensitizers in the Fig. 2 were discovered or confirmed during 1970 and 1975, and after that period, several new allergens, such as D&C yellow no. 11, artificial sandalwood (a mixture of bornyl methoxy cyclohexanol and other components), armoise oil, bay oil, spearmint oil, narcissus absolute, and Iso E super were found. As primary sensitizers D&C yellow no. 11, costus root oil and methylheptine carbonate were the first to be discovered, followed by damascone and damacenone. These primary sensitizers were not patch tested on the patients except for D & C yellow no. 11 because they were found to have been primary sensitizers at the stage of volunteer testing.

D & C yellow no. 11 was a primary sensitizer at 5% in a polyethyleneglycol base, but was continued to be patch tested especially on systemic lupus ery-

Table 1. Reactivity of ylang-ylang oil (5% in petrolatum, evaluated in 1974)

Reactions	Cosmetic dermatitis		Controls		Total
	Pigmented	Not pigmented	Other dermatoses	Healthy	
(+), (++)	9	4	3	0	16
? (+)	10	9	3	0	22
(–)	102	96	112	40	350
Subtotal	121	109	118	40	
Total	230		158		388

Cosmetic dermatitis vs. controls: $F = 11.10, p \leq 0.01$.

Table 2. Reactivity of D & C yellow no 11 (5% in polyethyleneglycol, evaluated up to 1979)

Reactions	Cosmetic dermatitis	SLE	Other diseases	Total
(+), (++)	4	5	1	10
? (+)	4	1	3	8
(–)	39	3	27	69
Total	47	9	31	87

themathosus (SLE) patients, for this reason it was regarded an important causation of SLE at that time (Table 2) [4]. D & C yellow no. 11 was prohibited to be used in cosmetics except for hair and nail preparations in 1980 by the Japanese Government, and after that there was a remarkable decrease in the frequency of severe cases of SLE in young women; therefore the patch test of D & C yellow no. 11 was regarded as unnecessary thereafter. It was after the introduction of D & C yellow no. 11 especially in lipsticks that there occurred a worldwide outbreak of SLE, a new disease after the World War II, and today young women with severe SLE are rare in Japan. Considering the fact that successive injection of D & C yellow no. 11 with complete adjuvant produces serum antinuclei antibody in rabbits with cutaneous erythema, yellow no. 11 was apparently one of most disastrous cosmetic allergens in the history of mankind. It is strongly recommended that D & C yellow no. 11 be prohibited worldwide [5].

As for fragrances, it was only hydroxycitronellal that produced several positive reactions in SLE patients, and they were not regarded as important allergens associated with SLE. On the other hand, patients with ordinary cosmetic dermatitis and pigmented cosmetic dermatitis (PCD) produced numerous positives with a variety of fragrances.

Common cosmetic sensitizers newly discovered by this project included jasmine absolute, ylang-ylang oil, cananga oil, sandalwood oil, artificial san-

Cosmetic contact allergens discovered or detected during 1970 and 1975

1970	1971	1972	1973	1974	1975
Hydroxycitronellal		Benzyl salicylate			Red-219 (D & C Red 31)
Jasmine oil		Methoxycitronellal			Isosafrol
α-Hexylcinnamic aldehyde			Benzyl propionate		
Patchouli oil			Benzyl alcohol		
Geranium oil			Methyl salicylate		
	Cananga oil				
	ylang ylang oil				
	Vetivers				
	Sandal wood oil				
	Costus root oil*				
	Methyl heptine carbonate*				

* Primary sensitizers

Fig. 2. Cosmetic contact allergens discovered or detected between 1970 and 1975

dalwood, benzyl salicylate, methoxycitronellal, geraniol, geranium oil, and hay green [1–3]. Hydroxycitronellal, which was reported as a causation of a case of occupational contact dermatitis by Saito [6], was also found to have been a common cosmetic sensitizer by this research project [1]. Rare cosmetic sensitizers newly discovered included vetivers, narcissus absolute, bay oil, armoise oil, spearmint oil, and eucalyptus oil.

Such discoveries in addition to the knowledge of fragrance allergens reported previously to this project, such as bergamot oil, rose oil, lavender oil, cinnamic derivatives and eugenol [7], enabled the group to perform an allergen control, the first trial in the world to eliminate all the conceivable and detected allergens from the soaps, shampoos, and cosmetics for the patients' contact environment, The system composed of patch test reagents, including fragrances, pigments such as D&C red 31 (Japanese name: R-219) [8, 9], D & C yellow no. 10 (Japanese name: Y-203), wool alcohols and methylparaben, Miniplaster, UV-A irradiator for photopatch testing, allergen-controlled soap (Minon) and cosmetics (Acseine) were at that time designated Allergen Control System (ACS) [1–3].

The introduction of ACS successfully disclosed the responsible contact sensitizers in soaps, shampoos and cosmetics for the pigmented and nonpigmented cosmetic dermatitis patients, and at the same time, could completely cure this disastrous cosmetic trouble at the rate of 75% by 1977 [3]. It was an epoche-making event in the field of contact hypersensitivity. The success strongly suggested that a close support of cosmetic industries and fragrance industry to dermatologists was most recommended to solve the contact dermatitis problems caused by cosmetics and toiletries.

Prevention

After the causative cosmetic sensitizers were confirmed by repeated study of patch testing and the effect of allergen control, it was natural that prevention of cosmetic dermatitis was planned in 1977. After this year efforts have been concentrated to find out not only new contact allergens in cosmetic materials but also materials which can be used by the cosmetic industries without causing cosmetic dermatitis and the secondary hyperpigmentation. Similar trials performed after 1977 resulted in the discoveries of a few new allergens, confirmation of already discovered allergens, and their cross-sensitizers, and also the discoveries of a number of fragrances which did not show positive reactions on either the cosmetic dermatitis patients or the controls even at high concentrations of 5%–10%. The latter were regarded as very safe materials even to the patients hypersensitive to various cosmetic components judging from clear negative results of patch testing. In 1980 the accumulated data enabled the classification of fragrant materials into four groups (see "Appendix"). The mixture of numerous class C and D fragrances actually eliminates all the common and rare sensitizers. It was the perfumers' skill that decided the nature of the fragrances they made for the products, having the notes such as bouquet, oriental, floral, etc. Hitoshi Hiroyama, an extraordinarily excellent perfumer of the Hasegawa Perfumery Company, Tokyo, could make a hypoallergenic jasmine oil using only class C and D fragrances. The results of patch testing performed by a project E-360 in eight countries (United States, Japan, Germany, Ireland, Switzerland, Sweden, Denmark, United Kingdom) showed no positives among 178 persons tested, while 16.9% positively reacted when jasmine absolute was patch-tested at the same concentration of 10% in petrolatum. It was amazing that even having a similar note of jasmine, the mixture of class C and D fragrances did not produce any positive reaction among most hypersensitive persons to fragrances in eight countries [10].

Less success was experienced with hypoallergenic ylang-ylang oil, presumably because it was not only dehydrodiisoeugenol but also cinnamic derivatives that were the contact sensitizers in it. Even with the use of class C and D fragrances 7.3% of the 192 internationally studied patients positively reacted to hypoallergenic ylang-ylang oil, while 17.2% of the same patients positively reacted to natural ylang-ylang oil at the same 10% concentration.

Since about 1980 some Japanese cosmetics companies have adopted the Guideline System, by which they can avoid the usage of class A fragrances

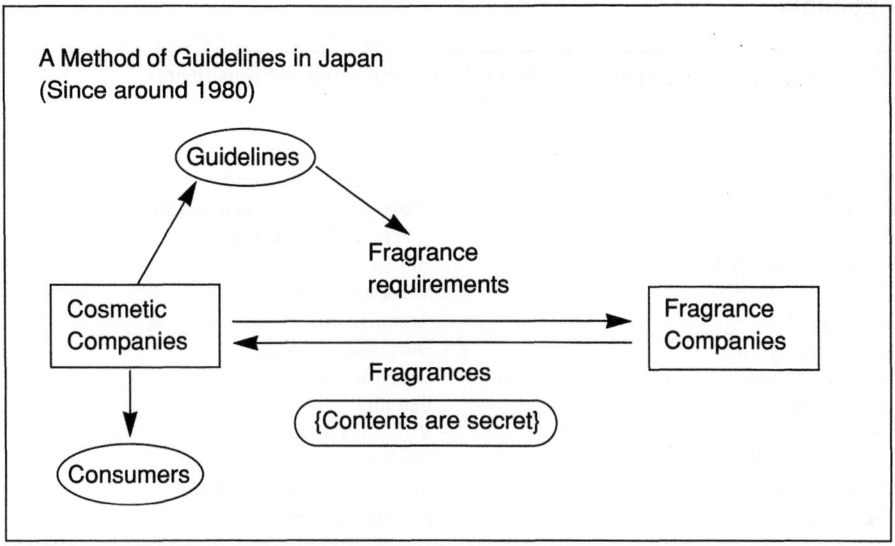

Fig. 3. The guideline method in use in Japan

(Fig. 3). This had resulted in the great decrease in the positive rates of common fragrance sensitizers. An international comparative study on the previously mentioned E-360 has demonstrated significantly lower positive rates in Japan than in the United States and Europe [10]. Apparently Japanese cosmetic companies had to use class B, C and D, whereas fragrance companies were honest enough to avoid the use of class A fragrance after the Guidelines were requested by cosmetic companies.

Conclusions

To decrease the incidence of certain allergens such as fragrance materials, their use can easily be avoided by using alternative materials. Guidelines to avoid them have already been set up by a part of the cosmetic industry. The history of discovering fragrance allergens and their substitutes over the past 26 years shows that it is important for us not only to discover contact sensitizers but also to discover substitutes for allergens by patch testing. The usage of class C and D fragrances are more highly recommended to the cosmetic industry than class A and B fragrances.

Appendix

Class A fragrances (common cosmetic sensitizers and primary* sensitizers)	
Hydroxycitronellal (*d* & *d*, *l*)	Geranium oil
Jasmine absolute	Sandalwood oil
Ylang-ylang oil	Artificial sandalwood
Cananga oil	(Bornyl methoxy cyclohexanol containing artificial sandalwood)
Cinnamic alcohol	Hay green
Cinnamic aldehyde	Musk ambrette
Eugenol	Armoise oil
Isoeugenol	Narcissus absolute
Benzyl salicylate	Lavender oil
Balsam of Peru	Bay oil
d-Carvone	Violet leaves absolute
l-Carvone	Methylheptine carbonate*
Costus root oil*	Methyloctine carbonate*
α-Damascone	β-Damascone*
Geraniol	

Class B fragrances (rare sensitizers)	
Amylis oil	Fir balsam absolute
Citral diethyl acetate	Nutmeg oil
l-Hydroxycitronellal	*d*-Methoxycitronellal
Vetiver oil	*cis*-3-Hexenyl acetate
α-Ionone	Acetivenol
β-Ionone	Allyl cyclohexyl propionate
Methylisoeugenol	Bourgeons de cassis absolute
Clove buds oil	β-Damacenone
Cedarwood oil	5-Cyclohexadecenone
Basil oil	Rose de May absolute
Cedramber	γ-Methylionone
Oakmoss absolute	α-Methylionone
Petitgrain citronnier	Others
Iso E super	

Class C fragrances (virtually nonsensitizing fragrances)	
Isoamyl salicylate	Gerany nitril
γ-Dodecalactone	Lyral
Guaiacyl acetate	Musk tibetene
6-Isobutyl quinoline	Ligustral
γ-Undecalactone	ε-Nonalactone
Neroli oil	Rosemary oil
Bergamot oil FL (furocoumanrinfree)	*p*-*tert*-Butyl cyclohexyl acetate
Tetrahydrogeraniol	Allyl amyl glycolate
ε-Decalactone	Allyl ionone
cis-3-Hexenol	Ambrette seed oil
Musk ketone	Bois de rose oil
Citral hexylene glycol acetal	Linalool

Class C fragrances (virtually nonsensitizing fragrances) (continued)	
Caraway oil	Mentyl acetate
Citronellyl acetate	Petigrain oil
Cumin oil	*l*-Nonanal
l-Methoxycitronellal	*l*-Decanal
Isobutyl salicylate	Bacdanol
Phenyl propyl alcohol	Others
Lavandin oil	

Class D fragrances (Considered as nonsensitizers)	
Linalool oxide	ε-Dodecalactone
Dihydro linalool	Phenylethyl isoamyl ether
Dihydro myrcenol	Mandarin oil
Myrcenyl acetate	Octyl dodecanol
Pentalide	Almond oil
Phenylethyl salicylate	Phenylacetaldehyde dimethylacetal
Tonka absolute	Jasmal
Tetrahydro linalool	δ-Nonalactone
Tetrahydromuguol	δ-Undecalactone
Tetrahydromyrcenol	γ-Nonalactone
Isopropyl myristate	γ-Decalactone
Hedione	δ-Dodecalactone
Citronellyl nitrile	Isobuthyl angelate
Lemon FL (furocoumarinfree)	*cis*-3-Hexenyl salicylate
Lime oil FL (furocoumarinfree)	Others

References

1. Nakayama H (1974) Perfume allergy and cosmetic dermatitis. Jap J Dermatol 84:659–667 (in Japanese)
2. Nakayama H, Hanaoka H, Ohshiro A (1974) Allergen controlled system 1–42. Kanehara Shuppan, Tokyo
3. Nakayama H, Matsuo S, Hayakawa K et al. (1984) Pigmented cosmetic dermatitis. Int J Dermatol 23:299–305
4. Inamoto N, Nakayama H, Hirai A (1979) Two cases of lupus erythematosus, allergic to Y-204. Rinsho-Hifuka 33:1075–1082 (in Japanese)
5. Nishiyama O, Suzuki A, Nakayama H (1988) A case of SLE acutely aggravated after the fifth day of the strong positive D&C yellow no.11 patch test. Hifu 30(4):113–121 (in Japanese with English abstract)
6. Saito F (1960) A case of perfume dermatitis. Hifuka-Rinsho 2:930–933 (in Japanese)
7. Fisher AA (1967) Contact dermatitis. Lea & Febiger, New York
8. Nakayama H, Harada R, Toda M (1976) Pigmented cosmetic dermatitis. Int J Dermatol 15:673–675
9. Kozuka T, Tashiro M, Sano S et al. (1979) Brilliant Lake Red R as a cause of pigmented contact dermatitis. Contact Dermatitis 5:297–304
10. Larsen W, Nakayama H, Lindberg M et al. (1996) Fragrance contact dermatitis: a worldwide multicenter investigation. I. Am J Contact Dermatitis 7:77–83

Are Major Components of Fragrances a Problem?

P. J. Frosch, on behalf of the European Environmental
and Contact Dermatitis Research Group (EECDRG)

The fragrance mix (FM), or perfume mix, as introduced for screening by Larsen [1] in 1977, contains eight basic constituents of perfumes commonly used at that time (eugenol, isoeugenol, oak moss, geraniol, hydroxycitronellal, α-amyl cinnamic aldehyde, cinnamic alcohol, and cinnamic aldehyde). Originally formulated at 16% in petrolatum (pet., 2% of each constituent), it frequently produced irritant reactions; therefore the FM was lowered to 8%. With this mix, the response rate in dermatological patients presently ranges worldwide from 4% to 11%: Germany, from 7.5% [2] to 11.2% [3]; Denmark, 5.5% [4]; Belgium 8.3% (A. Dooms-Goossens, personal communication); Portugal, 4.2% (329 children) [5]; Sweden, 5.6% [6]; and in Europe as a whole, 7.8% (2455 patients at eight centres [7]).

In most lists of frequent allergens, the FM ranges among the top five, usually number two after nickel sulfate. Although it is frequently stated that the FM often produces false-positive reactions, the European Environmental and Contact Dermatitis Research Group (EECDRG) was able to demonstrate in a large study on 702 patients that clinical relevance does exist in at least two thirds of positive patch test results [8]. The highest proportion of 2+ and 3+ reactions was found in the group with a positive fragrance history (55/82 = 67%). However, quite a few reactions were observed without a clear clinical history. The proportion of negative or doubtful relevance was particularly high in the group of 1+ (39/53) and doubtful reactions (57/70) (Table 1).

Table 1. Intensity of patch test reactions to the 8% fragrance mix and/or constituents in relationship to history (from [8])

Fragrance history	±/IR	+	++	+++	Total
Positive	13	14	39	16	82
Negative	52	25	26	0	103
Doubtful	5	14	18	2	39
Total	70	53	83	18	224

For this reason, testing with the current FM has been frequently criticised:

1. 'The sensitizing capacities of these eight constituents are well-known and no conscientious perfumer would compose such a "cocktail of super allergens" for one product'.
2. 'Institutions such as the International Fragrance Association (IFRA) and the Research Institute for Fragrance Materials (RIFM) have published recommendations regarding the safe usage of these and other fragrance components which are followed by most manufacturers (concentration limits and even bans on certain fragrances)' [9].
3. 'The overwhelming majority of fragrance constituents is either non-sensitizing or, if so, is used at such low concentrations that no risk for the consumer will ensue. Dermatologists do not test and therefore paint an unjustified, "negative picture" of the fragrance industry'.

Fenn [10] has examined the 'aroma chemical usage trends in modern perfumery' by detecting the top 25 materials in 'fine fragrances' (perfumes, toilet water, some creams), household products (fabric softener, cleaners) and soaps (bar, tablet). Each group included products commonly purchased in the United States. Fenn composed a list of the most frequently used fragrance materials in the year 1987/88, based on quantitative analysis (vol %).

Intrigued by this list, the EECDRG performed a patch test study with these Fenn Fragrances (FF). The major aims of this study were to answer the following questions:

1. Are dermatological patients sensitized to these materials?
2. If so, what is the clinical relevance of the reactions?
3. Can one or a series of FF replace the current fragrance mix for identifying fragrance-sensitive patients?

Materials and Methods

The details of this study have been published [11]. Briefly, a total of 48 fragrance constituents were tested in 11 centres on consecutive patients of the patch test clinic. A total of 1323 patients were examined, with testing consisting in most centres of a minimum of 100 patients exposed to a set of five chemicals. Concentrations ranged from 0.1% to 5% in petrolatum (most materials were tested at 1% and 5%). Concentration and vehicle were based on an initial study. Isopropyl myristate was found to be an unsuitable vehicle because of the high number of irritant reactions it triggered. Diethylphthalate was also not regarded as appropriate because reactivity was too low – allergic reactions were absent in cases where the same fragrance in petrolatum had produced strong reactions. All FF materials were of high-grade quality and kindly provided by Harmann and Reimer (Holzminden, Germany).

The 8% fragrance mix contained 5% sorbitan sesquioleate (SSO) as emulsifier; the eight constituents were tested at 1% with the addition of 1% SSO; the vehicle was petrolatum.

The standard patch test procedure was carried out with Finn chambers on Scanpore tape applied for 2 days to the back with readings on days 2 and 3 (or in some centres on days 2 and 4) as described by Wahlberg [12].

Results

An excerpt of the extensive data is given in Tables 2 and 3. The FF series produced only a few reactions, the majority of patients being negative to these materials. In contrast, the 8% FM caused allergic reaction at a frequency of 8.3% (ranging from 5% to 14% in nine centres). In the 'breakdown' the constituents of the mix were frequently positive: oak moss, isoeugenol and eugenol were among the top three.

Table 2. Results of patch tests with Fenn Fragrances (FF) (from [12])

	Concentration (%)	Positive/tested	Positive (%)
Allergic reactions[a]			
Amyl salicylate	5	1/100	1.0
Lyral	5	3/106	2.8
Lyral	1	1/106	0.9
Vertofix (acetyl cedrene)	1	1/100	1.0
Citronellol	1	1/100	1.0
Amyl salicylate	5	2/100	1.0
Eugenol	5	2/107	1.9
Hydroxycitronellal	5	1/107	0.9
Hydroxycitronellal	1	1/107	0.9
Iso E Super (1,1,6,7-tetra-methyl-6-acetyl decalene (isomers))	5	1/313	0.3
Iso E Super (1,1,6,7-tetra-methyl-6-acetyl decalene (isomers))	1	1/313	0.3
Cyclacet	5	1/313	0.3
DMBCA (dimethylbenzyl carbinyl acetate)	5	1/313	0.3
Doubtful of irritant reactions[b]			
Linalool	5	1/100	1
Linalool	1	1/100	1
Benzyl acetate	1	1/100	1
Benzyl salicylate	5	1/100	1

Table 2 (continued)

	Concentration (%)	Positive/tested	Positive (%)
Galaxolide 50 (1,3,4,6,7,8-hexahydro-4,6,6,7,8,8-hexamethyl-cyclopenta-gamma-2-benzopyran)	1	1/100	1
Citronellol	5	2/100	2
Citronellol	1	1/100	1
Amyl salicylate	5	1/100	1
Amyl salicylate	1	2/100	2
Vanoris (isononyl acetate)	0.1	1/192	0.5
Musk xylene	1	3/192	1.6
Musk xylene	0.1	2/192	1
Musk ambrette	0.1	1/192	0.5
Limonene	1	1/192	0.5
Citral (IFRA)	1	2/192	1
Citral (IFRA)	0.1	1/192	0.5
Lemon grass oil	0.1	1/95	1.1
Geranium o. B.	5	2/200	1
Methyl octine carbonate	1	1/205	0.5
Lavandin oil	5	1/205	0.5
Ionone alpha	5	1/205	0.5
Ionone beta	5	2/205	1
Alpha-isomethyl-ionone	5	1/205	0.5
Alpha-isomethyl-ionone	1	1/205	0.5
Negative reactions			
Linalyl acetate	5, 1	0/100	0
Phenyl ethyl alcohol	1	0/100	0
Benzyl acetate	5	0/100	0
Benzyl salicylate	1	0/100	0
Coumarin	5, 1	0/100	0
Terpineol	5, 1	0/100	0
Hedione (methyl dihydro-jasmonate)	5, 1	0/100	0
Hexyl cinnamic aldehyde	5, 1	0/100	0
Methyl ionone gamma	5, 1	0/106	0
Terpinyl acetate	5, 1	0/106	0
Lilial	5, 1	0/106	0
Geraniol	1, 0.1	0/106	0
Heliotropine	5, 1	0/106	0
Galaxolide 50	5	0/100	0
Vertofix (acetyl cedrene)	5	0/100	0
Musk ketone	5, 1	0/100	0
Eugenol	1	0/107	0
Vertenex	5, 1	0/107	0
Isobornyl acetate	5, 1	0/107	0
Amyl cinnamic aldehyde	5, 1	0/107	0
Tonalide	5, 1	0/313	0

Table 2 (continued)

	Concentration (%)	Positive/tested	Positive (%)
Cyclacet	1	0/313	0
DMBCA	1	0/313	0
Verdox	5, 1	0/313	0
Vanoris (isononyl acetate)	1	0/192	0
Musk ambrette	1	0/192	0
Limonene	0.1	0/192	0
Lemon grass oil	1	0/95	0
Isoamyl salicylate	5, 1	0/95	0
Cedarwood oil	5, 1	0/95	0
Jasmine absolute (Egypt)	5, 1	0/95	0
Salicylaldehyde	5, 1	0/95	0
Ethyl vanillin	5	0/200	0
Orange oil (Brasil)	5, 1	0/205	0
Methyl octine carbonate	0.1	0/205	0
Lavandin oil	1	0/205	0
Ionone alpha	1	0/205	0
Ionone beta	1	0/205	0

[a] In order to be classified an allergic reaction, material has to produce at least a 1^+ reaction.
[b] Materials with doubtful or irritant reactions.

Table 3. Results of testing with the 8% fragrance mix and its constituents (FM) in white petrolatum with 5% sorbitan sesquioleate (SSO) and with 1% SSO, respectively. Summary of nine centers with a total of 1072 patients (from [11])

Material	Conc. (%)	Irritant or ? +	Positive + to +++
FM	8	29 (2.71%)	89 (8.30%)
Oak moss	1	14 (1.31%)	24 (2.24%)
Isoeugenol	1	10 (0.93%)	20 (1.86%)
Eugenol	1	5 (0.47%)	13 (1.21%)
Cinnamic aldehyde	1	12 (1.12%)	10 (0.93%)
Geraniol	1	4 (0.37%)	8 (0.75%)
Hydroxycitronellal	1	5 (0.47%)	8 (0.75%)
Cinnamic alcohol	1	10 (0.93%)	6 (0.56%)
α Amyl cinnamic aldehyde	1	4 (0.37%)	5 (0.47%)
Sorbitan sesquioleate	20	15 (1.34%)	5 (0.47%)

In terms of the FF series, a total of 32 irritant or doubtful reactions were observed in the whole population. In only 12 cases were the reactions regarded as allergic, however; clinical relevance was not ascertained. The reactions to Iso E Super, Cyclacet, dimethylbenzyl carbinyl acetate (DMBCA), Vertofix, citronellal and amyl salicylate were recorded in patients without any history of fragrance sensitivity. In Barcelona, Lyral produced allergic reactions of possible clinical relevance in three patients. Two patients had a positive history of fragrance sensitivity and also reacted to a sunscreen and a massage lotion. However, it was not possible to obtain detailed information on the composition of the fragrances or whether Lyral in particular was one of the constituents.

Discussion

In two previous papers we have commented at length on the problems of patch testing with fragrances [8, 11]. The reader is referred to these papers which list many references on the subject. Moreover, an extensive literature review on fragrances prepared by de Groot and Frosch has just been published [13]. Important aspects may be summarized as follows.

One drawback of this 48-fragrance study is that at most centres only 100 consecutive patients of a given patch test clinic were tested with a set of five materials. The results might have been different if a *larger population* had been tested or if only patients with a *positive history of fragrance sensitivity* had been included. The main goal of this study was to obtain information on the sensitization frequency of dermatological patients to the 'Fenn materials'. We are aware of the fact that the figures do not represent sensitization rates, because there was no controlled exposure to the products tested. Therefore nothing can be said about the *sensitizing potential* of these products. As most 'Fenn materials' are frequently used for a number of years and most patients probably have had contact with them, it may be concluded with caution that there is no strong sensitizer among them. As already mentioned in conjunction with Lyral, it is often difficult to prove the clinical relevance of an observed positive reaction. Manufacturers of perfumes often remain secretive about their composition. With all due respect for professional confidentiality, we as physicians must ask for full cooperation in order to be of use to the patient. Only on the basis of a clear picture of the sensitization pattern, can the patient look for alternative products which do not contain the sensitizer(s). The fragrance industry must realize that nowadays a considerable portion of the normal population is sensitized to one or more fragrance constituents [13, 14]. These subjects neither want nor are able to avoid all perfumed products, given their present ubiquity. The current fragrance mix still seems to be the best screening tool for fragrance sensitive subjects, even if not ideal. A weakly positive or doubtful reaction may not be relevant, but a strong reaction is usually meaningful. According to our own experience there is only a small group of patients which is negative to the fragrance mix but reacts strongly to their own perfume(s). Further work on these patients is necessary to identify the causative agents. Lyral may be a promising candidate for screening because, apart of the suspected cases in our study, other groups have identified it as a relevant sensitizer [15, 16, 17].

In the guinea pig maximization test (Magnusson and Kligman), Lyral produced weak sensitization effects at 0.5%. In human studies according to Draize (repeated-insult patch test on normal skin) and Kligman (maximization test on irritated skin), no sensitizations were observed at induction concentrations of 1% and 10%, respectively [18]. However, as we know from experience with other fragrance materials, these can be negative in so-called predictive tests and still be sensitizers (e.g. hydroxycitronellal [19]). After being used by thousands of subjects, allergic contact dermatitis may be induced at a noticeable level. It is then the responsibility of the manufacturer to seek full cooperation with dermatologists and toxicologists in order to obtain more data on the safety of such a product. A risk-benefit ratio can only be determined if the number of exposures is compared to the number of sensitizations. This is still unknown for most fragrance constituents. It is an urgent task of the future. In a recent Swedish analysis of adverse reactions to cosmetics, fragrances were found to be the most frequent cause of contact allergies [20].

References

1. Larsen WG (1977) Perfume dermatitis. A study of 20 patients. Arch Dermatol 113: 623–626
2. Schnuch A,-Uter W, Lehmacher W et al. (1993) Epikutantestung mit der Standardreihe. Erste Ergebnisse des Projektes "Informationsverbund Dermatologischer Kliniken" (1VDK). Dermatosen 41: 60–70
3. Frosch PJ, Pilz B (1995) Kontaktallergene 1994. In: Plewig C, Korting HC (eds). Fortschritte der praktischen Dermatologie und Venerologie. Springer, Heidelberg Berlin New York, 14:7–14
4. Johansen JD, Mennd T (1995) The fragrance mix and its constituents: a 14-year material. Contact Dermatitis 32:18–23
5. Conøalo S, Conøalo M, Azenha A et al. (1992) Allergic contact dermatitis in children. A multicenter study of the Portuguese contact dermatitis group (GPEDC). Contact Dermatitis 26:112–115
6. Edman B, Möller H (1992) Contact allergy and contact allergens in atopic skin disease. Am J Contact Dermatitis 3:27–29
7. Wilkinson JD, Andersen KE, Camarasa JG et al. (1989) Preliminary results of effectiveness of two forms of fragrance mix as screening agents for fragrance sensitivity. In: Frosch PJ, Dooms-Goossens A, Lachapelle JM, Rycroft RJG, Scheper RJ (eds) Current topics in contact dermatitis. Springer, Heidelberg Berlin New York, pp 385–398
8. Frosch PJ, Pilz B, Burrows D et al. (1995) Testing with the fragrance mix – is the addition of sorbitan sesquioleate to the constituents useful? Contact Dermatitis 32:266–272
9. IFRA (lntemational Fragrance Association) (1983) Code of practice. Code de bons usages. Verfahrenscodex. Geneva
10. Fenn RS (1989) Aroma chemical usage trends in modern perfumery. Perfum Flavor 14:1–10

11. Frosch PJ, Pilz B, Andersen KE et al. (1995) Patch testing with fragrances: results of a multicenter study of the European environmental and contact dermatitis research group with 48 frequently used constituents of perfumes. Contact Dermatitis 33:333–342
12. Wahlberg JE (1995) Patch test guidelines. In: Rycroft RJG, Menné T, Frosch PJ (eds) Textbook of contact dermatitis, 2nd edn. Springer, Berlin Heidelberg New York, pp 241–268
13. De Groot AC, Frosch PJ (1997) Adverse reactions to fragrances. A clinical review. Contact Dermatitis 36:57–86
14. Nielsen NH, Menné T (1992) Allergic contact sensitization in an unselected Danish population. The Glostrup allergy study, Denmark. Acta Derm Venereol 72:456–460
15. Benke GM, Larsen WG (1984) Safety evaluation of perfumed shampoos: dose/response relationships for product use testing by presensitized subjects. J Toxicol Cut Ocul Toxicol 3:65–67
16. Handley J, Burrows D (1994) Allergic contact dermatitis from the synthetic fragrances Lyral and acetyl cedrene in separate underarm deodorant preparations. Contact Dermatitis 31:288–290
17. De Groot AC (1987) Contact allergy to cosmetics: causative ingredients. Contact Dermatitis 17:26–34
18. Ford RA (1992) Lyral. Monographs on fragrance raw materials. Food Chem Toxicol 30:49–51
19. Ford RA, Api AM (1988) Allergic contact sensitization potential of hydroxycitronellal in humans. Food Chem Toxic 26:921–926
20. Berne B, Boström A, Grahnén AF, Tammela M (1996) Adverse effects of cosmetics and toiletries reported to the Swedish medical products agency, 1989–1994. Contact Dermatitis 34:359–362

Quantitative Aspects in Patch Testing and Usage Tests

J.D. JOHANSEN

Introduction

In an unselected Danish population 1.1% reacted in patch testing to the fragrance mix [1]. This implies that at least 4 million people in the European community are sensitized to perfume materials. There is good reason to believe that this is actually an underestimate of the real problem as the consumption of cosmetics per inhabitant in Denmark is much lower than for other European countries. In Denmark 36 ECU were expended per inhabitant in 1994 while, for instance, in France and Germany 77 and 71 ECU were spent on cosmetics [2]. In studies of eczema patients perfume allergy is found to be the second most common cause of contact allergy [3, 4], and in several European countries an increasing trend in perfume allergy among eczema patients has been detected [3, 5].

Contact allergy is a chronic disease, but if elicitation of eczema can be prevented in those sensitized, the disease stays subclinical and has few or no socio-economic consequences. Recommendations for the safe use of sensitizing fragrance materials in different types of products are published by the International Fragrance Research Association (IFRA). However data supporting these recommendations in relation to elicitation of allergic fragrance contact dermatitis is lacking.

Threshold Responses in Sensitized Individuals

Eczema develops in sensitized individuals if exposure exceeds a certain individual threshold of response. A key determinant in this exposure is the concentration of allergen/unit skin. The threshold concentrations of allergen provoking eczema in sensitized individuals may be determined by testing with a serial dilution of the allergen in question. Few studies have been published providing such results for fragrance materials [6–9].

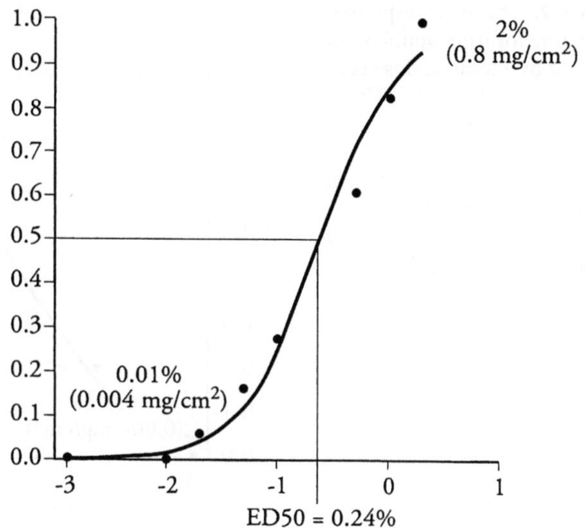

Fig. 1. The dose-response curve for cinnamic aldehyde obtained by a logistic dose response analysis [15]. The response frequency (*y-axis*) is given versus the $\log_{10}$ dose of cinnamic aldehyde (*x-axis*). ED_{50}, the dose eliciting a response in 50% of the test subjects

Serial Dilution Patch Tests

Basketter et al. studied 10 subjects sensitized to cinnamic aldehyde [6]. They were patch tested with a serial dilution of cinnamic aldehyde from 1%–0.1% in pet.; 60% still reacted to the lowest concentration of 0.1% [6]. In another study 22 cinnamic aldehyde sensitive individuals completed a study of patch testing with a serial dilution of cinnamic aldehyde in pet. from 2% to 0.01% [8]. The resulting dose-response curve is seen in Fig. 1.

A statistically significant dose-response relationship was found between exposure concentrations and the response frequency in the group of sensitized eczema patients. The dose eliciting a reaction in 50% of the test subjects was 0.24% and the level where no subjects reacted at patch testing was 0.01% cinnamic aldehyde. Isoeugenol has been studied by a similar method [9]. Twenty isoeugenol sensitive individuals were patch tested with a serial dilution of isoeugenol in petrolatum from 2% to 0.01% [9]; one was completely negative, leaving 19 subjects in the group. As with cinnamic aldehyde, a statistically significant dose-response relationship was found (Fig. 2).

The curve for isoeugenol was less steep but more to the left than the dose-response curve for cinnamic aldehyde (Fig. 1), with the result that the dose eliciting a response in 50% of the individuals was 0.08%, that is, three times lower than for cinnamic aldehyde. Of the isoeugenol-sensitive individuals, 20% still reacted to the lowest concentration of isoeugenol 0.01%. Epstein found a no effect level of 0.08% isoeugenol in 12 sensitized individuals patch tested with 8%, 0.8%, 0.08% and 0.008% isoeugenol in petrolatum [7].

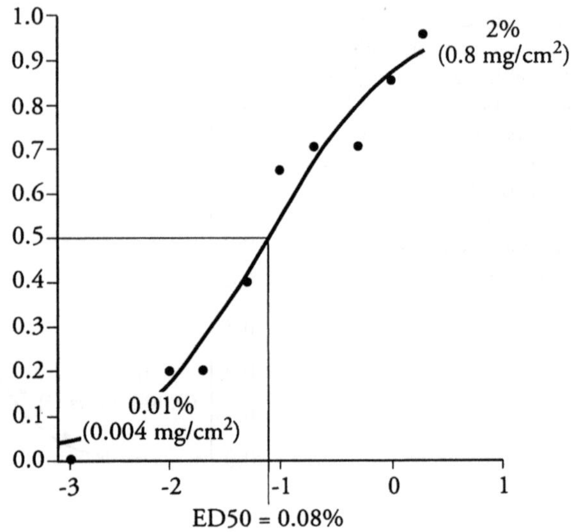

Fig. 2. The dose-response curve for isoeugenol obtained by a logistic dose response analysis [15]. The response frequency (*y-axis*) is given versus the $\log_{10}$ dose of cinnamic aldehyde (*x-axis*). ED_{50}, the dose eliciting a response in 50% of the test subjects

The effect levels demonstrated by patch testing may represent the worst case assumption since petrolatum is used as vehicle, and the test preparation is applied under occlusion. Occlusion may, however, be relevant to the use of cosmetics as deodorants and the patch test does not take into account that consumer products may be applied repeatedly and perhaps to damaged skin.

Effect levels determined by patch testing have been considered in safety assessment of metal salts in consumer products [10].

Usage Tests

In addition to patch testing the patients in three of the above-mentioned studies were asked to perform a usage test [7–9].

In the cinnamic aldehyde sensitive individuals three different concentrations of cinnamic aldehyde in ethanol were chosen based on information from industry [8]. The maximum concentration that may be used in creams or lotions is 0.02%, 0.1% is the usual concentration in perfumes, and 0.8% is the maximum concentration in perfumes [11]. The patients started to apply the weakest solution, 0.1 ml twice daily on a 5 × 5 cm area on the upper arm; ethanol was applied as vehicle control on the other arm [8]. The solution was applied for 14 days and in case of no reaction a higher concentration was applied for another 14 days. Of the 21 subjects, 13 developed eczema at the cinnamic aldehyde test site and had a negative ethanol control (Fig. 3): 62% (13/21) of those who completed the whole study but 72% (13/18) of those with a positive patch test to cinnamic aldehyde 2% in pet. A healthy control group

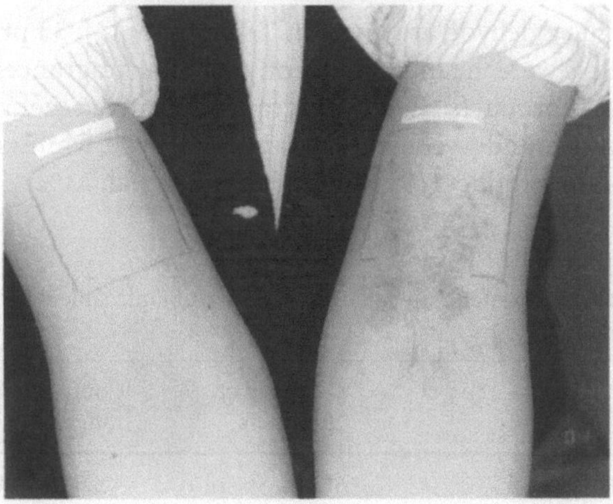

Fig. 3. A positive usage test to cinnamic aldehyde 0.1% in ethanol on one arm and a negative response to ethanol on the other. 0.1% cinnamic aldehyde is the usual concentration of cinnamic aldehyde in perfumes [11]

applied the maximum concentration of 0.8% for 14 days, and no eczema developed.

In the parallel study of isoeugenol only one concentration was applied, that is, 0.2% in ethanol, the maximum concentration that may be used in perfumes [9]. The test conditions were the same as described above except that the test period was 4 weeks. Here 12/19 (63%) developed eczema at the usage test site and were negative at the ethanol control site. None of the test subjects reacted beyond day 14; therefore a group of 20 healthy volunteers were asked to apply 0.2% isoeugenol for 14 days, and none reacted [9].

In the isoeugenol study by Epstein [7] a usage test was performed using 0.008, 0.08 and 0.8% in petrolatum, the anticubital fossa was used as test site and two of three applications were made per day. The test subjects started applying the weakest solution of 0.008 for 14 days, in case of no reaction the subjects rested 1 week and were exposed to the next concentration. Of the 12, 5 (42%) developed a positive usage test: one at 0.008%, two at 0.08% and one at 0.8%. A previous history of rash to perfumes has been demonstrated to be a powerful predictor of a positive usage test in fragrance sensitive individuals [12]. None of the test subjects in this study had a history of adverse skin reactions to perfumes, which may explain the fewer respondents in this study than in the above study, where all test subjects had previously experienced rash to perfumes [9]. It also emphasizes the importance of choosing test subjects for elicitation studies who have had a clinical problem.

Exposure Assessment

Few studies exist providing quantitative exposure information on fragrance materials. Data from two studies assessing exposure to isoeugenol and cinnamic aldehyde are given in Table 1 [13, 14]; 33 products were studied. Ten of these were the most frequently sold fine fragrances in Europe [14], and the rest were products used by fragrance-sensitive eczema patients [13]. No products were found to contain cinnamic aldehyde, while isoeugenol was found in 40% of the products (95% confidence interval: 23%–58%; Table 1).

Table 1. Content of isoeugenol and cinnamic aldehyde in a selection of 33 consumer products

	Number of products	Concentration range	Concentration mean
Isoeugenol	13	<0.001%–0.34%	0.1%
Cinnamic aldehyde	0		

Summary and Conclusions

It has been demonstrated that both isoeugenol and cinnamic aldehyde sensitive eczema patients react to the concentration of allergen that may be or are used in cosmetics. The dose eliciting a reaction at patch testing in 50% of isoeugenol-sensitive subjects was 0.08% isoeugenol. In comparison, 0.2% isoeugenol is the maximum concentration that may be used in perfumes and in a sample of cosmetics the mean concentration found was 0.1% isoeugenol (range <0.001–0.34%). Furthermore, 63% of the test subjects developed eczema when exposed to an 0.2% solution of isoeugenol in ethanol in an usage test.

In cinnamic aldehyde sensitive individuals 0.24% elicited a reaction in 50% of the test subjects in one study, and another study indicates that this may value may be even lower in other test populations as 60% reacted to 0.1% cinnamic aldehyde. In comparison 0.8% cinnamic aldehyde is the maximum concentration that may be used in perfumes according to informations of IFRA and 62% reacted to this or lower concentrations in an usage test. No cinnamic aldehyde was detected in a sample of cosmetics. It may be concluded that cinnamic aldehyde sensitive eczema patients react to concentrations of cinnamic aldehyde that may be used in cosmetics, and that isoeugenol sensitive eczema patients react to concentrations of isoeugenol that are used in cosmetics.

Serial dilution patch and usage testing contribute significant information regarding the safe use of fragrance allergens in cosmetics. More substances need to be described and the results considered in safety assessments.

References

1. Nielsen NH, Menné T (1992) Allergic contact sensitization in an unselected Danish population. Acta Derm Venereol 72:456-460
2. Colipa (1993/1994). European market review 1993/94. The European Cosmetic Toiletry and Perfumery Association, Brussels
3. Schnuch A, Geier J (1995) Die häufigsten Kontaktallergene im Jahr 1994. Dermatosen 43:275-278
4. Christophersen J, Menné T, Andersen KE, Brandrup F, Kaaber K, Osmundsen PE, Thestrup-Pedersen K, Veien NK (1989) Clinical patch test data evaluated by multivariate analysis. Contact Dermatitis 21:291-299
5. Johansen JD, Menné T (1995) The fragrance mix and its constituents a 14-year material. Contact Dermatitis 32:18-23
6. Basketter DA, Allenby CF (1991) Studies of the quenching phenomenon in delayed contact hypersensitivity reactions. Contact Dermatitis 25:160-171
7. Epstein WL (1982) The use test for contact hypersensitivity. Arch Dermatol Res 272:279-281
8. Johansen JD, Andersen KE, Rastogi SC, Menné T (1996) Threshold responses in cinnamic aldehyde-sensitive subjects: results and methodological aspects. Contact Dermatitis 34:165-171
9. Johansen JD, Andersen KE, Menné T (1996) Quantitative aspects of isoeugenol contact allergy assessed by use and patch tests. Contact Dermatitis 34:414-418
10. Basketter DA, Briatico-Vangosa G, Kaestner W, Lally C, Bontinck WJ (1993) Nickle, cobalt and chromium in consumer products: a role in allergic contact dermatitis? Contact Dermatitis 28:15-25
11. Opdyke DLJ (1979) Cinnamic aldehyde. Fragrance raw materials monographs. Food Cosmet Toxicol 17:253-57
12. Frosch PJ, Pilz B, Burrows D, Camarasa JG, Lachapelle JM, Lahti A, Menné T, Wilkinson JD (1995) Testing with fragrance mix. Is the addition of sorbitan sesquioleate to the constituents useful ? Contact Dermatitis 32:5:266-272
13. Johansen JD, Rastogi SC, Menné T (1996) Exposure to selected fragrance materials. A case study of fragrance-mix-positive eczema patients. Contact Dermatitis 34:106-110
14. Johansen JD, Rastogi SC, Menné T (1996) Contact allergy to popular perfumes assessed by patch test, use test and chemical analysis. Br J Dermatol 135:419-422
15. Vølund AA (1993) Potency evaluation of contact allergens. Statistical part. Nordiska Seminar og Arbejdsrapporter, p 570

d-Limonene – An Old Perfume Ingredient Introduced as a "Natural" Solvent in Industry: Is There a Risk of Sensitization?

A.-T. KARLBERG

d-Limonene (Fig. 1) is a monocyclic terpene and the main constituent of oil from several fruits of the genus *Citrus*, and also occurs in caraway, dill and celery. Its enantiomeric form *l*-limonene is found, for example, in turpentine and peppermint oil.

Production and Use

d-Limonene is obtained as a by-product from the citrus juice industry. Peel oil from the skins of the citrus fruits contains normally more than 95% *d*-limo-

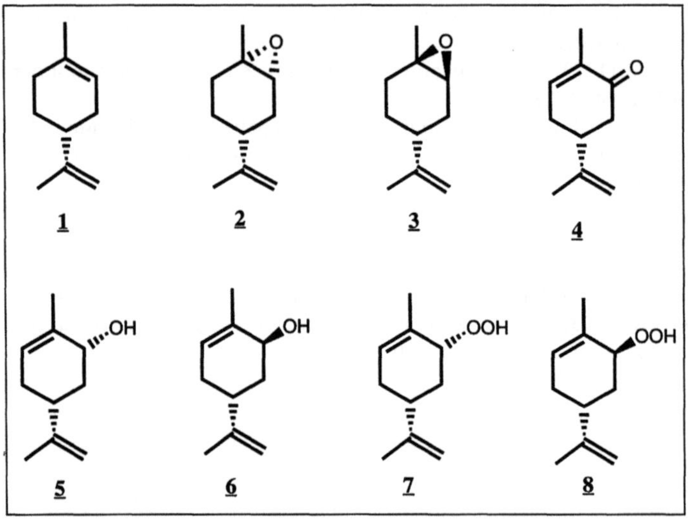

Fig. 1. *d*-Limonene and identified oxidation products of which *cis*- and *trans*-limonene oxide, (*R*)-(−)-carvone and *cis*- and *trans*-hydroperoxide were found to be sensitizers. *1*, *d*-limonene (*p*-mentha-1,8-diene); *2*, (+)-*cis*-limonene-1,2-oxide (1,2-epoxy-*p*-mentha-8-ene); *3*, (+)-*trans*-limonene-1,2-oxide (1,2-epoxy-*p*-mentha-8-ene); *4*, (*R*)-(−)-carvone (*R*)-(−)-6,8-*p*-mentha-diene-2-one]; 5, (−)-*cis*-carveol (*cis*-2-hydroxy-*p*-mentha-6,8-diene); *6*, (−)-*trans*-carveol (*trans*-2-hydroxy-*p*-mentha-6,8-diene); *7*, *cis*-limonene-2-hydroperoxide (*cis*-2-hydroperoxy-*p*-mentha-6,8-diene); *8*, *trans*-limonene-2-hydroperoxide (*trans*-2-hydroperoxy-*p*-mentha-6,8-diene)

nene and small amounts of other monoterpenes such as α- and β-pinene, sabinene and myrcene [1, 2]. The main usage of *d*-limonene is listed below:

- Perfume (concentration: 0.005% – 1%)
- Perfume additive
- Penetration enhancer
- Insecticide
- Antifungal agent
- Solvent in paint
- For cleaning assemblies and printing machines (concentration: 20% – 100%)
- For histological preparations
- In hand cleansers (concentration: 10%)

Traditionally, *d*-limonene is used for flavouring and as perfume in household products in low concentrations. It is also used by the fragrance industry as a perfume additive because of its declared effect to reduce the allergenic effect of other fragrance components, for example, cinnamic aldehyde and citral [3]. It is used as a penetration enhancer in transdermal delivery systems [4]. The use of *d*-limonene as an insecticide and antifungal agent, for example, in baths for cats and dogs has been reported [5]. During the past decade, *d*-limonene and synthetically produced dipentene, containing both *d*- and *l*-limonene, have gained increased use as defatting and cleaning agents in industry. The interest of the industry is due to the importance of replacing chlorinated hydrocarbons, chlorofluorocarbons and other organic solvents with substances considered to be less toxic and more environmentally friendly [6].

Oxidation of d-Limonene Creates Strong Contact Allergens

d-Limonene is rapidly oxidized in contact with air [7, 8]. Samples of *d*-limonene with a purity of 96% were handled and exposed to air in such a way as to mimic handling of such products in industry. After 10 weeks the content of *d*-limonene was less than 50% of the original amount in all samples [9]. The oxidation products formed polymerize leading to changes in the technical properties of the solution [10]. Antioxidants, such as butylated hydroxytoluene (BHT), are therefore often added to the commercial products. We have shown that BHT prevents autoxidation for a time, but that the stability depends on the purity of *d*-limonene and on the temperature [9]. Once the antioxidant is consumed, the oxidation starts immediately (Fig. 2). Sample 2, in which the antioxidant was consumed most rapidly, was identical with sample 1. The autoxidation of sample 2 started after a month of summer weather, during which the temperature in the laboratory rose to 25 °C, which might have increased the

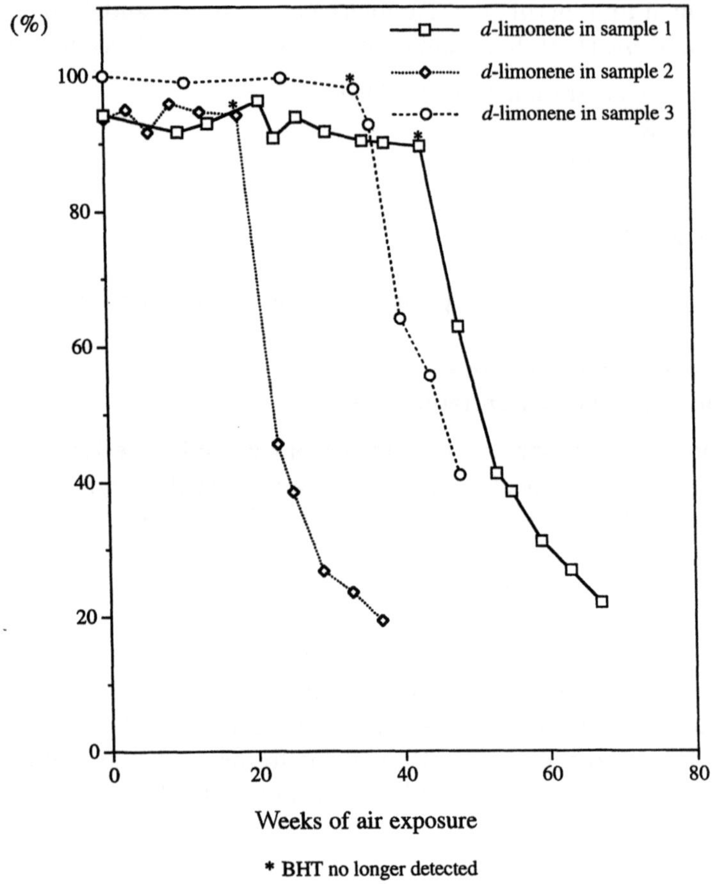

Fig. 2. Samples of *d*-limonene with BHT added were handled in the laboratory at room temperature to mimic handling in industry. Decrease in content of *d*-limonene was analysed with GC. *Sample 1*, *d*-limonene, 96% purity, addition of 0.2% BHT, air exposed for 67 weeks; *sample 2*, *d*-limonene of the same quality as sample 1, addition of 0.2% BHT, air exposed for 37 weeks; *sample 3*, *d*-limonene, 99% purity, addition of 0.1% BHT, air exposed for 48 weeks. (From [9], with permission)

oxidation rate and thus resulted in a more rapid consumption of BHT. The lower content of contaminants in sample 3 leads to a higher stability and a slower consumption of the antioxidant.

d-Limonene in high concentrations gives skin irritation [11, 12], but the reports on its allergenic activity diverge [13–15]. According to our experience *d*-limonene itself has a very low allergenic activity [16]. However, the major compounds formed at air oxidation are *cis*- and *trans*-limonene oxide, (R)-(–)-carvone, *cis*- and *trans*-carveol and limonene hydroperoxides (Fig. 1). Of these, all but carveol are strong sensitizers (Table 1) [17, 18]. The diverging

Table 1. The sensitizing potential of *d*-limonene and its oxidation products according to Freund's complete adjuvant test method

Substance (induction conc.)	No. sensitized/ no. exposed	Test conc.	*p* (exp/co)	Ref.
d-Limonene (5%)[a]	2/15	5%	n.s.	16
(+) Limonene oxide (5%)[a]	13/15	1%[c]	<0.001	17
(+) Limonene oxide (5%)[a]	15/15	1%[c]	<0.001	18
(R) (–)-Carvone (5%)[b]	13/14	0.2%[c]	<0.001	17
(–)-Carveol (5%)[b]	3/14	5%	n.s.	17
d-Limonene hydroperoxides (1.5%)[a]	8/15	0.3%[c]	<0.01	18
d-Limonene hydroperoxides (1.5%)[a]	13/15	0.5%[c]	<0.001	18

[a] *n* exposed animals = 15; *n* controls = 15.
[b] *n* exposed animals = 14; *n* controls = 14.
[c] Tested minimum dose that exhibited significant reactivity.

results seen in literature from experimental sensitization studies on *d*-limonene [13–15] could well be explained by a variation in the content of oxidation products in the samples investigated. The purity of the compound was not taken into account in those experiments. Our results are in line with the results from the studies on Δ^3-carene in the 1950s. Unidentified hydroperoxides of this compound were reported to be responsible for the main allergenic effect of turpentine [19, 20]. The results are also in accordance with results from studies on the allergenic activity of colophony (rosin) in which oxidation products of the diterpenoids abietic acid and dehydroabietic acid are found to be the major allergens [21, 22].

In order to be a contact allergen a compound must have the ability to react with epidermal macromolecules to form a complete antigen. Thus, from a mechanistic point of view, it is logic that the limonene itself is a weak sensitizer, while the oxidation products are strong sensitizers. The oxygen atom introduced into the molecule, attracts the electrons from the adjacent carbon atoms. These are deficient of electrons and available for a nucleophilic attack from electron-rich sites, for example, in proteins, to form covalent bonds and create an antigen. Regarding the hydroperoxides, the formation of covalent bonds is very likely to occur via a radical mechanism (Fig. 3) [23, 24].

Screening with Oxidized *d*-Limonene in Addition to the Standard Series

Air exposed *d*-limonene with an original purity of 96% was added to the standard series for patch testing of dermatitis patients at the Department of Environmental and Occupational Dermatology, Karolinska Hospital, Stock-

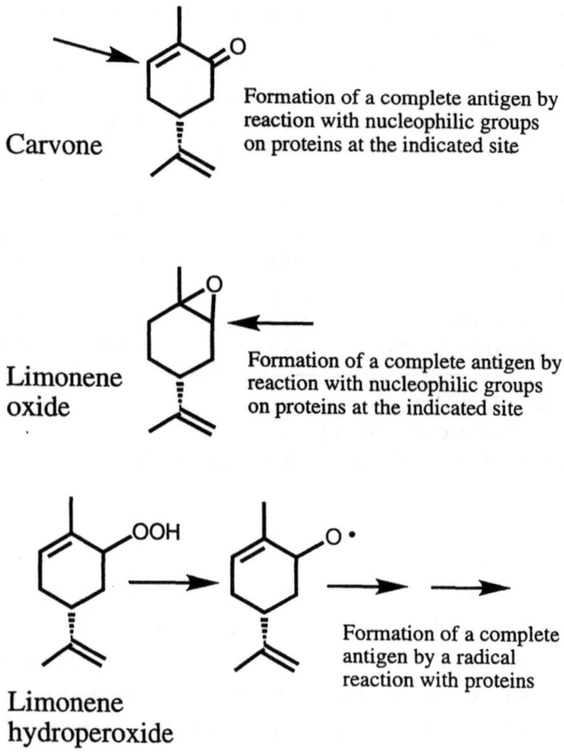

Fig. 3. Mechanisms of antigen formation from oxidation products of *d*-limonene.

holm and at the Department of Dermatology, University Hospital, Leuven. Two batches of autoxidized *d*-limonene, 3% in petrolatum, were tested at the clinics. More patients were tested with batch II than with batch I, and a better accordance of the results from the two clinics was seen for batch II. More doubtful reactions were recorded in Stockholm than in Leuven, which could be due to a difference in the interpretation (Table 2). The frequency of positive reactions to oxidized *d*-limonene was comparable to that seen for common contact allergens such as formaldehyde [25]. Extended studies on the most adequate test concentration and vehicle are in progress.

In June 1996 the commission working group on the classification and labelling of dangerous substances for health effects within the European Union suggested that *d*-limonene should be classified as allergenic due to its ability to form allergenic oxidation products.

Table 2. Screening with oxidized *d*-limonene in consecutive dermatitis patients

	Stockholm					Leuven				
		Positive		Doubtful			Positive		Doubtful	
	Tested	*n*	%	*n*	%	Tested	*n*	%	*n*	%
Batch I	153	4	2.6	3	2.0	216	2	0.9	0	0
Batch II	413	8	1.9	13	3.1	953	14	1.6	5	0.5

Conclusions

d-Limonene itself has a low sensitizing capacity. However, it is easily oxidized at air exposure and the oxidation products formed are strong sensitizers. The frequency of allergic reactions to *d*-limonene containing oxidation products is comparable to that of common allergens such as formaldehyde. Increased occupational exposure to *d*-limonene will increase the prevalence of allergic contact dermatitis.

References

1. Opdyke DLJ (1975) Monographs on fragrance raw materials. Food Cosmet Toxicol 13 [Suppl II]:825–826
2. Kirk-Othmer (1969) Encyclopedia of chemical technology, vol 19. Wiley, New York, pp 803–838
3. Opdyke DLJ (1976) Inhibition of sensitization reactions induced by certain aldehydes. Food Cosmet Toxicol 14:197–198
4. Williams AC, Barry BW (1991) Terpenes and the lipid-protein-partitioning theory of skin penetration enhancement. Pharm Res 8:17–24
5. Hooser SB, Beasley VR, Everitt JI (1986) Effects of an insecticidal dip containing d-limonene in the cat. J Am Vet Med Assoc 189:905–908
6. Karlberg A-T, Lindell B (1993) Limonene. In: Beije B, Lundberg P (eds) Criteria document from the Nordic Expert Group 1993. Arbete och Hälsa, Nordic Council of Ministers, National Institute of Occupational Health, Solna no 35, pp 207–276
7. Grayson DH (1990) Monoterpenoids. Natural Product Reports 7:327–347
8. Royals EE, Horne Jr SE (1955) Observations on the rate of autoxidation of d-limonene. J Am Chem Soc 77:187–188
9. Karlberg A-T, Magnusson K, Nilsson U (1994) Influence of an anti-oxidant on the formation of allergenic compounds during auto-oxidation of d-limonene. Ann Occup Hyg 38:199–207
10. Nilsson U, Bergh M, Shao LP, Karlberg A-T (1996) Analysis of contact allergenic compounds in oxidized d-limonene. Chromatographia 42:199–205
11. Falk A, Fischer T, Hagberg M (1991) Purpuric rash caused by dermal exposure to *d*-limonene. Contact Dermatitis 25:198–199

12. Okabe H, Obata Y, Takayama K, Nagai T (1990) Percutaneous absorption enhancing effect and skin irritation of monocyclic monoterpenes. Drug Design Delivery 6:229–238
13. Greif N (1967) Cutaneous safety of fragrance material as measured by the maximization test. Am Perfumer Cosmet 82:54–57
14. Klecak G, Geleick H, Frey JR (1977) Screening of fragrance materials for the allergenicity in the guinea pig. I. Comparison of four testing methods. J Soc Cosmet Chem 28:53–64
15. Maisey J, Miller K (1986) Assessment of the ability of mice fed on vitamin A supplemented diet to respond to a variety of potential contact sensitizers. Contact Dermatitis 15:17–23
16. Karlberg A-T, Boman A, Melin B (1991) Animal experiments on the allergenicity of *d*-limonene – the citrus solvent. Ann Occup Hyg 35:419–426
17. Karlberg A-T, Magnusson K, Nilsson U (1992) Air oxidation of *d*-limonene (the citrus solvent) creates potent allergens. Contact Dermatitis 26:332–340
18. Karlberg A-T, Shao LP, Nilsson U, Gäfvert E, Nilsson JLG (1994) Hydroperoxides in oxidized *d*-limonene identified as potent contact allergens. Arch Dermatol Res 286:97–103
19. Hellerström S, Thyresson N, Blohm SG, Widmark G (1955) On the nature of the eczematogenic componenet of oxidized Δ^3-carene. J Invest Dermat 24:217–224
20. Pirilä V, Siltanen E (1958) On the chemical nature of the eczematogenic agent in oil of turpentine (III) Dermatologica 117:1–8
21. Karlberg A-T, Bohlinder K, Boman A, Hacksell U, Hermansson J, Jacobsson S, Nilsson JLG (1988) Identification of 15-hydroperoxyabietic acid as a contact allergen in Portuguese colophony. J Pharm Pharmacol 40:42–47
22. Karlberg A-T, Boman A, Hacksell U, Jacobsson S, Nilsson JLG (1988) Contact allergy to dehydroabietic acid derivatives isolated from Portuguese colophony. Contact Dermatitis 19:166–174
23. Gäfvert E, Shao LP, Karlberg A-T, Nilsson U, Nilsson JLG (1994) Contact allergy to resin acid hydroperoxides. Hapten binding via free radicals and epoxides. Chem Res Toxicol 7:260–266
24. Lepoittevin JP, Karlberg A-T (1994) Interactions of allergenic hydroperoxides with proteins: A radical mechanism? Chem Res Toxicol 7:130–133
25. Karlberg A-T, Dooms-Goossens A (1997) Contact allergy to oxidized *d*-limonene among dermatitis patients. Contact Dermatitis 36:201–206

Contents of Sensitizing Fragrance Materials in Natural Ingredient Based Cosmetics

S.C. Rastogi

Introduction

Perfumes are one of the major causes of allergic contact dermatitis (Adam and Maibach 1985; De Groot 1987; Larsen et al. 1992). Over 3000 fragrance materials are used to compound various types of perfumes, which may themselves contain from 10 to 300 chemicals. The fragrance materials may be natural products, i.e., essential oils, they may be nature identical chemicals, for example, synthetic linlool, which is also found in many essential oils, or they may be non-natural (synthetic) substances, for example, α-hexylcinnamic aldehyde. A large number of perfume allergy cases can be diagnosed by patch testing with the fragrance mix composed of geraniol, hydroxycitronellal, cinnamic aldehyde, cinnamic alcohol, eugenol, isoeugenol, α-amylcinnamic aldehyde and oak moss absolute. All of these substances except hydroxycitronellal may be present in essential oils used for compounding perfumes. These fragrance mix constituents, with the exception of oak moss absolute, are now chemically synthesized and used in the formulation of various perfumes. Johansen et al. (1996a) demonstrated that rather low levels of fragrance mix substances present in cosmetics used by patients with perfume allergy were associated with allergic contact dermatitis in the sensitized patients.

The use of cosmetics based on natural ingredients is becoming increasingly popular for reasons of environmental safety and animal welfare. These products may also contain fragrance mix substances originating from essential oils used in the formulation. The present study sought to investigate the levels of fragrance mix substances and some other known fragrance sensitizers in cosmetics based on natural ingredients, in order to evaluate the risk of developing allergic contact dermatitis by the use of such products.

Target Fragrance Substances

The 12 fragrance substances selected for the present study included the constituents of the fragrance mix with the exception of oak moss absolute (Table 1). Oak moss absolute was not included because it is itself a mixture of

Table 1. Target fragrance substances

Fragrance substance	CAS Reg. No.	Chemical structure
Geraniol	106-24-1	3,7-Dimethyl-2,6-octadien-1-ol
Cinnamic alcohol	104-54-1	3-Phenyl-2-propen-1-ol
Cinnamic aldehyde	14371-10-9	3-Phenyl-2-propenal
Hydroxycitronellal	107-75-5	3,7-Dimethyl-7-hydroxy octanal
Eugenol	95-53-0	2-Methoxy-4-(2-propenyl) phenol
Isoeugenol	97-54-1	2-Methoxy-4-(1-propenyl) phenol
α-Amylcinnamic aldehyde	122-40-7	2-Phenylmethylene heptanal
α-Hexylcinnamic aldehyde	101-86-0	2-Phenylmethylene octanal
Coumarin	91-64-5	2H-1-benzopyran-2-one
Dihydrocoumarin	119-84-6	3,4-Dihydro 2H-1-benzo-2-pyranone
Citronellal	106-23-0	3,7-Dimethyl-6-octenal
Citral	5392-40-5	3,7-Dimethyl-2,6-octadienal

several substances. Citral, coumarin and dihydrocoumarin were included as they are known as potent contact allergens (Malten et al. 1984, Larsen et al. 1992). α-Hexylcinnamic aldehyde was included because it is chemically similar to the fragrance mix constituent, α-amylcinnamic aldehyde, and is found in more than 50% of all cosmetic products (Fenn 1989). Citronellal was included because it is related to the fragrance mix constituent hydroxycitronellal. Besides target fragrance substances, a number of non-target fragrance substances present in the investigated perfumes could also be identified (see "Results and Discussion").

Materials and Methods

Cosmetic Products

The present study analyses 22 perfumes and 20 other cosmetic products, purchased at retail outlets in Denmark. The products were made by 20 cosmetic companies in Europe and the United States. According to manufacturers' information, all of the products were based on natural ingredients or nature identical substances. The perfumes represented various scents: camomile, lavender, jasmine, sandalwood, vanilla, primrose, strawberry, and so on. The other cosmetic products included shampoo, gel, cream, lotion, balm, deodorant, face water, stress buffer and massage oil.

Analysis

A gas chromatography (GC)–mass spectrometric (MS) method for the analysis of fragrance substances in cosmetic products described previously

(Rastogi 1995) was used in the present study. Prior to analysis, the perfumes were appropriately diluted in methanol. Analysis of perfumes diluted 1:10 and serial dilutions up to 1:1000 were required for the identification and quantification of all of the target fragrance substances. Fragrance materials from other cosmetics were extracted by silica gel column chromatography of sample solutions (2 g sample/25 g methanol) as described elsewhere (Rastogi 1995).

Results And Discussion

Cosmetic products were analysed by GC-MS to ascertain the identification of the target fragrance substances. The GC-MS analysis also provided the opportunity to identify other substances present in these samples. A mixture of target fragrance substances in methanol was analysed every day to check system suitability. The separation of target fragrance substances from a mixture containing 83 ppm (0.0083 %) of each of these is shown in Fig. 1. The detection limit for each of the target fragrance substances was approximately 1 ppm, except for citral. The detection limit for citral was 5 ppm. Analysis of undiluted perfumes revealed that they contain high amounts of several substances which interfere with the identification and quantification of the target fragrance materials. The perfumes were therefore diluted at least 1:10 prior to GC-MS analysis. Thus, the detection limit for the target fragrance substances in these products was approximately 10 ppm (0.001 %). Dilution up to 1:1000 was necessary for some perfumes in order to attain a satisfactory GC-MS analysis with respect to identification and quantification of the target fragrance substances.

A typical example of perfume analysis is shown in Fig. 2. Several non-symmetrical and unresolved GC peaks in the chromatogram are mainly due to overloading the GC column with relatively high concentrations of some substances present in a 1:10 diluted sample (Fig. 2 A). A MS library search indicated the presence of dipropylene glycol, benzyl alcohol, methyl benzoate, linalool and phenethyl alcohol in the area between scan no. 750 and scan no. 1000 and the presence of benzyl acetate, linalyl acetate + geraniol, hydroxycitronellal, cinnamic alcohol, α-amylcinnamic aldehyde and α-hexylcinnamic aldehyde + benzylbenzoate in GC peaks with scan nos. 1074, 1320, 1397, 1451, 2182 and 2131, respectively (Fig. 2 A). Coumarin and eugenol present in relatively low concentrations in this perfume could be identified and quantified at 1:10 dilution (Fig. 2 A). Hydroxycitronellal and cinnamic aldehyde were satisfactorily identified and quantified when a 1:500 diluted sample was analysed (Fig. 2 B), and a 1:1000 dilution of the sample was required for the proper identification and quantitification of α-amylcinnamic aldehyde and α-hexylcinnamic aldehyde. Geraniol in the sample was identified only by the analysis

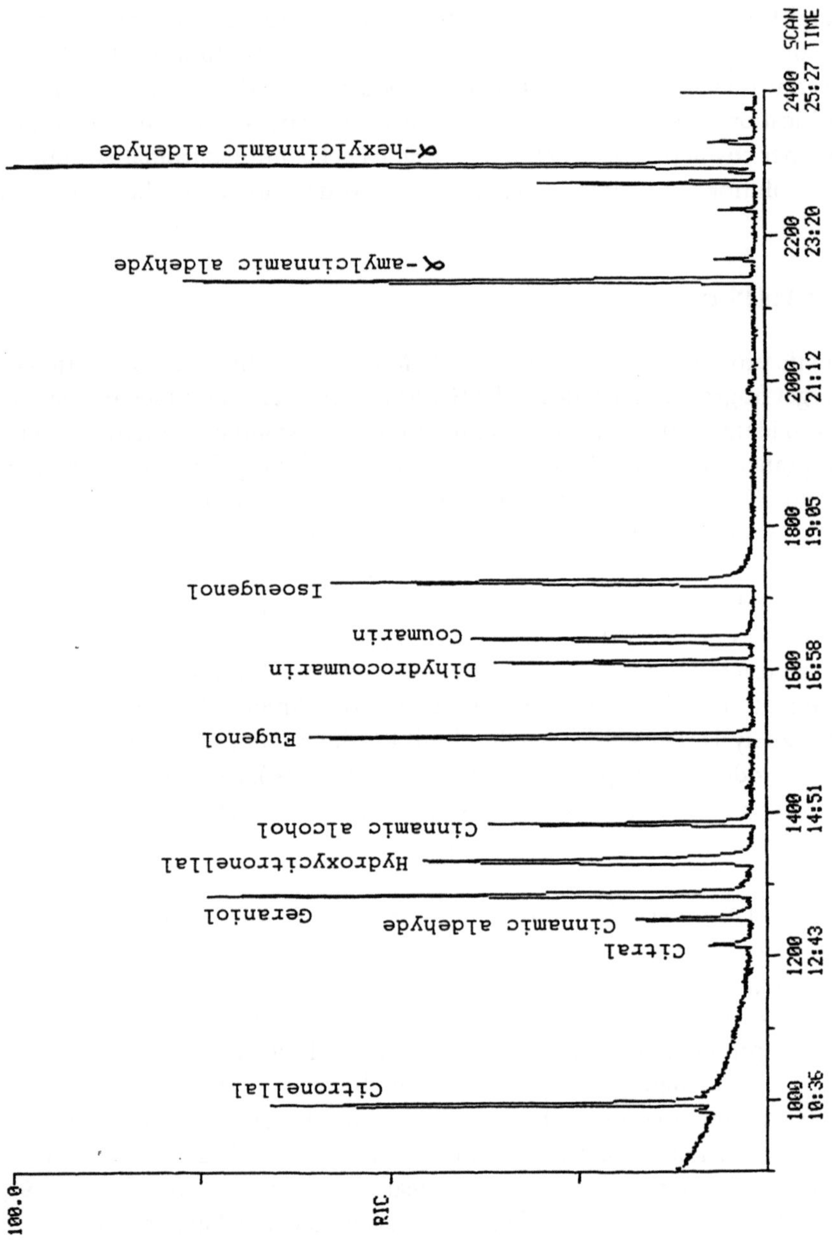

Fig. 1. GC-MS analysis of a mixture containing 83 ppm of each of the target fragrance substances

Fig. 2A–C. GC-MS analysis of a perfume. A In a dilution of 1:10, the area between scan no. 1620 and scan no. 1670 is enlarged to show the presence of coumarin. Geraniol was identified in a part (scan nos. 1312–1313) of the large peak of linalyl acetate (scan no. 1320) and eugenol was identified in the peak with scan no. 1508. Indications of the presence of

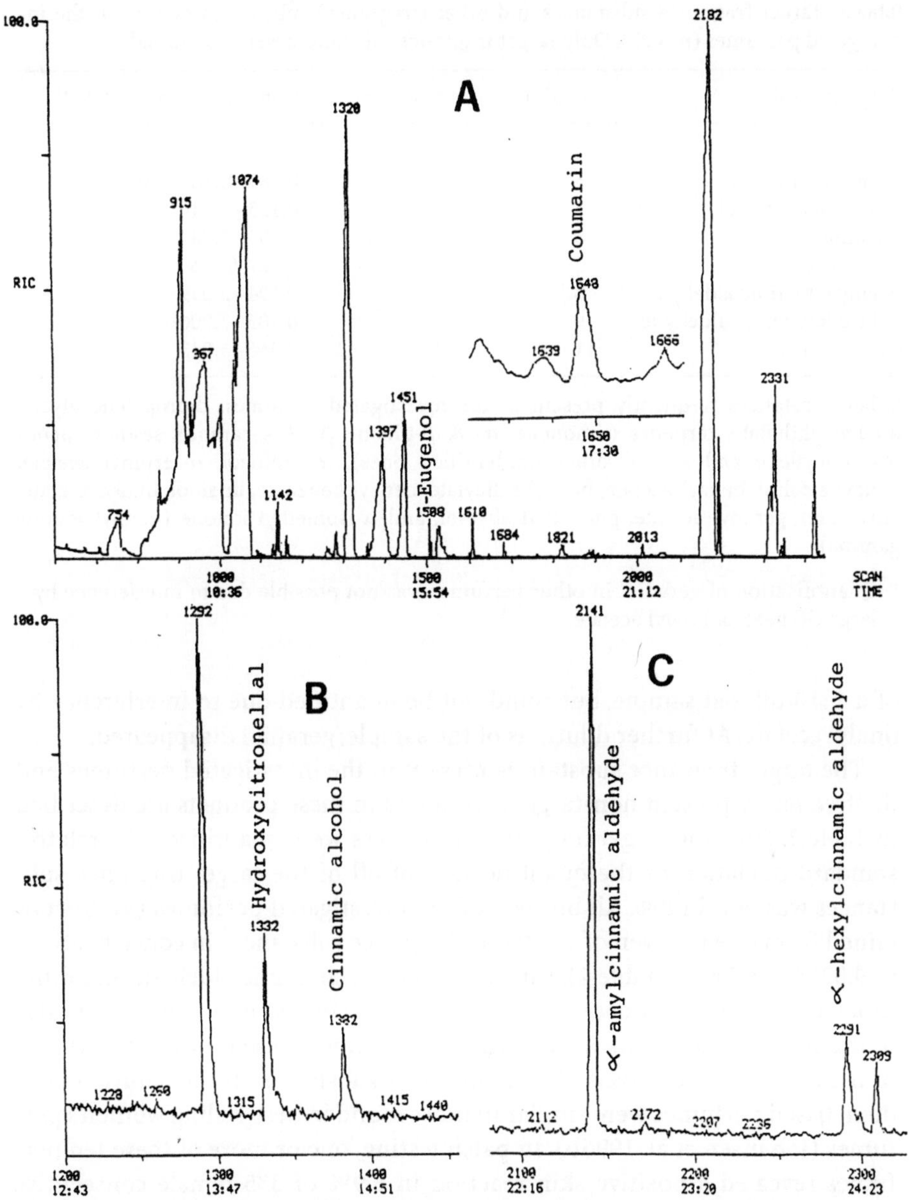

hydroxycitronellal and cinnamic alcohol were found in the broad peak with scan no. 1397, α-amylcinnamic aldehyde in the peak with scan no. 2182 and α-hexylcinnamic aldehyde in the peak with scan no. 2331. **B** Hydroxycitronellal and cinnamic alcohol were satisfactorily identified and quantified by the analysis of a 1:500 diluted sample. **C** A 1:1000 diluted sample was analysed for α-amylcinnamic aldehyde and α-hexylcinnamic aldehyde without the interference of neighbouring peaks. The sample contained 1.158% hydroxycitronellal, 2.101% cinnamic alcohol, 0.169% eugenol, 0.155% coumarin, 3.039% α-amylcinnamic aldehyde and 1.015% α-hexylcinnamic aldehyde

Table 2. Target fragrance substances and other (fragrance) substances present in the investigated perfumes ($n = 22$). Only target fragrance substances were quantified

Fragrance substance	No. of products found in	Concentration (%) (W/V)
Geraniol	14	1.191[a]
Cinnamic alcohol	3	0.089, 0.109, 2.101
Hydroxycitronellal	5	0.135–6.044
Eugenol	8	0.035–2.289
Isoeugenol	2	0.027, 0.139
α-amylcinnamic aldehyde	8	0.194–3.039
α-hexylcinnamic aldehyde	9	0.105–7.706
Coumarin	11	0.046–6.043

Other substances frequently present in the investigated perfumes: dipropylene glycol, diethyl phthalate, terpenes (limonene, α- & β-pinene, 3- & 4-carene), sesquiterpenes (caryophyllene and several other unidentified ones), α-terpineol, α-terpinyl acetate, benzyl alcohol, benzyl acetate, benzyl salicylate, benzyl benzoate, linalool, linalyl acetate, citronellol, geranyl acetate, phenethyl alcohol, and α-isomethyl ionone (methyl ionone gamma).

[a] Quantification of geraniol in other perfumes was not possible due to interference by a large GC peak of linalyl acetate.

of a 1:10 diluted sample, but could not be quantified due to interference by linalyl acetate. At further dilutions of the sample, geraniol disappeared.

The target fragrance substances present in the investigated perfumes and the frequently present non-target substances in these products are described in Table 2. Only the target fragrance substances were quantified. The relative standard deviation of the quantification of all of the target fragrance substances was within 8%. All but two of the investigated perfumes (91%) contained from one to seven of the target fragrance substances in concentrations of 0.027%–7.706% (Table 2). Citronellal, citral, cinnamic aldehyde and dihydrocoumarin were not detected in any of the perfumes. Between one and five of the synthetic constituents of fragrance mix were present in 18 of 22 (82%) of the perfumes. The levels of fragrance mix substances in the natural ingredient based perfumes were similar to those found in best-selling women's perfumes (Johansen et al. 1996b). In patch testing, one or more of these ten perfumes revealed a positive skin reaction in 6.9% of 335 female consecutive eczema patients. This indicates that exposure to fragrance mix constituents cannot be avoided by using natural ingredient based perfumes, and consumers using these products may run a similar risk of developing allergic contact dermatitis as those using other popular perfumes.

Among other investigated cosmetics, seven of 20 (35%) of the products were found to contain between one and three of the target fragrance substances (Table 3). These products contain 3–820 ppm of the following fra-

Table 3. Contents of target fragrance substances in the investigated non-perfume cosmetic products ($n = 20$)

Fragrance substance	No. of products found in	Concentration (%) (w/v)
Geraniol	1	0.0163[a]
Cinnamic alcohol	1	0.0036
Cinnamic aldehyde	1	0.0745
Eugenol	1	0.0186
Isoeugenol	1	0.0127
α-amylcinnamic aldehyde	1	0.082
α-hexylcinnamic aldehyde	3	0.0007-0.0543
Coumarin	2	0.0003, 0.0130

[a] Identification of geraniol in other products was not possible due to interference by a large GC peak of linalyl acetate.

grance substances: geraniol, cinnamic aldehyde, cinnamic alcohol, eugenol, isoeugenol, α-amylcinnamic aldehyde, α-hexylcinnamic aldehyde and coumarin.

Hydroxycitronellal and α-hexylcinnamic aldehyde are synthetic chemicals which have not yet been shown to be present in natural products. Presence of hydroxycitronellal and α-hexylcinnamic aldehyde in five and nine of the investigated perfumes, respectively, demonstrates that synthetic fragrance substances are added to perfumes claimed to be based on natural ingredients. Synthetic α-hexylcinnamic aldehyde was also present in three of the other cosmetic products investigated. Non-natural substances like α-isomethyl ionone (methyl ionone gamma), diethyl phthalate and dipropylene glycol were also frequently identified in the investigated perfumes as well as in other cosmetics. Thus, it is rather misleading to claim that a cosmetic product is based on natural ingredients when it contains synthetic chemicals such as surfactant, preservative, sunscreen, perfume, and/or colourant.

Acknowledgements. I am grateful to Dr. J.D. Johansen for her suggestions on the preparation of this chapter.

References

Adam RM, Maibach HI (1985) A 5-year study of cosmetic reactions. J Am Acad Dermatol 13:1062–1069

De Groot AC (1987) Contact allergy to cosmetics: causative ingredients. Contact Dermatitis 17:26–34

Fenn RS (1989) Aroma chemical usage trends in modern perfumery. Perfumer & Flavorist 14:2–10

Johansen JD, Rastogi SC, Menné T (1996a) Exposure to selected sensitizing fragrance materials – a case study of fragrance mix positive eczema patients. Contact Dermatitis 34:106–110

Johansen JD, Rastogi SC, Menné T (1996b) Contact allergy to popular perfumes; assessed by patch test, use test and chemical analysis. Brit J Dermatol 135:419–422

Larsen WG, Jackson EM, Barker MO, Bednarz RM, Engasser PG, O'Donoghue MN, Strauss JS (1992) A primer on cosmetics. J Am Acad Dermatol 27:469–484

Malten KE, VanKetel WG, Nater JP, Liem DH (1984) Reactions in selected patients to 22 fragrance materials. Contact Dermatitis 11:1–10

Rastogi SC (1995) Analysis of fragrances by gas chromatography–mass spectrometry. J High Resolut Chromatogr 18:653–658

RIFM Activities in the Safety Assessment of Systemic Effects of Fragrance Materials

E. A. Pfitzer

The Research Institute for Fragrance Materials (RIFM) maintains a computerized database of the world literature on the safe use of fragrance ingredients, that is, the individual scented chemicals that go into formulations for cosmetics and household products. RIFM does not test or maintain data on finished products. This chapter covers activities for the safety assessment of systemic effects from fragrance ingredients, while other papers cover dermal effects, in vitro research on percutaneous absorption and how RIFM data and recommendations are used by the International Fragrance Association (IFRA).

The potential for systemic effects from chemicals can be understood on the basis of some "first principles" in toxicology. One is that essentially all chemicals, including fragrance ingredients, can be absorbed into the body to some degree. The principal route for absorption of fragrance ingredients is the skin. While there is potential for absorption by the lungs after inhalation, the pulmonary route is quantitatively very minor compared with the skin. The oral route is also minor for scented cosmetics or household products. Another "first principle" is that, once absorbed, chemicals can cause toxic effects at some site of toxic action in the body to some degree if at sufficiently high concentration, that is, "the dose makes the poison".

What is important is that the known or suspected systemic toxic effects would occur only under conditions sufficiently in excess of expected use conditions to provide for adequate safety. To accomplish this for a fragrance ingredient the challenge is: (a) to estimate levels in the body that cause adverse effects and levels at which the effects are absent, (b) to estimate exposure to the skin under conditions of use, and (c) to estimate percutaneous absorption into the body.

For a new chemical without available toxicity data, the suspected systemic toxicity may be inferred by analogy to known toxicants. For many years RIFM has used the decision tree approach of Cramer et al. (1978) that includes structure-activity relationships, but also estimates of absorption and metabolism. This decision tree approach is used generally for systemic effects and the publications of Ashby and Tennant (1991), Ashby and Paton (1993) and Ashby

(1994) are also used for potential for carcinogenicity and mutagenicity. In vitro tests may also assist with estimating toxicity and metabolism, but are very valuable for estimating absorption.

With guidance from structure-activity and other data, the steps for obtaining data on potential systemic effects from animal tests progress as follows: (a) determine the toxicity profile of the chemical in animals, usually at quite high doses, show the absence of these effects at some lower dose, described as the "no observed adverse effect level" (NOAEL), and (b) apply an appropriate safety factor to the animal data for extrapolation to humans (the factor may vary depending upon the nature of the adverse effects).

It is then necessary to know that the exposure for humans under the conditions of use does not exceed the estimated safe dose. To estimate the exposure to the skin the following questions must be answered:

- What is the nature of the product (body lotion, cologne, etc.)?
- How much is applied to the skin and how often is it applied?
- Does some of the product wash-off as with a shampoo or toilet soap?
- What is the concentration of the specific fragrance ingredient in the final product?

This information is obtained from surveys of in-use experience conducted by the cosmetic industry and from the analysis of the composition of products conducted by the fragrance industry.

The next step is to estimate the potential for percutaneous absorption into the body. In vitro techniques using excised skin provide one estimate. A more specific technique is to conduct in vivo studies applying radiolabeled chemical to the skin of human volunteers or animals. With humans systemic absorption can be estimated from measurements in blood, urine and feces, and local adherence to the skin can be estimated with successive tape strippings after wash-off. With animals more complete information is obtained for absorption, distribution throughout the body, excretion and, often, metabolism. The best estimate of per cent percutaneous absorption can then be applied to the exposure estimate to determine the expected level in the body. This level is compared with the previously determined safe level in the body for the assessment of overall safety for use of the fragrance ingredient.

Five fragrance ingredients that have had extensive testing for systemic toxicity in past years are described here as illustrative examples. For two of these, musk ambrette and acetylethyltetramethyltetralin (AETT, Versalide), the results of tests led to a decision by the International Fragrance Association to prohibit their use as fragrance ingredients.

Musk ambrette caused hind limb weakness when administered in the diet or applied to skin of rats for periods up to 12 weeks (Spencer et al. 1984). This was associated with primary demyelination and distal axonal degeneration in selected regions of the central and peripheral nervous system. Although it was possible to demonstrate a NOAEL for musk ambrette for neurotoxicity, IFRA initially restricted its use, but after observations that it was also a photosensitizer, established a prohibition of use. Subsequently Ford et al. (1990) conducted 90-day dermal studies to show that the neurotoxicity with musk ambrette did not occur with other closely related fragrance ingredients, namely, musk ketone, musk xylene, musk tibetene and moskene.

AETT also caused damage to the nervous system when applied to the skin of rats (Spencer et al. 1984). However the chemical structure is quite different from musk ambrette and the neuropathological responses were also different in that the changes with AETT were considered to be irreversible. The RIFM Expert Panel judged that there were insufficient data to demonstrate an acceptable risk and its use was first suspended in 1977 and then prohibited in 1980.

Phenyl ethyl alcohol (PEA; Mankes et al. 1983; Ford 1990) and *para*-tertiary butyl-methylhydrocinnamaldehyde (BMHCA; Pfitzer 1992; Pfitzer 1995) were found to cause reproductive effects at high doses in animals by the oral route. PEA caused developmental effects and BMHCA caused testicular effects. In both cases extensive studies comparing oral and dermal routes of exposure, and absorption in rats and humans were conducted. It was possible to demonstrate adequate margins of safety and IFRA has not issued any restrictions on their use.

Mouse liver tumors have been reported with musk xylene in B6C3F1 mice (Maekawa et al. 1990), although musk xylene has been shown to be nongenotoxic (Api et al. 1995). Careful metabolic studies, including enzyme induction, demonstrated that musk xylene acts in the mouse liver in a way similar to phenobarbital, and the mouse liver tumors are considered to be due to secondary mechanisms that would not apply to humans under use conditions (Lehman-McKeeman 1995). No IFRA restrictions have been issued.

RIFM continues to look for new ways to estimate the potential for fragrance ingredients to cause systemic effects and to then conduct the research appropriate for the controls to ensure safe use.

References

Api AM, Ford RA, San RHC (1995) An evaluation of musk xylene in a battery of genotoxicity tests. Food Chem Toxicol 33:1039–1045

Ashby J (1994) Two million rodent carcinogens? The role of SAR and QSAR in their detection. Mutat Res 305:3–12

Ashby J, Tennant RW (1991) Definitive relationships among chemical structure, carcinogenicity and mutagenicity for 301 chemicals tested by the US NTP. Mutation Res 257:229–306

Ashby J, Paton D (1993) The influence of chemical structure on the extent and sites of carcinogenesis for 522 rodent carcinogens and 55 different human carcinogen exposures. Mutat Res 286:3–74

Cramer GM, Ford RA, Hall RL (1978) Estimation of toxic hazard – a decision tree approach. Food Cosm Toxicol 16:255–276

Ford RA (1990) Metabolic and kinetic criteria for the assessment of reproductive hazard. In: Volans GF, Sims J, Sullivan FM, Turner P (eds) Basic science in toxicology. Taylor & Francis, New York, pp 59–68

Ford RA, Api AM, Newberne PM (1990) 90-Day dermal toxicity study and neurotoxicity evaluation of nitromusks in the albino rat. Food Chem Toxicol 28:55–61

Lehman-McKeeman LD (1995) Enzyme induction studies with musk xylene. In: Proceedings from the Seventh International Information Exchange. Research Institute for Fragrance Materials, Hackensack, pp 79–84

Maekawa A, Matsushima Y, Onodera H, Shibutani M, Ogasawara H, Kodama Y, Kurokawa, Y, Hayashi Y (1990) Long-term toxicity/carcinogenicity of musk xylol in B6C3F1 mice. Food Chem Toxicol 28:581–586

Mankes RF LeFevre R, Bates H, Abraham R (1983) Effects of various exposure levels of 2-phenylethanol on fetal development and survival in Long-Evans rats. J Toxicol Environ Health 12:235–244

Pfitzer EA (1992) Recent studies with para-tertiary butyl-alpha-methylhydrocinnamaldehyde (BHMCA). In: Proceedings from the Sixth International Information Exchange. Research Institute for Fragrance Materials, Hackensack, pp 84–88

Pfitzer EA (1995) BHMCA: an evaluation of risk assessment. In: Proceedings from the Seventh International Information Exchange. Research Institute for Fragrance Materials, Hackensack, pp 93–96

Spencer PS, Bischoff-Fenton MC, Moreno OM, Opdyke DL, Ford RA (1984) Neurotoxic properties of musk ambrette. Toxicol Appl Pharmacol 75:571–575

Absorption of Fragrance Ingredients Using In Vitro Models with Human Skin

S. A. M. Hotchkiss

The Cutaneous "Life Cycle" of a Fragrance Chemical

Historically, the skin has been regarded as an inert structure which acts as a relatively impervious barrier to the inward movement of chemicals. However, it is now accepted that the skin is not a complete barrier, but is, in fact, an important route of entry of xenobiotics into the systemic circulation. The passage of a chemical from outside the skin into the body can be described as its topical fate or "life cycle". In order to assess the risk associated with the use of fragrance chemicals, it is desirable to have knowledge concerning their "life cycle", including the rate and extent of percutaneous absorption and the factors affecting this process. Following topical exposure to a fragrance chemical, some may be lost from the surface via the processes of evaporation, sweating, washing, abrasion and bacterial degradation. However, some may be absorbed into the skin, the extent to which depends upon a number of factors such as the physicochemical nature of the compound in question (including its lipophilicity, octanol/water partition coefficient, volatility and molecular volume), the dose and concentration applied, the vehicle of application, the surface area and region of application, the time of skin contact, occlusion of the skin surface, the extent of skin hydration, skin temperature and the degree of skin barrier compromisation by disease or physical damage. The precise site of application is also a factor determining the rate and extent of skin absorption, as is the age of the skin and structural differences such as its thickness and the number of hair follicles. During the percutaneous absorption process, the compound may be sequestered in the lipid-rich stratum corneum, forming a reservoir, or may diffuse deeper into the skin where it may be subject to metabolism by enzymes present in the epidermis and the dermis. Subsequently, the fragrance chemical and/or its metabolites may be absorbed into the systemic circulation via the dermal microvasculature, and be distributed to distant sites of the body (Hotchkiss 1995a).

Assessment of Fragrance Chemical Absorption

The skin disposition of a number of fragrance chemicals has been studied using a variety of in vivo techniques. In particular a skin absorption model or "SAM" system has been validated as an appropriate model for in vivo absorption in both rat and human skin (Hotchkiss et al. 1990 a, b, 1992 a, b). In the in vitro SAM system, freshly obtained circles of rat or human skin are placed into flow-through diffusion cells and surface temperature is maintained at 32 °C. The radiolabelled test compound is applied to the skin surface, and the skin is either occluded with a teflon cap or left open to the atmosphere. A buffer or tissue culture medium flows across the underside of the skin to aid the maintenance of skin viability, and this receptor fluid is collected at hourly intervals for up to 72 h and assayed for penetrated parent compound and metabolites by liquid scintillation spectrometry and/or HPLC. At the end of the experiment, the skin surface is washed to remove any unabsorbed material, and the skin is digested to assess residual radioactive material (parent compound and/or metabolites). Besides being economical with animal and human tissue, the SAM system is rapid, reproducible and relatively inexpensive.

Structure–Activity Relationships in Skin Absorption

Percutaneous absorption data on some 24 fragrance compounds has been gathered to date, with the aim to correlate the extent of absorption with the structure and physicochemical properties of the compound. A knowledge of so-called structure–activity relationships (SARs) will be of value for the future prediction of systemic exposure after skin contact with fragrance chemicals.

The fundamental basis for defining SARs in percutaneous absorption relies upon an understanding of the constitution of the skin membrane, and the interactions between the chemical and its surrounding cutaneous environment. In essence, for a chemical to enter the lipid-rich stratum corneum it must be lipophilic in nature: hydrophilic substances are generally relatively poorly absorbed. However some degree of aqueous solubility is also required since the chemical must then be absorbed from the stratum corneum into the relatively aqueous viable tissue. The size of the molecule is also an important factor in percutaneous absorption, although considerably less so than lipid solubility. Increasing molecular weight or molecular volume, above a threshold, will have an inverse affect on absorption, with low molecular weight/volume compounds being better absorbed, generally, than those of higher molecular weight or volume.

From in vitro studies in human skin with 24 structurally unrelated chemicals, we have been able to construct some crude relationships between structure and percutaneous absorption. For this series, optimal absorption through human skin is observed when the octanol-water partition co-efficient, Log $P_{o/w}$ is within the range 1.3 – 2.0. For example, the fragrance chemical coumarin, with Log P = 1.41 is extremely well absorbed (60%), whilst *d*-limonene with Log P = 4.35 is only 3% absorbed. However, such simplistic relationships are never likely to provide a complete answer for all chemicals because the complex nature of the stratum corneum and other contributory factors such as skin metabolism. For more informative and predictive models, further, more rigorous analyses are required.

In Vitro–In Vivo Correlations in Fragrance Chemical Absorption

The percutaneous absorption of a number of fragrance chemicals has been assessed in human, rat and/or mouse skin using the in vitro SAM system, and the values compared with in vivo data obtained from the literature and other sources (Chidgey et al. 1987; Bronaugh and Stewart 1985; Bronaugh et al. 1985, 1990). For most chemicals (e.g. benzoic acid, benzyl acetate, cinnamyl anthranilate, coumarin, diethyl phthalate, dimethyl phthalate, eugenol, *d*-limonene, 2-phenylethanol, musk xylene, isoeugenol) there appears to be relatively good agreement between the extent of absorption observed in vitro and that observed in vivo, although there is little standardization of methods between various laboratories' studies in terms of parameters such as dose, exposed surface area, vehicle, occlusion, skin contact time and time of collection. However, the in vitro absorption of dibutyl phthalate and diphenyl ether is considerable less than that seen in vivo. This poor in vitro–in vivo correlation may reflect inter-laboratory differences in experimental procedure or the compounds' high lipophilicity (log P > 4) and poor aqueous solubility which make diffusion from the skin into the aqueous receptor fluid difficult in the in vitro SAM model. Conversely, for 2-phenoxyethyl isobutyrate, the in vitro absorption is greater than that in vivo, which may reflect the shorter application time used in the in vivo studies, as well as differences in dose and vehicle.

The Skin Reservoir

It is now well documented that the skin may act as a reservoir for topically applied chemicals, into which the chemicals may be rapidly taken up and from which they may be only slowly released into the systemic circulation (Hewitt et al. 1993). Such a cutaneous reservoir has potential toxicological significance in terms of continued systemic exposure after dermal application has ceased. We have investigated the phenomenon of reservoir formation for a range of fragrance chemicals, including coumarin, eugenol, benzyl acetate and three phthalic acid esters (dimethyl phthalate, diethyl phthalate, dibutyl phthalate).

The uptake of all chemicals into rat skin is very rapid, with substantial cutaneous levels after only 3 min and maximum skin levels within 4–6 h. This rapid absorption from the skin surface into the tissue is in contrast to the relatively delayed absorption through the skin and into the receptor fluid. Interestingly, it has been observed that essentially the entire dose of each chemical to which the systemic circulation is subsequently exposed has already partitioned into the skin by 4–6 h.

Using a range of skin sectioning and "stripping" techniques we have been able to demonstrate the precise location of the cutaneous depot for fragrance chemicals, and in the main this would appear to reside within the outer region of the skin, the stratum corneum. For example, after topical application of benzyl acetate to rat skin in vitro, 10 μm frozen sections were taken and assayed for radioactivity, and at all times, the majority of the recovered material was present in the first three or four sections, i. e. equivalent to the stratum corneum. Very little material was recovered in the remaining epidermis and dermis. In contrast, for coumarin, tape stripping experiments revealed that at 2 h, relatively little (13%) was located within the outer stratum corneum and considerably more (37%) was present within the viable tissue (epidermis and dermis). Hence, comparatively speaking, coumarin does not appear to form a substantial stratum corneum reservoir, because its physicochemical characteristics ensure that it rapidly partitions from the stratum corneum into the viable epidermis, dermis and receptor fluid (S. A. M Hotchkiss et al. – unpublished observations, 1997).

Factors Affecting Fragrance Chemical Absorption

As indicated above, a variety of factors may affect the percutaneous absorption of topically applied fragrance chemicals, including dose, vehicle, skin exposure time, occlusion and skin metabolism.

Occlusion. Occlusion of the skin surface after topical exposure has been documented to alter the permeation kinetics of certain fragrance chemicals (Hotchkiss et al. 1992c). The mechanisms via which this occurs may include reduction in the loss of volatile fragrance agents by evaporation, increased skin hydration and increased skin temperature, all of which may enhance absorption. Using the in vitro SAM system, we have studied the effect of occlusion on the percutaneous absorption of a number of fragrance chemicals through rat and human skin. In the rat, occlusion of the skin surface was observed to increase the percutaneous absorption of five of the 16 fragrance chemicals studied, namely *l*-menthol, cinnamyl anthranilate, cinnamaldehyde, cinnamyl alcohol and 2-phenylethanol. However, occlusion did not significantly enhance the absorption of the remaining 11 chemicals (Table 1). In

Table 1. Inter-species comparison and effect of occlusion on the percutaneous absorption of fragrance chemicals through rat and human skin in vitro

Compound	Amount absorbed at 72 h (% dose)			
	Rat		Human	
	Unoccluded	Occluded	Unoccluded	Occluded
Diphenyl ether	0.3	0.3	0.2	0.2
l-Menthol (48 h)	1	3[a]		
2-Methoxynaphthalene	2	2	2	2
d-Limonene	6	6	3	5
Cinnamic acid (48 h)	9	7		
Dibutyl phthalate	12	10	0.4	0.5
Dimethyl phthalate	26	17	4	4
Cinnamyl anthranilate(48 h)	30	38[a]		
Eugenol	34	40		
Cinnamaldehyde	34	42[a]	24	52[a]
Cinnamyl alcohol (48 h)	37	56[a]		
Diethyl phthalate	38	23	5	4
2-Phenoxyethyl isobutyrate	41	46	5	5
Coumarin	57	64	46	60[a]
Benzyl acetate	58	59	12	12
2-Phenylethanol (48 h)	64	70[a]		

[a] Significantly different ($p < 0.05$) from unoccluded data.

human skin, occlusion served to enhance the absorption of only two of the ten fragrance chemicals studied, namely cinnamaldehyde and coumarin, although there was no effect upon the absorption of the other seven chemicals (Table 1). Hence for most fragrance chemicals, occlusion does not appear to alter absorption, although any effects that do occur are compound and species specific.

Species. Skin from various species may be used for percutaneous absorption studies. However, in order to make reliable judgements for risk extrapolation to humans, it is important to have a clear understanding of how absorption may vary between animals and humans. We have studied species differences in absorption for a number of fragrance chemicals through occluded and occluded rat and human skin (Beckley-Kartey and Hotchkiss 1995; Garnett et al. 1994; Mint and Hotchkiss 1993; Mint et al. 1994). In unoccluded human skin, percutaneous absorption is generally either less than (benzoic acid, benzyl acetate, cinnamaldehyde, dimethyl phthalate, diethyl phthalate, dibutyl phthalate, 2-phenoxyethyl isobutyrate) or sometimes the same as (coumarin, diphenyl ether, *d*-limonene, 2-methoxynaphthalene) the absorption through unoccluded rat tissue (Table 1). The magnitude of the species difference is compound dependent and is greatest for dibutyl phthalate where a 30-fold difference was observed (12% rat; 0.4% human). When the skin is occluded, the same species differences are apparent for all chemicals with the exception of cinnamaldehyde and benzoic acid, where the absorption is greater through human skin than through rat tissue (Table 1). The rank order of increasing fragrance chemical absorption is similar in both species, although there is not complete concordance. These marked differences in absorption between rat and human skin suggest that care should be taken when relying on animal data to provide an accurate model for human absorption.

Dose. The dose of a fragrance chemical applied to the skin surface may affect the rate and amount that is absorbed. For example, for benzyl acetate in the rat, absorption at 48 h is a fixed proportion (50%) of the applied dose up to a dose rate of 33 mg/cm^2. However, thereafter absorption efficiency decreases with each dose to only 7% at 331 mg/cm^2. A similar relationship is observed between dose and absorption for the phthalate esters in human skin, where absorption linearly increases with dose up to 10 – 20 mg/cm^2, but is non-linear thereafter. The absorption of eugenol and anethole through rat skin is also linearly dose-related up to a dose level of 15 mg/cm^2. Hence the relationship between the applied dose and the extent of absorption is both compound and species specific. These data highlight the requirement for care when extrapolating from data derived by other laboratories without knowledge of dose effects.

Vehicle. Fragrance chemicals will generally come into contact with the skin, not as the neat material, but as a formulated product containing additional constituents. The effect of formulation or vehicle on the percutaneous absorption of a range of fragrance chemicals has been investigated using the SAM system. For benzyl acetate, an ethanol vehicle enhances absorption through rat skin at early times after application (6 h) but this effect is short lasting and is not observable at 48 h. 2-Phenylethanol and dimethyl sulfoxide both enhance benzyl acetate absorption at all times after application. Similarly, with eugenol, an ethanol vehicle enhances absorption through rat skin at early times, although not at 72 h. The extent of absorption of coumarin at 48 h and 72 h is unaffected by application in a vehicle of ethanol or ethanol/diethyl phthalate (75:25), although the rate of absorption at early times is enhanced more than 2-fold when ethanol is used. Ethanol is a well documented skin penetration enhancer, and is often employed therapeutically in transdermal delivery systems for this purpose. Its mechanism of action is complex, but may involve transient damage to the stratum corneum lipid matrix, altered solubility and partitioning of coumarin between the vehicle and the skin (Hotchkiss et al. 1992c).

Skin Metabolism

There is now considerable evidence that the skin is a living tissue, containing many of the xenobiotic metabolizing enzymes previously identified in the liver (Hotchkiss 1992, 1995b; Hewitt et al. 1996). These enzymes can catalyze so-called phase 1 or "functionalization" reactions including oxidation, reduction and hydrolysis as well as phase 2 or "conjugation" reactions. The presence of these cutaneous enzymes is generally thought to play a beneficial role in catalysing the detoxification of potentially harmful chemicals. In fact, cutaneous esterases may be so efficient that topically applied esters may be completely metabolized during skin absorption. In contrast, other cutaneous enzymes such as cytochromes P_{450}, although generally less active, may serve to convert certain relatively harmless substances into potentially toxic metabolites. Although the specific activities of individual skin enzymes may be low (generally <10% liver activities), the considerable mass of tissue with its extensive surface area (about 2 m^2), suggests that cutaneous metabolism may play a significant role in the biotransformation of topically applied fragrance chemicals.

Studies in freshly excised human and rodent skin in the in vitro SAM system and cultured epidermal keratinocytes, suggest that the skin is able to metabolize certain fragrance chemicals, but not others, during absorption (Beckley-Kartey et al. 1997; Nasseri-Sina et al. 1997). The extent to which such metabolism occurs depends on the chemical itself and the precise nature of the enzymes systems involved. Esterase activity is particularly high in skin, explaining the fact that after topical application of benzyl acetate to full thickness rat skin in vitro there is rapid and complete hydrolysis to benzyl alcohol (97%) with some further oxidation to benzoic acid (3%). In human skin, benzyl acetate is also extensively, but not completely, hydrolysed (99%), with 1% of the absorbed material recovered as the parent compound (Garnett 1992). The phthalic acid esters are also extensively metabolized during percutaneous absorption in human and rat skin (Mint 1995). Similarly, hydroxycitronellal is completely metabolized during absorption through rat skin, with oxidation to the corresponding acid (catalyzed by cutaneous aldehyde dehydrogenase; ALDH) and reduction to the alcohol (catalyzed by alcohol dehydrogenase; ADH) (Tonge 1995). In these cases, systemic exposure after topical application in vivo will be to the metabolites, and not to the parent fragrance chemical. However, other fragrance compounds, particularly cytochrome P_{450} substrates, are not metabolized significantly during absorption. For example, topically applied coumarin is absorbed through human, rat and mouse skin essentially unchanged, suggesting a lack of the cytochrome P_{450} isoforms responsible for hydroxylation in these species (Beckley-Kartey et al. 1997). Systemic exposure after topical application of unmetabolized fragrance

Table 2. Metabolism of fragrance chemicals during percutaneous absorption

Chemical	Species	Extent of skin metabolism (%)	Metabolites
Benzyl acetate	Rat Human	100 99	Benzyl alcohol and benzoic acid
Dimethyl phthalate and diethyl phthalate	Rat and human	100	Monoester and phthalic acid
Dibutyl phthalate	Rat Human	100 93	Monoester and phthalic acid
Cinnamaldehyde	Rat	100	Cinnamic acid and cinnamic alcohol
Hydroxycitronellal	Rat	100	Acid and alcohol
Coumarin	Rat, mouse, and human	0	–

Data drawn from Garnett 1992, Mint 1995, Tonge 1995, and Beckley-Kartey et al. 1997.

chemicals such as coumarin in vivo is thus likely to be to the parent compound and not to its metabolites (Table 2).

Cutaneous metabolism during percutaneous absorption may be of relevance for fragrance chemical toxicity, both at the local (skin) and systemic level (Hotchkiss 1995b). The sensitizer, cinnamaldehyde is rapidly converted to cinnamic acid and cinnamyl alcohol in human skin. Since all the available evidence suggests that it is the parent aldehyde that is the reactive moiety (Majeti and Suskind 1977; Weibel and Hansen 1989), one might hypothesise that the enzymes responsible for its metabolism to cinnamic acid (ALDH) and cinnamyl alcohol (ADH) in skin, might catalyze a reduction in the availability of the aldehyde within the tissue, therefore reducing cutaneous sensitization. Similarly, the contact sensitizer hydroxycitronellal undergoes extensive cutaneous oxidation and reduction by ALDH and ADH, respectively, to the corresponding carboxylic acid and alcohol, both in human skin homogenates and after topical application to full-thickness rat skin in SAM diffusion cells. This cutaneous metabolism may also serve to detoxify the reactive aldehyde (Table 2).

Cutaneous Toxicity

The ability of a fragrance chemical to elicit cutaneous toxicity is dependent upon three factors: (1) skin absorption (2) skin metabolism and (3) interaction with target sites e.g. skin macromolecules. As indicated above, hydroxycitronellal is a skin sensitizing agent in humans, and in order for this toxicity to occur it must first be absorbed from the skin surface into the epidermis, where it can be presented to the immune system. For small molecular weight haptens (<1 kDa) such as hydroxycitronellal, association with proteins in the skin is a likely pre-requisite for immune recognition. Haptens are generally electrophilic molecules, and as such they are able to bind covalently with the nucleophilic groups of protein amino acids, mainly amine groups (NH_2) in lysine (and arginine and histidine), and thiol groups (SH) in cysteine. Hydroxycitronellal is a reactive aldehyde capable of direct protein conjugation via free amino and/or thiol groups, the former leading to a Schiff's base formation. The hapten-modified protein then acts as an immunogen via antigen presenting cells (Langerhans cells) in the epidermis, a classic type 4 delayed hypersensitivity reaction. However, if a fragrance chemical is not directly reactive it may be metabolized by cutaneous enzymes to a reactive metabolite (the hapten) which, in turn, forms conjugates with skin protein.

We have confirmed experimentally that hydroxycitronellal is well absorbed after topical application to full-thickness rat skin in SAM cells, with approx. 30% absorbed into the receptor fluid and 30% remaining within the skin at 72 h (Tonge 1995). We have also employed immunochemical and cellular approaches to investigate the covalent binding of hydroxycitronellal to skin proteins. Using a fully characterized polyclonal antibody raised in our laboratory against hydroxycitronellal-modified protein, we have detected hydroxycitronellal protein adducts in full-thickness rat and human skin and skin homogenates by ELISA. Reducing conditions would appear to be critical for the development of these adducts in skin, possibly because reducing conditions are required to stabilise Schiff's bases. The formation of hydroxycitronellal-conjugates in full-thickness skin is dose-dependent and three distinct protein targets have been identified by Western blotting. Three polypeptides with molecular weights from 45 kDa to 65 kDa were most intensely labelled, and these proteins could be considered as candidate immunogens skin sensitization elicited following topical exposure to hydroxycitronellal (Tonge et al. 1994).

Summary

Our studies have shown clearly that all fragrance chemicals are absorbed into the skin to some extent, although this varies with the chemical from very low (e.g. dibutyl phthalate <1%) to extremely high (e.g. coumarin 70%). Skin absorption is affected by many factors, including dose, vehicle, duration of exposure and occlusion of the skin site. In addition, the skin acts as a reservoir for many fragrance chemicals into which they are rapidly taken up from the skin surface, but only slowly released into the systemic circulation. Furthermore, the skin is metabolically active and although some fragrance chemicals may be absorbed essentially unchanged (e.g. coumarin), others may be entirely metabolized during absorption (e.g. diethyl phthalate). Once absorbed into the skin, reactive fragrance chemicals are able to covalently modify skin proteins and form adducts that may be responsible for cutaneous toxicity such as skin sensitization. Thus, in gaining a detailed understanding of the mechanisms underlying the skin absorption, cutaneous metabolism and dermal toxicity of fragrance chemicals, a more accurate assessment may be made of the safety of such compounds after skin contact in humans.

Acknowledgements. The research described in this paper was conducted by members of the Dermal Toxicology Research Group: Annette Garnett, Philip Hewitt, Andrew Mint, Pari Nasseri-Sina, Robert Tonge, Senam Beckley-Kartey and Julie-Ann Ashcroft. We are grateful to the Research Institute for Fragrance Materials (RIFM) for its financial support.

References

Beckley-Kartey SAJ, Hotchkiss SAM (1995) The percutaneous absorption of coumarin through fresh human and rat skin in vitro. In: Brain KR, Hadgraft J, James VJ, Walters KA (eds) Prediction of percutaneous penetration: methods, measurements and modelling, vol 4b. STS, Cardiff, pp 299–302

Beckley-Kartey SAJ, Capel M, Hotchkiss SAM (1997) Comparative in vitro skin absorption and metabolism of coumarin (1,2-benzopyrone) in human, rat and mouse. Toxicol Appl Pharmacol (in press)

Bronaugh RL, Stewart RF (1985) Methods for in vitro percutaneous absorption studies. IV. The flow-through diffusion cell. J Pharm Sci 74:64–67

Bronaugh RL, Stewart RF, Wester RC, Bucks D, Maibach HI (1985). Comparison of percutaneous absorption of fragrances by humans and monkeys. Food Chem Toxicol 23: 111–114

Bronaugh RL, Wester RC, Bucks D, Maibach HI, Sarason R (1990) In vivo percutaneous absorption of fragrance ingredients in rhesus monkeys and humans. Food Chem Toxicol 28:369–373

Chidgey MAJ, Kennedy JF, Caldwell J (1987) Studies on benzyl acetate III. The percutaneous absorption and disposition of [methylene-^{14}C] benzyl acetate in the rat. Food Chem Toxicol 25 (7):521–525

Garnett A (1992) Investigation of the in vitro percutaneous absorption and metabolism of benzyl acetate and related compounds. PhD Thesis, University of London

Garnett A, Hotchkiss SAM, Caldwell J (1994) Percutaneous absorption of benzyl acetate through rat skin in vitro. 3. A comparison with human skin. Food Chem Toxicol 32 (11):1061–1065

Hewitt PG, Hotchkiss SAM, Caldwell J (1993) Cutaneous reservoir formation and localization after topical application of 4,4′-methylene-bis-(2-chloroaniline) and 4,4′-methylenedianiline to rat and human skin in vitro. In: Brain KR, James VJ, Walters KA (eds) Prediction of percutaneous penetration: methods, measurements and modelling, vol. 3b. STS, Cardiff, pp 638–645

Hewitt P, Hotchkiss SAM, Perkins JM, Rowe RR (1996) Transdermal metabolism of fluroxypyr 1-methylheptyl ester during percutaneous absorption through fresh human and rat skin in vitro. In: Brain KR, James VJ, Walters KA (eds) Prediction of percutaneous penetration: methods, measurements and modelling, vol 4b. STS, Cardiff, pp 303–306

Hotchkiss SAM (1992) The skin as a xenobiotic metabolizing organ. In: GG Gibson (ed) Progress in drug metabolism, vol 13. Taylor & Francis, London, pp 217–262

Hotchkiss SAM (1995a) Skin absorption of occupational chemicals. In: Handbook of Occupational Hygiene, instalment 46. Croner, Kingston upon Thames, vol 1, part 2.1.8, pp 1-38

Hotchkiss SAM (1995b) Cutaneous toxicity: kinetic and metabolic determinants. Toxicol Ecotoxicol News 2(1):10-18

Hotchkiss SA, Chidgey MAJ, Rose S, Caldwell J (1990a) Percutaneous absorption of benzyl acetate through rat skin in vitro. 1. Validation of an in vitro model against in vivo data. Food Chem Toxic 28:443-447

Hotchkiss SA, Fraser S, Chidgey MAJ, Caldwell J (1990b) An in vitro skin diffusion technique for the prediction of in vivo absorption: a case study with benzyl acetate. In: Scott RC, Hadgraft J, Guy R (eds) Prediction of percutaneous penetration: methods, measurements and modelling, I.B.C., London, pp 123-128

Hotchkiss SAM, Hewitt P, Caldwell J, Chen WL, Rowe RR (1992a) Percutaneous absorption of nicotinic acid, phenol, benzoic acid and triclopyr butoxyethyl ester through rat and human skin in vitro. Further validation of an in vitro model by comparison with in vivo data. Food Chem Toxicol 30:891-899

Hotchkiss SA, Hewitt P, Caldwell J, Chen WL, Rowe RR (1992b) Absorption of nicotinic acid, phenol and benzoic acid through rat and human skin in vitro. In: Scott RC, Hadgraft J, Guy R (eds) Prediction of percutaneous penetration: methods, measurements and modelling, vol 2. I.B.C., London, pp 472-482

Hotchkiss SAM, Miller JM, Caldwell J (1992c) Percutaneous absorption of benzyl acetate through rat skin in vitro. 2. Effect of vehicle and occlusion. Food ChemToxicol 30:145-153

Majeti VA, Suskind RR (1977) Mechanism of cinnamaldehyde sensitization. Contact Dermatitis 3:16-18

Mint A (1995) Investigation into the topical disposition of the phthalic acid esters dimethyl phthalate, diethyl phthalate and dibutyl phthalate in rat and human skin. PhD Thesis, University of London

Mint A, Hotchkiss SAM (1993) Percutaneous absorption of dimethyl phthalate and di-n-butyl phthalate through rat and human skin in vitro. In: Brain KR, James VJ, Walters KA (eds) Prediction of percutaneous penetration: methods, measurements and modelling, vol 3b. STS, Cardiff, pp 646-657

Mint A, Hotchkiss SAM, Caldwell J (1994) Percutaneous absorption of diethyl phthalate through rat and human skin in vitro. Toxic in Vitro, 8(2):251-256

Nasseri-Sina P, Hotchkiss SAM, Caldwell J (1997) Cutaneous xenobiotic metabolism: glycine conjugation in human and rat keratinocytes. Food Chem Toxicol 35:409-416

Tonge RP (1995) The cutaneous disposition of the sensitizing chemicals hydroxycitronellal and dinitrochlorobenzene. PhD Thesis, University of London

Tonge RP, Kenna JG, van Pelt FNAM, Hotchkiss SAM (1994) An immunochemical investigation into covalent binding of hydroxycitronellal to human skin proteins in vitro. J Invest Dermatol 102(4):637

Weibel H, Hansen J (1989) Interaction of cinnamaldehyde (a sensitizer in fragrance) with protein. Contact Dermatitis 20:161-166

Synthetic Musk Fragrances in Human Fat and Their Potential Uptake by Dermal Resorption

G.G. Rimkus

Introduction

Animal fragrances have a long history of application by mankind. Musk is one of the most important and often used fragrances in perfumery. The odorous components in natural musk originate from the musk deer (*Moschus moschiferus* L.). Because of its thick, oily, jelly-like natural musk, the musk deer is the most desired, although untamed animal of Tibet and Siberia. Both the male and female deer have a musk gland (pod) under the tail; in addition, the adult male also has a pouch on the abdomen. Each musk pod contains about one ounce of liquid. The natural extracts contain macrocyclic ketones, alcohols and pyridine derivatives. Musk deers are still hunted for their musk, but not as much as in the past [1]. Moreover, due to the high cost and uncertainty of supply of natural musk and great expense and complexity involved in the chemical synthesis of the original musk compounds, natural musk has been replaced by synthetic musks with fragrance and other properties similar to those of the natural substances. The phenomenal growth demand for musk has created a world-wide synthetic musk industry. Today almost all of the musks used in cosmetics and fragrance products are synthetic.

Baur had already introduced musk xylene as the first synthetic musk compound from the group of nitro musks in the last century [2]. This was followed by several similar nitroaromatic compounds. Table 1 presents the chemical names, CAS numbers, and chemical structures of the most important nitro musk compounds. These artificial musks do not occur in nature, and there is no chemical or structural relationship of the trinitro and dinitro benzenes with the natural musk compounds. They impart desirable musk-like odours to various consumer products and are used on a grand scale as fragrance fixatives and materials in personal-care and household products such as cosmetics, soaps, laundry detergents, fabric softeners, household cleaning products, air fresheners, and so on. Synthetic nitro musks are of great industrial importance, especially since they are easy and inexpensive to produce. Their world-wide production in 1987 was estimated to be about 2,500 tons per year [1]. China and India are the leading producers of nitro musks for the world

Table 1. Chemical names, common names, CAS numbers, and chemical structures of five nitro musk compounds

Chemical Name	Trivial Name	CAS No.	Chemical structure
1-*tert*-Butyl-3,5-dimethyl-2,4,6-trinitrobenzene or 2,4,6-Trinitro-1,3-dimethyl-5-*tert*-butylbenzene or 2,4,6-Trinitro-5-*tert*-butyl-1,3-xylene	Musk xylene, Musk xylol	81–15–2	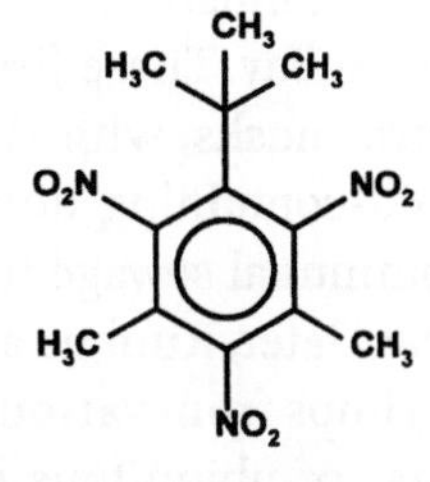
1-*tert*-Butyl-3,5-dimethyl-2,6-dinitro-4-acetylbenzene or 4-*tert*-Butyl-3,5-dinitro-2,6-dimethylacetophenone	Musk ketone	81–14–1	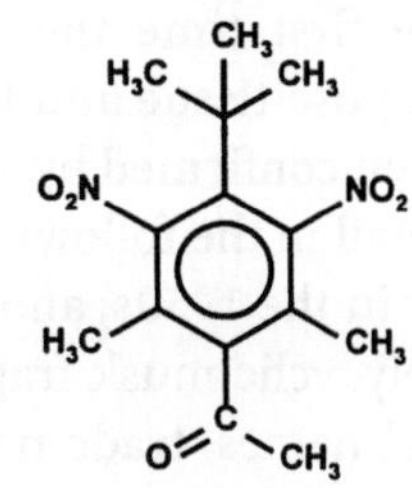
1-*tert*-Butyl-2-methoxy-4-methyl-3,5-dinitrobenzene or 4-*tert*-Butyl-2,6-dinitro-3-methoxytoluene	Musk ambrette	83–66–9	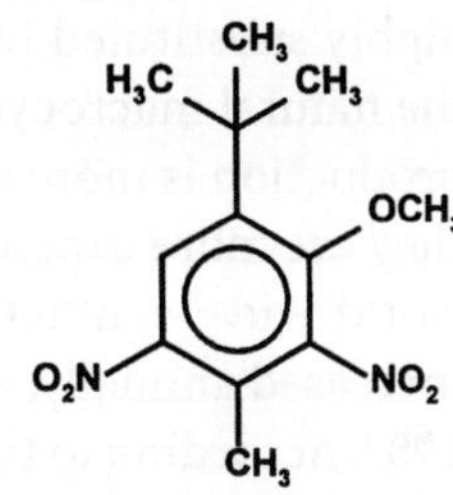
1-tert-Butyl-3,4,5-trimethyl-2,6-dinitrobenzene	Musk tibetene	145–39–1	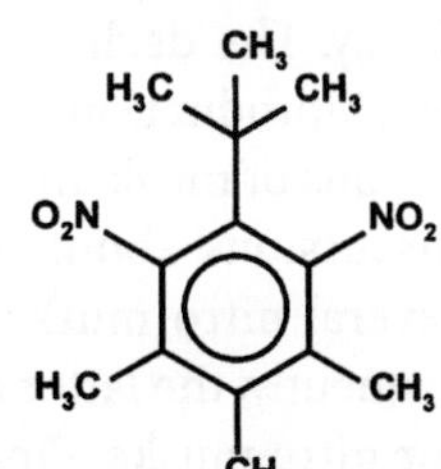
1,1,3,3,5-Pentamethyl-4,6-dinitroindane	Musk moskene	116–66–5	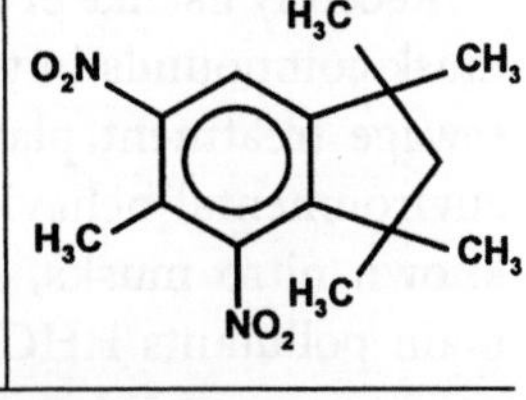

market [3, 4]. In 1991, there was even a reported increase of about 29% in Chinese musk xylene production [3].

In 1981 Yamagishi et al. [5, 6] identified for the first time musk xylene and musk ketone in the aquatic environment. They analysed these nitro aromatics in fish, mussels, and water collected from the Japanese river Tama and the Tokyo Bay. These first results indicated the lipophilic and persistent nature of nitro musks, with their strong tendency to bioaccumulate in fish and other lipid-containing aquatic organisms. They identified the effluents of some communal sewage treatment plants as the cause of contamination. About ten years later, Rimkus and Wolf [7–9] analysed nitro musks in fish, mussels, and shrimps from various locations and started a broad discussion about this new class of ubiquitous environmental contaminants in aquatic ecosystems. For the first time they also unambiguously detected nitro musks in human adipose tissue and human milk [10–12]. In the meantime, their results have been confirmed by various studies; they will be summarized and discussed in detail in the following paragraphs.

In the 1950s, another important group of synthetic musk compounds, the polycyclic musk fragrances, were introduced. Table 2 summarizes the chemical names, trade names, CAS names and numbers, and the chemical structures of seven polycyclic musk compounds. These polycyclic musks are highly substituted indane and tetraline derivatives and they do not resemble the natural macrocyclic musk components in their chemical structures. Their production is more complex and, therefore, in comparison to the nitro musks, they are more expensive. Nevertheless, according to the data of a study on the world-wide synthetic musk market [1], polycyclic musk production has increased annually, with a world-wide production of about 4,300 tons a year in 1987. According to this study, polycyclic musks accounted for about 61% of the total world market of synthetic musk fragrances in 1987, with an upward tendency. The decline in nitro musk production and the increase in polycyclic musk production is based primarily on the restrictions on the use and applications of musk ambrette [1]. Furthermore, it may be assumed that the critical discussions about some environmental and toxicological characteristics of several nitro musks promoted their replacement by polycyclic musks. Consequently, the latter are used as substitutes not only for natural musk, but also for nitro musks – mainly musk xylene and musk ketone – in the same way in personal-care and household products as mentioned above.

Recently Eschke et al. [13, 14] also identified for the first time the polycyclic musk compounds in water and fish from the river Ruhr and some municipal sewage treatment plants. Their findings indicated some similarities in the environmental behaviour of these compounds with the comparatively well-known nitro musks, even though the environmental concentrations of the main pollutants HHCB and AHTN seem to exceed to some extent those of

Table 2. Chemical names, trade names, CAS names, CAS numbers, and chemical structures of seven polycyclic musk compounds

Chemical name (abbreviation)	Trade name(s)	CAS name	CAS no.	Chemical structure
1,3,4,6,7,8-Hexahydro-4,6,6,7,8,8-hexamethyl-cyclopenta[g]-2-benzo-pyrane (HHCB)	Galaxolide Abbalide Pearlide	1,3,4,6,7,8-hexahydro-4,6,6,7,8,8-hexamethyl-cyclopenta[g]-2-benzopyrane	1222–05–5	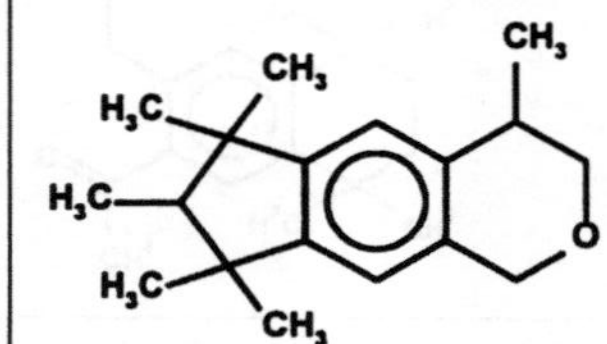
7-Acetyl-1,1,3,4,4,6-hexamethyltetrahydro-naphthalene (AHTN)	Tonalide Fixolide	1-(5,6,7,8-tetrahydro-3,5,5,6,8,8-hexamethyl-2-naphthalenyl)-ethanone	1506–02–1	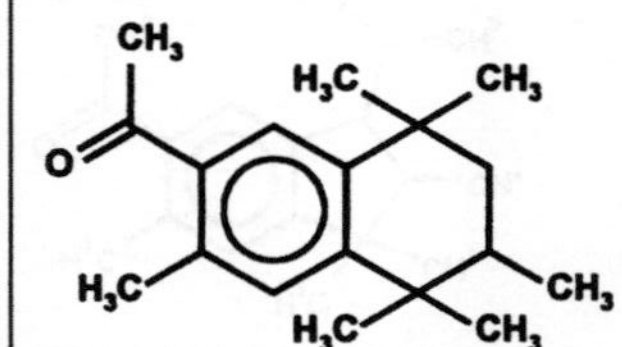
4-Acetyl-1,1-dimethyl-6-*tert*-butyldihydroindene (ADBI)	Celestolide Crysolide	1-[6-(1,1-dimethylethyl)-2,3-dihydro-1,1-dimethyl-1H-inden-4-yl]-ethanone	13171–00–1	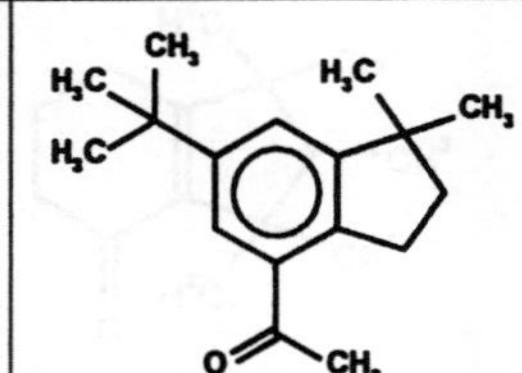
6-Acetyl-1,1,2,3,3,5-hexamethyldihydroindene (AHDI)	Phantolide	1-(2,3-dihydro-1,1,2,3,3,6-hexamethyl-1H-inden-5-yl)-ethanone	15323–35–0	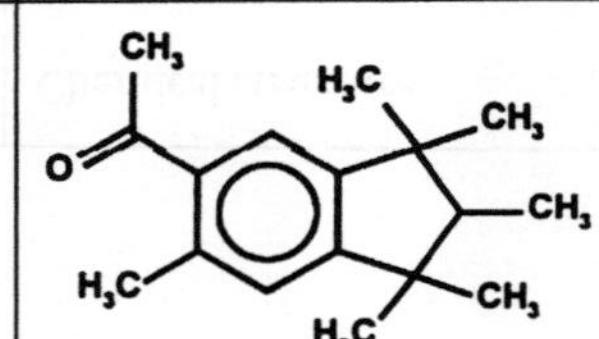

Table 2 (continued)

Chemical name (abbreviation)	Trade name(s)	CAS Name	CAS so.	Chemical structure
6,7-Dihydro-1,1,2,3,3-pentamethyl-4(5H)indanone (DPMI)	Cashmeran	1,2,3,5,6,7-hexahydro-1,1,2,3,3-pentamethyl-4H-inden-4-one	33704–61–9	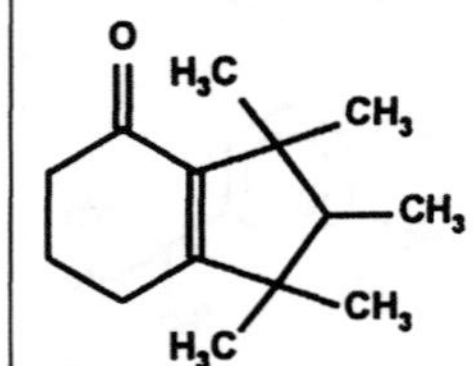
5-Acetyl-1,1,2,6-tetramethyl-3-iso-propyl-dihydroindene (ATII)	Traseolide	1-[2,3-dihydro-1,1,2, 6-tetramethyl-3-(1-methyl-ethyl)-1H-inden-5-yl]-ethanone	68140–48–7	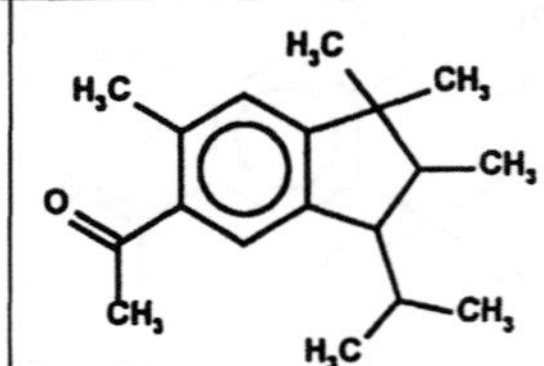
7-Acetyl-1,1,4,4-tetramethyl-6-ethyl-tetrahydronaphthalene (ATTN)	Versalide	1-(3-ethyl-5,6,7,8-tetra-hydro-5,5,8,8-tetramethyl-2-naphthalenyl)-ethanone	88–29–9	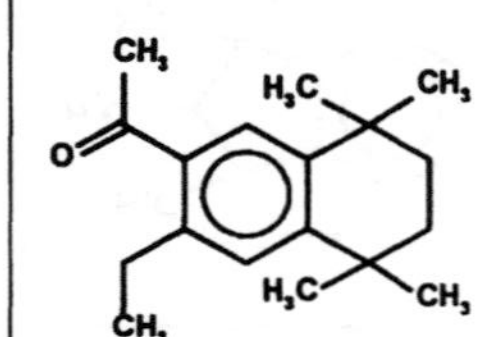

musk xylene and musk ketone. These synthetic musk compounds were recently also found in human fat samples [15–17]; the results will be summarized and extensively discussed in the following.

The aim of this chapter is to summarize all published data available on the contamination of human fat, especially of human adipose tissue and human milk, by synthetic musk compounds. The results will be critically discussed in detail, with special emphasis on potential dermal resorption and the chronic toxicity of synthetic musks.

Results

The residue analysis of the relatively nonpolar and lipophilic nitro musk fragrances in human samples is carried out similarly to and together with the well-known routine analysis of organochlorine pesticides and polychlorinated biphenyls (PCBs) [11]. They are completely extracted from the human tissue together with the lipid fraction, the cleaned extracts are analysed by capillary gas chromatography and detected with the equivalent current dipoles (ECDs), together with the chlorinated pesticides and PCBs. The nitro musk are identified and confirmed by various techniques of mass spectrometry [11].

The concentrations of musk xylene and musk ketone in human milk, human adipose tissue, and human blood that have been reported in the literature to date are summarized in Table 3. Most of the studies were carried out in Germany, and some further data were reported from Switzerland. Due to the world-wide production and use of nitro musks, it is assumed that comparable contamination levels in human samples from other geographical sites exist. In almost all analysed samples, musk xylene and musk ketone were found, with the levels in human milk ranging from 0.005 to 1.22 mg/kg lipid for musk xylene and from less than 0.001 to 0.24 mg/kg lipid for musk ketone. The contamination of human adipose tissue was comparable: 0.005–0.288 mg/kg lipid for musk xylene and from less than 0.001 to 0.22 mg/kg lipid for musk ketone. Irrespective of the various studies, there is a relatively close correlation between all the mean values of musk xylene and musk ketone. In most of the samples the musk xylene concentrations exceeded those of musk ketone significantly. Musk xylene was also detected in blood plasma and blood lipid [23, 24]. The musk xylene concentrations could be compared with those of some organochlorine pesticides such as lindane, β-HCH or dieldrin detected in the same samples [11]. In a few samples musk ambrette and musk moskene were also detected at very low levels [11, 17, 18]. Musk tibetene could not be detected at all.

The analysis of the lipophilic polycyclic musk compounds in human tissue samples is similar to the routine analysis of chlorinated pesticides [16]. In con-

Table 3. Concentrations of musk xylene and musk ketone in human milk, human adipose tissue and human blood (mg/kg lipid)

Material (origin)	Musk xylene			Musk ketone			Reference
	Sample (*n*)	$x_{min} - x_{max}$ [a]	[b]	Sample (*n*)	$x_{min} - x_{max}$ [a]	[b]	
Human milk (Germany, Schleswig-Holstein, 1992–93)	23	0.02–0.19	0.08	23	0.01–0.09	0.03	[10, 11]
Human milk (Germany, Schleswig-Holstein, 1992/95)	5	0.01–0.03		5	0.005–0.015		[16]
Human milk (Germany, South Bavaria)	391	0.01–1.22	0.10	391	< 0.01–0.24	0.04	[18]
Human milk (Germany, Baden-Württemberg)	68	0.005–1.00					[19]
Human milk (Germany, Freiburg)	87	0.005–0.27					[20]
Human milk (Germany, Essen)	2	0.029–0.056		2	0.007–0.021		[15]
Human milk (Germany, Middle Hesse)	55	0.011–0.252	0.057	55	< 0.001–0.102	0.020	[21]
Human milk (Switzerland)	10	–0.25					[22]
Human adipose tissue (Germany, Schleswig-Holstein, 1992, females)	13	0.02–0.22	0.09	13	0.01–0.22	0.035	[10, 11]
Human adipose tissue (Germany, Schleswig-Holstein, 1995, females)	8	0.005–0.030	0.013	8	0.05–0.010	0.006	[16]
Human adipose tissue (Germany, Schleswig-Holstein, 1993, males)	19	0.02–0.09	0.05	19	0.01–0.03	0.02	[11]
Human adipose tissue (Germany, Schleswig-Holstein, 1993/95, males)	6	0.020–0.050	0.027	6	0.005–0.030	0.016	[16]
Human fat (Germany, Essen)	2	0.026–0.080		2	0.004–0.005		[15]
Human adipose tissue (Switzerland, females)	10	0.0067–0.106	0.038	10	0.0028–0.173	0.026	[17]
Human adipose tissue (Switzerland, males)	5	0.013–0.288	0.082	5	< 0.001–0.011	0.0039	[17]
Human blood (Switzerland)	11	0.012–0.049					[23]
Human blood (Germany, Erlangen/Nürnberg)	72	< 0.1–1.12 [c]	0.24 [c,d]				[24]

[a] minimum and maximum concentration; [b] mean value; [c] g/l plasma; [d] median concentration.

trast to the nitro musks, the polycyclic musk compounds cannot be detected with sufficient sensitivity by capillary gas chromatography with an ECD due to their chemical structure. On the other hand, mass spectrometry can be used for identification and routine analysis [16]. Hitherto, in three studies from Germany and Switzerland, polycyclic musk compounds have been analysed in a total of 38 samples of human milk and human adipose tissue. Table 4 summarizes the reported concentrations of HHCB, AHTN and ADBI in human samples. In all analysed samples HHCB and AHTN were unambiguously detected and quantified. The levels ranged from 0.012 to 0.360 mg/kg lipid for HHCB and from 0.001 to 0.290 mg/kg lipid for AHTN. The ADBI concentrations were significantly lower, and only in some samples could AHDI and ATII also be detected at very low levels [15, 16]. None of the samples contained detectable traces of DPMII and ATTN [15, 16]. In all samples HHCB and AHTN were the main compounds within the group of polycyclic musks having the highest contamination levels. In all three studies the contents of musk xylene and musk ketone were also analysed in parallel; in most of the samples the levels of HHCB exceeded those of the nitro musks significantly. All these analysed concentrations in human tissues seem to correlate directly with the industrial production numbers and the usage rates of the individual musk fragrances.

Discussion

In all human samples of the several independent studies analysed to date, residues of nitro musks and polycyclic musk compounds were unambiguously detected and quantified. These synthetic musk fragrances represent a new group of ubiquitously distributed contaminants in human fat and milk, comparable with the contamination by some polyhalogenated compounds such as certain pesticides, PCBs and dioxins. In-depth statistical evaluations of these first results have not yet been carried out because of the limited number of analysed samples taken in conjunction with the rather large and typical variation of residue levels in human tissues. Furthermore, it does not yet appear possible to correlate meaningfully these residue concentrations with various biological parameters of the donors or with concentrations of other (polyhalogenated) contaminants. In order to understand which parameters affect these levels in human tissues, further extensive and systematic investigations with a higher number of samples together with detailed information about the donors of the samples are urgently needed.

In the discussion of the primary route of human contamination by organohalogenated compounds it is generally proven and accepted that the main route of uptake is performed by food, especially by food of animal origin. Until now the synthetic musk compounds have been identified only in organisms of

Table 4. Concentrations of three polycyclic musk compounds in human milk and human adipose tissue (mg/kg lipid)

Material (origin)	*n*	HHCB	AHTN	ADBI	Reference
Human milk (Germany, Schleswig-Holstein)	5	0.016–0.108 [a] (0.049) [b]	0.011–0.058 (0.026)	0.001–0.018 (0.007)	[16]
Human milk (Germany, Essen)	2	0.310–0.360	0.250–0.290	0.020–0.024	[15]
Human adipose tissue (Germany, Schleswig-Holstein, females)	8	0.039–0.133 (0.072)	0.008–0.031 (0.020)	< 0.001–0.003 (0.002)	[16]
Human adipose tissue (Germany, Schleswig-Holstein, males)	6	0.028–0.189 (0.095)	0.008–0.033 (0.018)	< 0.001–0.002 (0.001)	[16]
Human fat (Germany, Essen)	2	0.145–0.149	0.056–0.072	0.003–0.009	[15]
Human adipose tissue (Switzerland, females)	10	0.012–0.171 (0.065)	0.001–0.013 (0.006)	0.00012–0.0035 (0.0011)	[17]
Human adipose tissue (Switzerland, males)	5	0.012–0.135 (0.070)	0.0011–0.023 (0.014)	0.00024–0.002 (0.001)	[17]

[a] minimum and maximum concentration.
[b] mean value.

the aquatic environment such as fish and mussels (summary in [25]). In other food of animal origin, such as milk and dairy products, eggs, and meat/fat of cattle or pigs they have not been detected [25]. Moreover, the relatively low average fish consumption in Germany consists mainly of North Sea and Atlantic fish with very low or even non-detectable concentrations of synthetic musk fragrances [25]. Only samples of freshwater fish from polluted rivers or aquacultures showed higher contamination levels. Thus the average oral uptake of musk compounds has to be assumed to be relatively low and, therefore, negligible. Due to this assumption, another contamination route besides food consumption was already suggested in the first publications about nitro musks in human fat and milk [10, 11]. It was assumed that the synthetic musk compounds, due to their high lipophilicity and due to their frequent and intensive dermal contact as fragrances in cosmetics and washed/softened textiles, would be percutaneously resorbed and bioaccumulated in human fat. In the meantime this hypothesis about the dermal resorption of synthetic musks has been supported by several studies and various arguments.

For this reason, 72 human blood samples were recently analysed in order to determine the musk xylene concentrations within the general population [24]. The subjects were asked about their fish consumption habits. In almost all samples musk xylene was detected, but any statistical relationship between musk xylene concentrations and fish consumption habits – which should be expected if the primary uptake route had been by food – could not be found. Kokot-Helbling et al. [26] calculated from the reported musk xylene concentrations in human adipose tissue, together with an average human fat content of 25%, a total body burden of 1.75 mg musk xylene on the basis of 70 kg body weight. Moreover, they determined that musk xylene has a half-life in human blood of about 100 days. From these data they calculated an average daily uptake of musk xylene of about 11 μ/person or 160 ng/kg body weight. In this context, Ford et al. [27] reported an estimated maximum exposure to nitro musks from their use in fragrances to be 40–320 μg/kg body weight per day. Kokot-Helbling et al. [26], as well as Brunn and Rimkus [28], calculated that only one portion of extremely contaminated fish can lead to an oral uptake of about the average daily uptake. On the other hand the use of cosmetics and household detergents with high musk xylene contents, together with an estimated dermal absorption of 5% can easily exceed the calculated daily uptake. In comparison the uptake of musk xylene by inhalation seem to be quantitatively negligible [26].

Studies with rats [27, 29] and in vitro tests with skin [30] also support the argument of dermal resorption of synthetic musk compounds. Subchronic dermal and dietary treatment of male and female rats with musk ambrette induced the same neurotoxic effects [29]. Another detailed study [27] confirmed that obviously identical results with similar doses were caused regardless whether the route of exposure was oral or dermal. Similar results were also reported with ATTN [31]. Recently a FDA study measured the percutaneous absorption of musk xylene in vitro in human and in hairless guinea pig skin [30]. For comparison, musk xylene was applied to skin in an oil-in-water emulsion or in the volatile solvent methanol. After 24 h, total absorption of musk xylene in hairless guinea pig skin was 55% from the emulsion and 45% from methanol. Permeation of musk xylene into human skin from both solvents decreased to 22% of the applied dose. The data suggested that most of the absorbed musk xylene in the skin at 24 h will be systemically absorbed in vivo within 1 week. Throughout the 24 h study, absorbed musk xylene was not metabolised. A permeability constant for musk xylene permeation through hairless guinea pig skin of 6.86×10^{-5} cm/h was calculated. The amount of musk xylene absorbed through human skin from soap, body lotion and perfume was estimated. The highest absorption resulted for body lotion because it is applied to large areas of the body and remains on the skin for relatively long periods. Products such as soaps and shampoos which are removed a few minutes after application resulted in much less penetration of musk xylene.

All these cited studies may be an evidence that dermal resorption of synthetic musk fragrances is probably the main route of contamination. In this context it should be mentioned that this is apparently in contrast to the contamination of humans by polyhalogenated compounds. Recently some lipophilic sunscreen agents from cosmetic products were also analysed for the first time in human milk samples [32]. It seems that the human skin is not such a total barrier to some lipophilic compounds from cosmetics as had been previously assumed. Further extended studies are urgently needed in order to assess the contamination and elimination routes (including their mechanisms) of synthetic musk compounds in humans in more detail.

For the time being there is only very limited knowledge about the chronic toxicity of these artificial fragrances. Despite the high production figures, the world-wide use of these compounds, and their presence as pollutants in the aquatic environment and in humans, little has been reported about their toxic and possibly other adverse biological effects. Studies of adverse human health effects have primarily focused up to now on photosensitivity and dermal reactions. Musk ambrette showed photoallergenic, neurotoxic, and mutagenic effects and, therefore, its usage in cosmetics has been banned in the European Community since 1995 [33]. ATTN also demonstrated strong neurotoxic effects [31] and for that reason world-wide production was discontinued in 1980. The few toxicological data available are summarized and evaluated by a number of reviewers [28, 34–38]. All reviewers came to the conclusion that due to the lack of appropriate toxicological data, it is not yet possible to make an assessment of a resulting health risk. In 1995 the International Agency for

Research on Cancer (IARC) came to the overall evaluation that musk xylene and musk ambrette were not classifiable as to their carcinogenicity to humans (Group 3). There is a strong need for further investigations to gain sufficient toxicological data for risk assessment, to identify the main sources of human exposure and to establish pharmacokinetic data for the estimation of the daily absorbed dose and bioaccumulation [17]. In terms of prospective health protection these contaminations from cosmetics in human tissues are not desirable. Irrespective of the final toxicological assessment, strong efforts are urgently needed to reduce and avoid such contamination in humans. Due to their high bioaccumulation potential in humans and in the aquatic environment, their general persistence, lipophilicity, dermal permeability and insufficiently assessed toxicity, these synthetic musk fragrances should be immediately replaced in cosmetics and detergents by other compounds which are toxicologically and ecologically harmless.

References

1. Barbetta L, Trowbridge T, Eldib IA (1988) Musk aroma chemical industry. Perfum Flavor 13:60–61
2. Baur A (1891) Studien über den künstlichen Moschus. Ber Dtsch Chem Ges 24:2832
3. Qinghua Z (1993) China's perfumery industry picks up. Perfum Flavor 18:47–48
4. Srinivasan SK, Om Reddy G (1993) GC-MS analysis of the nitration products in the preparation of the nitro musk. Indian Perfum 37:344–363
5. Yamagishi T, Miyazaki T, Horii S, Kaneko S (1981) Identification of musk xylene and musk ketone in freshwater fish collected from the Tama river, Tokyo. Bull Environ Contam Toxicol 26:656–662
6. Yamagishi T, Miyazaki T, Horii S, Akiyama K (1983) Synthetic musk residues in biota and water from Tama river and Tokyo bay (Japan) Arch Environ Contam Toxicol 12:83–89
7. Rimkus G, Wolf M (1993) Rückstände und Verunreinigungen in Fischen aus Aquakultur, 2. Mitteilung: Nachweis von Moschus Xylol und Moschus Keton in Fischen. Dtsch Lebensm Rundsch 89:71–175
8. Rimkus GG, Wolf M (1995) Nitro musk fragrances in biota from freshwater and marine environment. Chemosphere 30:641–651
9. Rimkus GG, Butte W, Geyer HJ (1997) Critical considerations on the analysis and bioaccumulation of musk xylene and other synthetic nitro musks in fish. Chemosphere (in press)
10. Rimkus G, Wolf M (1993) Nachweis von Nitromoschusverbindungen in Frauenmilch und Humanfett. Dtsch Lebensm Rundsch 89:103–107
11. Rimkus G, Rimkus B, Wolf M (1994) Nitro musks in human adipose tissue and breast milk. Chemosphere 28:421–432
12. Rimkus GG (1995) Comments on the extraction of fat from human milk for analysis of contaminants. Answer to the letter to the editor from Prof. Dr. R. G. Jensen. Chemosphere 31:4200–4202
13. Eschke HD, Traud J, Dibowski HJ (1994) Untersuchungen zum Vorkommen polycyclischer Moschus-Duftstoffe in verschiedenen Umweltkompartimenten – Nachweis und Analytik mit GC/MS in Oberflächen-, Abwässern und Fischen (1. Mitteilung). UWSF-Z Umweltchem Ökotox 6:183–189

14. Eschke HD, Dibowski HJ, Traud J (1995) Untersuchungen zum Vorkommen polycyclischer Moschus-Duftstoffe in verschiedenen Umweltkompartimenten. 2. Mitteilung: Befunde in Oberflächen-, Abwässern und Fischen sowie in Waschmitteln und Kosmetika. UWSF-Z Umweltchem Ökotox 7:131–138
15. Eschke HD, Dibowski HJ, Traud J (1995) Nachweis und Quantifizierung von polycyclischen Moschus-Duftstoffen mittels Ion-Trap GC/MS/MS in Humanfett und Muttermilch. Dtsch Lebensm Rundsch 91:375–379
16. Rimkus GG, Wolf M (1996) Polycyclic musk fragrances in human adipose tissue and human milk. Chemosphere 33:2033–2043
17. Müller S, Schmid P, Schlatter C (1996) Occurrence of nitro and non-nitro benzenoid musk compounds in human adipose tissue. Chemosphere 33:17–28
18. Liebl B, Ehrenstorfer S (1993) Nitro musks in human milk. Chemosphere 27: 2253–2260
19. Hahn J (1993) Untersuchungen zum Vorkommen von Moschus-Xylol in Fischen. Dtsch Lebensm Rdsch 89:175–177
20. Kypke-Hutter K (1993) Schadstoffgehalte in Humanmilch aus Süddeutschland – Ursachen, Trends, Bewertung. In: Schlumpf M, Lichtensteiger W (eds) Kind und Umwelt – Humanmilch – Daten zur Belastung mit PCB, Dioxinen, Pestiziden und Moschus-Xylol, vol 2. pp 49–72
21. Ott M, Failing K, Georgii S, Brunn H (1997) Chlorinated pesticides and PCB congeners in human milk in Middle Hesse, Germany from 1984/85, 1990/91, 1995 and current contamination with nitro musks. Chemosphere (in press)
22. Meier W, Sedlacek H (1993) Organochlorpestizide und PCB in Humanmilch – Analytik und Resultate 1992. In: Schlumpf M, Lichtensteiger W (eds) Kind und Umwelt – Humanmilch – Daten zur Belastung mit PCB, Dioxinen, Pestiziden und Moschus-Xylol, vol 2. pp 25–47
23. Helbling KS, Schmid P, Schlatter C (1994) The trace analysis of musk xylene in biological samples: problems associated with its ubiquitous occurrence. Chemosphere 29:477–484
24. Angerer J, Käfferlein HU (1997) A GC/ECD method for the determination of musk xylene in human blood samples – biological monitoring of the general population. J Chromatogr B693:71–78
25. Rimkus G, Brunn H (1996) Synthetische Moschusduftstoffe – Anwendung, Anreicherung in der Umwelt und Toxikologie. Teil 1: Herstellung, Anwendung, Vorkommen in Lebensmitteln, Aufnahme durch den Menschen. Ernaehr Umschau 43:442–449
26. Kokot-Helbling K, Schmid P, Schlatter C (1995) Die Belastung des Menschen mit Moschus-Xylol – Aufnahmewege, Pharmakokinetik und toxikologische Bedeutung. Mitt Geb Lebensm Hyg 86:1–13
27. Ford RA, Api AM, Newberne PM (1990) 90-Day dermal toxicity study and neurotoxicity evaluation of nitromusks in the albino rat. Food Chem Toxicol 28:55–61
28. Brunn H, Rimkus G (1997) Synthetische Moschusduftstoffe – Anwendung, Anreicherung in der Umwelt und Toxikologie. Teil 2: Toxikologie der synthetischen Moschusduftstoffe und Schlußfolgerungen. Ernaehr Umschau 44:4–9
29. Spencer PS, Bischoff-Fenton MC, Moreno OM, Opdyke DL, Ford RA (1984) Neurotoxic properties of musk ambrette. Toxicol Appl Pharmacol 75:571–575
30. Hood HL, Wicket RR, Bronaugh RL (1996) In vitro percutaneous absorption of the fragrance ingredient musk xylol. Food Chem Toxicol 34:483–488
31. Spencer PS, Sterman AB, Horoupian DS, Foulds MM (1979) Neurotoxic fragrance produces ceroid and myelin disease. Science 204:633
32. Hany J, Nagel R (1995) Nachweis von UV-Filtersubstanzen in Muttermilch. Dtsch Lebensm Rundsch 91:341–345

33. 18. Richtlinie 95/34/EG der Kommission vom 10. Juli 1995 zur Anpassung der Anhänge II, III, VI und VII der Richtlinie 76/768/EWG des Rates zur Angleichung der Rechtsvorschriften der Mitgliedstaaten über kosmetische Mittel an den technischen Fortschritt, ABl L 167:19–21
34. Liebl B, Ehrenstorfer S (1993) Nitromoschusverbindungen in der Frauenmilch. Gesund Wes 55:527–532
35. Ippen H (1994) Nitromoschus, Teil I. Bundesgesundhbl 37:255–260
36. Schlatter J, Hunyady G (1993) Moschus-Xylol in Lebensmitteln und Kosmetika. Bull BAG 30:546–549
37. Geyer HJ, Rimkus G, Wolf M, Attar A, Steinberg C, Kettrup A (1994) Synthetische Moschus-Duftstoffe und Bromocyclen – Neue Umweltchemikalien in Fischen und Muscheln bzw. Muttermilch und Humanfett. UWSF-Z Umweltchem Ökotox 6:9–17
38. IARC monographs on the evaluation of carcinogenic risks to humans (1996) Printing processes and printing inks, carbon black and some nitro compounds. 65:477–497

Part IV
Safety Assessment – Predictive Assays for Irritation and Sensitization

A Reappraisal of the Guinea Pig Maximization Test

A. M. Kligman

Introduction

The human maximization test was described 30 years ago, in 1966, followed 3 years later by the guinea pig maximization test [1,2]. Owing to limited access to human volunteers, it is the guinea pig test which has been far more frequently used. Although alternative animal models are receiving appreciable attention, the guinea pig maximization test is still the gold standard for assessing allergenicity.

It will be recalled that it was the failure of repeated insult tests in rabbits to identify well known human contact allergens that stimulated the search for a more sensitive model. This was accomplished by "maximizing" the exposures so as to boost the immune responses allowing even weak and marginal allergens to be identified. An extensive experience has demonstrated that the enhanced sensitivity has greatly reduced the possibility of false negative outcomes, in which weaker allergens are not detected. On the other hand, new problems have arisen which Magnusson and Kligman failed to appreciate. For example, a problem opposite to the original one of false negatives has emerged, namely, false positives in which irritants are misidentified as allergens. This is not uncommon and has generated new controversies regarding the reliability of the test. Thus, the specificity of the maximization procedure has been challenged. Moreover an enormous experience in laboratories of toxicology around the world has raised up disturbing questions about substantial inter-laboratory differences and the all too frequent occurrence of labeling irritants as allergens. Much of this new awareness of the limitations of the guinea pig maximization procedure lies buried in the private files of manufacturers of topical chemicals and skin care products.

Kligman and Basketter have recently addressed the above issues in detail and have suggested guidelines for avoiding unreproducible and false positive results [3]. The Bundesgesundheitsamt (BGA) has voiced similar concerns and has amended the maximization test to improve both sensitivity and specificity [4]. Others have recently been drawn into the vexing problem of false positives. Buehler, a prominent figure in cutaneous toxicology, has called attention to the fact that even common vehicles widely accepted as innocent materials, can give rise to inflammatory reactions at the time of challenge [5]. Magnusson and Kligman were completely unaware of false positive responses and inappropriately scored erythematous reactions, even patchy ones, as allergic responses. Thus are inventors seduced by their own creations!

Andersen et al. have recently suggested strategies for interpreting weak patchy erythematous reactions so as to avoid mislabeling of irritants as allergens [6].

These new cautions have improved the credibility of the guinea pig model. For interested investigators, the aforementioned papers furnish full technical details which are not pertinent to this review.

This chapter deals with more general conceptual issues which relate to our understanding of the biology of cutaneous inflammatory reactions. This is an appropriate place to review some of the problems which have plagued investigators concerned with developing procedures for identifying and rating the allergenicity of topical substances.

The Angry Back Phenomenon

This term was created by Mitchell in 1975 [7]. It received immediate, enthusiastic and universal acceptance. Mitchell observed that when multiple patches were positive in the diagnostic workup, many became negative when tested one at a time at a later time. This led him to create the catchy concept that "eczema creates eczema". His definitive statement, comprising the central tenet of his concept was: "A single strong patch test reaction creates an angry back which is hyper-reactive to other patch test applications. Concomitant false positive reactions are thus obtained." While he did not investigate the phenomenon experimentally, his clinical observations were correct, as far as they went.

Maibach, realizing that the whole integument, not just the back, was hyper-reactive expanded the concept into the "excited skin syndrome" [8].

It turns out that the excited skin syndrome, also known as hyper-irritable skin, has a long history by distinguished masters of dermatology. Already in 1921 von Zumbusch reported that patients with eczema reacted to multiple materials which were nonirritating to normals [9]. In 1924 Bloch introduced the term "status eczematicus" for the same phenomenon [10]. Geiger too in 1924 warned about nonspecific reactions in eczema patients [11]. He found that only 4% of normals reacted to 60% turpentine in contrast to 90% in eczema patients. Bjornberg in 1968 clearly understood hyper-irritable skin. In his classic paper on hand dermatitis he realized that patches that were positive when the dermatitis was active became negative when the eruption cleared [12].

Kligman and Gollhausen went to considerable pains to demonstrate in normal human volunteers that a single strongly positive patch test, whether irritant or allergic, had no effect on concomitant patch tests, whether allergic or irritant, regardless of whether the patches were nearby or distant [13]. Their studies contravened the generalized concept that eczema creates eczema.

Mitchell found that 42% of positive patch tests were lost upon repatching later [7]. Lost positives turn up frequently in the literature. Bruynzeel noted a 44% rate of loss upon retesting 3 weeks later [14]. The record is held by Luderschmidt et al. with a loss rate of 62% [15]. Even 4^+ severe reactions sometimes became negative on later retesting.

There is no doubt that the excited skin syndrome and the Angry back are clinical realities. The dispute centers around the interpretation.

The resolution of this controversy lies in recognizing that multiple reactions are common when patients attending patch test clinics are tested with 20 or more common allergens. When 4 or 5 patches are strongly positive, one should instantly suspect false positives. This phenomenon, as pointed out by Kligman and Gollhausen, cannot be experimentally demonstrated in normal subjects. It is the presence of a long standing dermatitis that creates the hyper-irritable state. It is precisely the patients with a stubborn or undiagnosable dermatitis who are subjected to batteries of patch tests. When such patients are successfully treated, the multiple positive reactions fade into insignificance. It is the clearing of the dermatitis and the passage of time that accounts for the conversion of positives to negatives.

This is not the place to speculate about mechanisms, but it seems very likely that a number of circulating cytokines, especially tumor necrosis factor and interleukins underlie the phenomenon of hyper-irritability [16].

With this human background we can now return to the celebrated guinea pig and to the experimental findings of Kligman and Basketter [3].

Firstly, these investigators were able to induce the hyper-irritable state by performing maximization tests to substances which are unequivocally known to be irritants and not allergens, viz., a cationic surfactant, benzalkonium chloride, and a hair dye, henna.

With the former at a concentration of 0.2% they found that 7 of 20 animals showed a positive challenge reaction. Upon rechallenge 3 weeks later, only one of 20 animals reacted. It has been our consistent experience, in humans as well, that false positive irritant reactions routinely become negative upon rechallenge 3–4 weeks later. Andersen et al. also recommend rechallenge as a way of identifying false positives [17]. By contrast in truly allergic reactions, positive reactions are demonstrable for at least 2–3 months after the original exposure. Sometimes weakly positive reactions may be relatively transient with some conversions to negative after 1–2 months. It is the commonly encountered grade 1, weakly positive reactions that poses the greatest challenge to the operator. Unfortunately up to this time, there is no practical way, clinically or histologically, to differentiate weakly positive allergic reactions from irritant ones. Thus rechallenge is decisive in rendering a final judgment. When in doubt the entire procedure should be repeated.

Kligman and Basketter, as well as the German G BA have proposed a modification which attempts to minimize the problem of false positives. A matched group of animals is added in which the skin is deliberately inflamed to a similar degree as for the test agent. This is accomplished by injecting an additional control group with Freund's adjuvant along with a pure irritant such as SLS. Then, this group which has been deliberately brought to the hyper-irritable state is challenged with the test substance. Equivalent erythematous reactions indicate a false positive result. This strategy is an attempt to factor in nonspecific hyper-irritability in performing maximization tests. Of course this adds to the expense and labor of the procedure.

Mitchell has reacted furiously to this proposal in a letter to the editor of the *journal of Contact Dermatitis* entitled "Egregious Blunder of Maximization by Angry Back and a Note on Unconfirmed Ergodata" [18]. He argues that attaining an equivalent angry back in the control group is a fundamental error and the statement that it can be achieved is "extraordinary and reckless". Evidently this is still a very hot issue!

Hazard and Risk Assessment

Magnusson and Kligman emphasized caution in converting maximization results into policies, especially regulatory edicts. It must be realized that the test assay only estimates the *potential* for inducing contact sensitization. It rates test substances along a spectrum ranging from low to high allergenicity, under the conditions of the assay. Toxicologists define this as a statement of hazard. It does not predict what will happen in the real world. The common parlance of calling these tests "predictive" leads to serious misunderstandings. It is true that a negative result conveys a sense of safety that widespread use will not result in prohibitive rates of sensitization. On the other hand, strongly allergenic substances should not automatically be discarded as posing too great a risk. It is the business of risk assessment to take into account the many factors which ultimately influence the actual rates of sensitization when the substance is released into the channels of commerce. These include concentration, duration and intensity of exposure, leave on or rinse off, application to normal or diseased skin, and others. One should not abandon a highly allergenic substance which has valuable properties whether a drug, cosmetic, toiletry or industrial chemical without a professional risk assessment. It must be remembered that the exposure conditions during induction are unusually intensified, designed to reduce the likelihood of missing even weak allergens.

Intensified exaggerated exposures will unavoidably raise the allergenicity scores all along the spectrum. The practical danger is that the maximization test exaggerates the risk and deters the manufacturer from commercial exploitation. There are a number of compelling examples in which nearly all of the test animals become sensitized to a given agent. Nonetheless these same materials are acceptable under normal conditions of use.

For example, benzoyl peroxide, used in acne treatment for half a century, sensitizes 100% of the guinea pigs. Similar results are obtained in the human maximization assay. Yet, sensitization in acne sufferers who may use this product daily for years is very low, probably not more than one in ten thousand. Why the dramatic discrepancy between testing and usage? The fact is that benzoyl peroxide is an unstable substance which quickly degrades to benzoic acid when it hits the skin. Moreover, it is applied openly, not occlusively, and in much lower concentrations therapeutically than in the guinea pig test. In the present regulatory climate one wonders whether benzoyl peroxide would have been marketed if the original producers could have known about its capacity to sensitize 100% of the test animals!

Ethanol 95% is likewise over-rated in the maximization test. About 30% of guinea pigs become sensitized. In humans the corresponding value is 20% [3]. Ethanol is a very rare sensitizer, worthy of a case report when it occurs. The low risk of sensitization is easily explained by the fact that ethanol evaporates rapidly after application, an event that is prevented under the occlusive exposure conditions of the test. Other examples in which the test results generate unnecessary worry are cinnamic aldehyde (a fragrance used in low concentrations), *p*-phenylenediamine (a hair dye mainly applied to hair not the scalp), and Kathon CG (a preservative which is used in low concentrations mainly in brief contact rinse off materials).

It must be conceded that the maximization test is hard and unpleasant for the guinea pigs. The mouse lymph node assay is much simpler, faster and less onerous for the animals. The guinea pig maximization test will become obsolete when it is shown conclusively with this model that weak allergens can be detected and false positives eliminated. So far, this has not been achieved.

References

1. Kligman AM (1966) The identification of contact allergens by human assay. J Invest Derm 47:369
2. Magnusson B, Kligman AM (1969) The identification of contact allergens by animal assay. The guinea pig maximization test. J Invest Derm 52:268
3. Kligman AM, Basketter DA (1995) A critical commentary and updating of the guinea pig maximization test. Contact Dermatitis 32:129
4. Schlede VE, Eppler R (1993) Prüfung auf Hautsensibilisierung nach den Kriterien des Chemikaliengesetzes am Beispiel des Magnusson-Kligman-Tests. Bundesgesundheitsamt 12:519

5. Buehler EU (1996) Non-specific hypersensitivity: false positive responses with the use of Freund's adjuvant. Contact Dermatitis 34:111
6. Andersen KE, Frankild S, Wahlberg JE, Boman A (1996) Nonspecific hyper-reactivity related to the use of Freund's Adjuvant. Contact Dermatitis 35:2:127
7. Mitchell J (1975) The angry back syndrome: eczema creates eczema. Contact Dermatitis 1:193
8. Maibach HE (1981) The excited skin syndrome. In: Ring J, Burg G (eds) New trends in allergy. Springer Berlin Heidelberg New York, pp 208–221
9. von Zumbusch L (1921) Über die Behandlung des Ekzems. Munchner Med Wochenschr 68:408
10. Bloch B (1924) Pathogenesis des Ekzems. Archiv Dermatol Syphol 145:34
11. Geiger R (1929) Unspezifische Desensibilisierungs-Versuche an Ekzematikern mit Tarpentinol auf perkutanem Wege. Archiv Dermatol Syphol 158:76
12. Bjornberg A (1968) Skin reactions to primary irritants in patients with hand eczema. Thesis, University of Goteberg Doctoral. Oscar Isacion
13. Kligman AM, Gollhausen R (1986) The "angry back": a new concept or old confusion. Br J Derm 115[Suppl 31]:93
14. Bruynzeel DP, van Ketel WG, von Blomberg BME, van der Flees, Schepes RD (1983) Angry back or the excited skin syndrome. J Am Acad Derm 8:392
15. von Luderschmidt C, Heilgemier R, Ring J, Burg G (1982) Polyvalente Kontaktallergie versus "angry back". Allergologie 5:262
16. Pasche-koo F, Hauser C (1992) How to better understand the angry back syndrome. Dermatology 184:237
17. Andersen KE, Bruee M, Karlberg DT, Wahlberg JE, Voland A (1994) How to do sensitization tests in guinea pigs. Contact Dermatitis 81:278
18. Mitchell JC (1996) Egregious blunder of maximization by the angry back and a note on unconfirmed ergodata. Contact Dermatitis 35:131–132

The Hydroxycitronellal Story: What Can We Learn from It?

R. R. Suskind

Introduction

What is the character and size of the database for this fragrance molecule? A computer review of the database – provided by A. M. Api of RIFM reveals 241 references in which the range of subjects includes animal studies, toxicity, diagnostic evaluation using patch tests, and safety assessment. These have been carried out over a period of almost 25 years. This compound, which is 7-hydroxy-3,7-dimethyloctan-1-al, is shown in Fig. 1. Between 1973 and 1980, 14 human maximization tests were carried out to determine the sensitizing potential of hydroxycitronellal. This is shown in Table 1.

Initially in 1973 when what was regarded as ten times the use level, 5%, in petrolatum elicited no allergic sensitization reactions. This was repeated by Epstein in 1976 who also elicited no reactions. In the same year Kligman using 10% hydroxycitronellal on subjects who were also being tested with cinnamic alcohol produced two sensitization reactions to the hydroxycitronellal. When this was repeated 2 years later with the same concentration, no reactions in 25 subjects were elicited. In the same year Epstein, using the same concentration, produced four reactions in 27 subjects. One year later, using a Japanese-

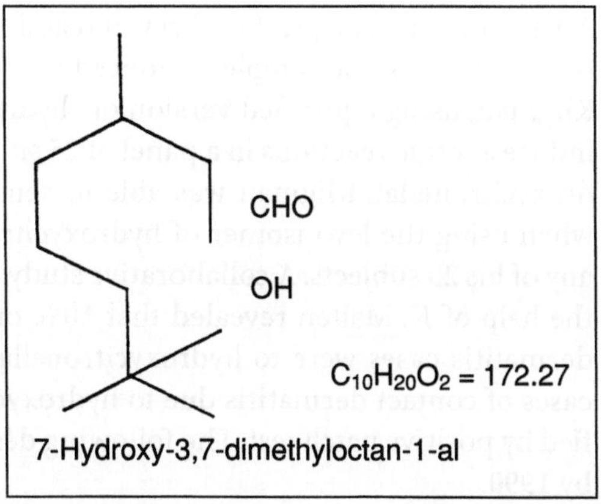

Fig. 1. Hydroxycitronellal (From Suskind 1992)

Table 1. Summary of human maximization testing for hydroxycitronellal sensitization potential (from Suskind 1992)

Sample	Source	Reference	Concentration	Results
A	Y	Kligman 1973	5% PET	0/25 male
B	X	Epstein 1976	5% PET	0/26
C	X	Kligman 1976	10% PET	2/25 [a]
C	X	Kligman 1976	10% PET	0/25 [b]
D	W	Kligman 1978	12% PET	0/25
E	W	Epstein 1978	12% PET	4/27
F	Z	Epstein 1979	12% PET	7/26 [c]
F	Z	Epstein 1979	12% PET	6/26 [d]
G [e]	W	Kligman 1979	12% PET	0/25
H [f]	W	Kligman 1979	12% PET	3/25
I [g]	W	Kligman 1979	12% PET	0/25
J [h]	W	Kligman 1979	12% PET	1/25
K [i]	Z	Epstein 1980	12% DEP	2/22
L [j]	Z	Epstein 1980	12% DEP	1/26
M	W	Epstein 1980	12% DEP	2/21 [k]

DEP, 25% diethyl phthalate was the vehicle; PET, petrolatum USP was the vehicle.

[a] Two subjects reacted to hydroxycitronellal and cinnamic alcohol.

[b] Sample C retested by itself in a virgin panel.

[c] Japanese-American panel.

[d] Sample F retested in a Caucasian panel.

[e] A purified version of Hydroxycitronellal from α-pinene.

[f] *d*-Hydroxycitronellal purified.

[g] *l*-Hydroxycitronellal purified.

[h] pseudo Hydroxycitronellal.

[i] Lower boiling fraction.

[j] Higher boiling fraction.

[k] Tested on same panel with washed cinnamic alcohol.

American panel, he produced seven reactions in 26 subjects, and in that same year, with the same sample, produced six reactions in 26 Caucasian subjects. Kligman, using a purified version of "hydroxy" from α-pinene was unable to induce allergic reactions in a panel of 25 subjects. In the same year, using dihydroxycitronellal, Kligman was able to sensitize three out of 25 subjects but when using the levo isomer of hydroxycitronellal, he was unable to sensitize any of his 25 subjects. A collaborative study conducted in the Netherlands with the help of K. Malten revealed that 10% of all positive test reactions among dermatitis cases were to hydroxycitronellal. Beginning in the middle 1970s, cases of contact dermatitis due to hydroxycitronellal were reported and verified by positive patch test. The following describes the status of the compound by 1990.

Status in 1990

1. No conclusive evidence 1 stereoisomer is less sensitizing than racemic *dl.*
2. Vehicle ethanol (ETOH; 75%)/diethyl phthalate (DEP; 25%) influenced frequency and degree of sensitization when compared with DEP alone.
3. 5% in a single phase HRIPT induced sensitization in 36% of subjects.

At that point also there was uncertainty that 1% hydroxycitronellal in ETOH/DEP induced sensitization. In a single phase HRIPT using 5% in the ETOH/DEP vehicle 36% of subjects were sensitized. In DEP alone 5% hydroxycitronellal produced no sensitization. In a two phase HRIPT, 2.5% hydroxycitronellal sensitized more than 20% of the subjects. In one HRIPT using 1% in ETOH/DEP, one of 52 panelist exhibited a questionable sensitization reaction. When repeated using 1%, positive elicitation responses were produced in three subjects considered at the time to be an irritant rather than sensitization reactions. Hence, it appears that there was no clear cut evidence that 1% in ethanol/DEP induced sensitization in humans under test conditions. However, the data was considered definitive enough to regard this as a "no effect" level (NOEL). It was apparent that use tests were now indicated. The results were quite revealing. The tests involved the six month long use of a bar soap containing a fragrance with 0.05% hydroxycitronellal followed by a three month use of moisturizing lotion containing a fragrance with 0.03% hydroxycitronellal. The final phase of the use test which lasted four months involved the use of four different cologne type products containing a perfume with 0.05% to 1% hydroxycitronellal.

The panels of subjects in the first use test included 41 previously sensitized in an HRIPTs, 18 subjects previously not sensitized in an HRIPTs, and 26 naive subjects. Prior to the start of the program all of the 85 subjects were patch tested to eight materials. After the completion of the use program, the panelists were patch tested again to the same materials. The materials were:

- A: 5% *dl*-Hydroxycitronellal in 75% ethanol/25% diethyl phthalate.
- B: 5% *l*-Hydroxycitronellal in 75% ethanol/25% diethyl phthalate.
- C: 5% *d*-Hydroxycitronellal in 75% ethanol/25% diethyl phthalate.
- D: 1% aqueous solution of the bar soap containing hydroxycitronellal.
- E: 1% aqueous solution of the bar soap without hydroxycitronellal.
- F: 1% aqueous solution of the bar soap base without perfume.
- G: 75% ethanol/25% diethyl phthalate.
- H: Distilled Water.
- I: 1% Perfume without hydroxycitronellal in 75% ethanol/25% diethyl phthalate.

The subjects ($n=85$) used a standard bar soap containing 0.05% hydroxycitronellal, at least once daily on the arms and forearms with the use being recorded in a diary. Evaluation examinations by the physician were made after two and four weeks of use. At 4 weeks a whole-body examination was conducted; following that the subjects were instructed to use the soap for all showering and bathing at least once daily for 6 months. The subjects returned every 4 weeks for review and whole-body examination. After three months of such use, a moisturizing lotion containing 0.03% hydroxycitronellal was used on the hands and forearms at least once daily. No clinical reactions were observed with that use program even in previously sensitized individuals who were patch test positive to hydroxycitronellal.

The results of this initial diagnostic patch test among the 41 sensitized panelists were as follows (Table 2): 51% reacted to 5% *dl*-hydroxycitronellal, 32% reacted to 5% *l*-hydroxycitronellal, 56% reacted to 5% *d*-hydroxycitronellal, 10% reacted mildly to the bat soap containing a fragrance with hydroxycitronellal and the same percentage to the bar soap containing a fragrance without hydroxycitronellal (Table 2). One panelist reacted to the 1% bar soap aqueous solution alone without a fragrance. None of the nonsensitized panelists reacted to these patch test materials; among the naive panelists, a few reacted mildly to the soap solutions which could be regarded as irritating.

Diagnostic patch tests with the same materials as were used in the pre-use program were carried out at the end of the second phase of this use program. A ninth material, however, was added which was a 1% perfume formulation, Parfum du Rhone, without hydroxycitronellal in ETOH/DEP. Thirty-four sensitized panelists were available for post use tests. The results are shown in Table 3.

The last phase of the use test involved cologne formulations. The subjects were the same as those participating in the bar soap-lotion use program. Thirty-one subjects in the sensitized group completed the program. Prior to entrance into the use test phase of the study, each subject had a whole body examination by the study dermatologist.

As previously described, the subjects were exposed to a different test material for each of four months. The test materials consisted of four different

Table 2. Hydroxycitronellal use test, preuse diagnostic patch test, 41 previously sensitized panelists (from Suskind 1992)

	No. of reactions	Reactions (%)
A	21	51
B	13	32
C	23	56
D	4	10
E	4	10
F	1	2
G	0	0
H	0	0

Table 3. Hydroxycitronellal use test, final diagnostic patch test, sensitized panelists ($n = 34$; from Suskind 1992)

	Positive reactions	Reactions (%)
A	15	47
B	10	29
C	20	59
D	2	6
E	1	3
F	3	9
G	0	0
H	0	0
I	1	3

Table 4. Cologne materials (from Suskind 1992)

1	0.05%	Hydroxycitronellal
2	0.1%	Hydroxycitronellal
3	0.3%	Hydroxycitronellal
4	1.0%	Hydroxycitronellal
5	0%	Hydroxycitronellal
6	Only 90%	Ethanol + 10% water

cologne type products identified as products 1, 2, 3 and 4, shown in Table 4. Two additional test materials (products 5 and 6) were reserved for usage in cases of severe reactions, as dictated by the protocol.

Each subject received a supply of test material to last one month, at which time the product was returned and a new product was issued. Applications of the test material were made three times a day to the proximal volar surface of the forearm with a cotton swab. The area of application was approximately 5 cm in diameter. A period of at least 4 h elapsed between each application. The subject recorded the date and time of each application on the diary sheet. The test lasted for 4 months.

The results were as follows: there was one reactor to the cologne containing 0.05% hydroxycitronellal among 31 patch test positive panelists. Positive reactions were elicited in 3 sensitized panelists with the cologne containing 1% hydroxycitronellal. Diagnostic patch tests were performed after the completion of cologne usage with six materials listed in Table 5, along with results in those who completed the test ($n = 29$).

The two remaining panelists of the 31 participants were not patch tested because one had reacted clinically to 0.05% hydroxycitronellal in cologne during the use program and another to 1% in cologne. The other 2 panelists who reacted to 1% in cologne were among the 29 tested. One of the naive panelists was observed to have a mild reaction to D, which is water. None of the nonsensitized previously used panelists reacted to the patch tests.

Table 5. Diagnostic test materials and percentage positive reactions (from Suskind 1992)

Sample	Substance	Positive reactions (%)
A	5% *dl*-Hydroxycitronellal in 3:1 ethanol:diethyl phthalate	34
B	3:1 Ethanol:diethyl phthalate	6
C	5% *l*-Hydroxycitronellal in 3:1 ethanol:diethyl phthalate	26
D	Distilled water	3
E	5% *d*-hydroxycitronellal in 3:1 ethanol:diethyl phthalate	40
F	9% Parfum du Rhone without hydroxycitronellal in 3:1 ethanol:diethylphthalate	9

After reviewing all of the data, the RIFM Expert Panel was of the opinion that additional studies for the safety of hydroxycitronellal were not indicated. One percent hydroxycitronellal is not likely to induce allergic sensitization in humans with repeated exposure. In other words, the risk is minimal. However, if a person is already sensitized, they do run the risk of developing clinical allergic reactions to concentrations as low as 0.05% in a cologne. It appears from the recent studies that there is little risk for person already sensitized reacting to concentrations of 0.05% in a bar soap or 0.03% in a moisturizing lotion.

What have we learned? The story of hydroxycitronellal indicates that, for an important fragrance, in-depth studies involving safety appraisals are imperative. Depending upon the circumstances of the evaluation (type of panels, quality of the studies, etc.), one can, as in the case of hydroxycitronellal, get mixed and even contradictory results. For hydroxycitronellal a careful review and interpretation of the enormous database provides a no effect level for induction of allergic skin sensitization as well as safe use levels in lotions and soaps for person already sensitized.

References

Epstein W (1976) Report to Research Institute for Fragrance Materials, Inc.
Epstein W (1978) Report to Research Institute for Fragrance Materials, Inc.
Epstein W (1979) Report to Research Institute for Fragrance Materials, Inc.
Epstein W (1980) Report to Research Institute for Fragrance Materials, Inc.
Kligman A (1973) Report to Research Institute for Fragrance Materials, Inc.
Kligman A (1976) Report to Research Institute for Fragrance Materials, Inc.
Kligman A (1978) Report to Research Institute for Fragrance Materials, Inc.
Kligman A (1979) Report to Research Institute for Fragrance Materials, Inc.
Suskind RR (1992) Hydroxycitronellal. "The Whole and Final? Story". Proceedings of the Sixth International Information Exchange of the Research Institute for Fragrance Materials. Princeton, New Jersey, 19-20 November, pp 75-83

The Value of Animal Assays and the Quenching Phenomenon

D. Basketter

Introduction

In the absence of in vitro models for the identification of skin sensitizers and for estimation of their potency, animal models still provide the foundation for risk assessment in this area of toxicology. In this chapter, the most commonly used models are briefly described, particularly with respect to their use in defining the potency of a particular skin sensitizer. The important points are demonstrated by a consideration of sensitizing fragrance ingredients and the quenching phenomenon.

Animal Tests for Skin Sensitization

Guinea Pig

For many years, the guinea pig has been the species of choice for the conduct of predictive skin sensitization tests. The principles of the methods and details of their conduct have been extensively reviewed (Maurer 1983; Andersen and Maibach 1985; Botham et al. 1991; Basketter 1994). Almost without exception the methods use the same approach, attempted induction of sensitization by injection and/or topical application of the test substance, followed, after a rest period, by challenge to elicit evidence of skin sensitization. The presence of skin sensitization is judged by the subjective assessment of the skin reaction, primarily erythema. The most commonly used protocols are the occluded application test of Buehler (Buehler 1965; Ritz and Buehler 1985) and the maximization test (Magnusson and Kligman 1970). The efficiency of these methods for the detection of known skin sensitizers has been extensively documented (Wahlberg and Boman 1985; Basketter and Chamberlain 1995; Basketter and Gerberick 1996). On this basis, it is reasonable to assume that they will also be able to serve as appropriate assays for the predictive identification of the sensitization potential of novel substances or combinations of substances (preparations). Consequently, the methods are recommended in various regulatory guidelines (EC 1992; OECD 1993). However, it is important to point out that the methods are far from standardized and have been reported to give quite variable results (Robinson et al. 1990; Botham et al. 1991). Careful interpretation of data and use of controls is thus essential.

Mouse

The last decade has seen the development of the mouse as an alternative to the guinea pig as the species of choice for predictive skin sensitization tests. This has been due largely to the development of the local lymph node assay (LLNA; Kimber and Weisenberger 1989; Kimber and Basketter 1992). The method measures cell proliferation in lymph nodes draining the skin site to which a test substance has been applied; details of the standard procedure are given elsewhere (Kimber and Basketter 1992). The ability of the LLNA to detect skin sensitizers has been extensively reported (reviewed in Kimber et al. 1994; Basketter et al. 1996) and it has undergone full international validation (Chamberlain and Basketter 1996).

The LLNA offers a number of animal welfare advantages over the guinea pig methods, notably in reduction of animal numbers and in the refinement of their use (Basketter et al. 1996). Furthermore, it provides an objective quantitative endpoint which is unaffected by coloured test substances. Importantly, it does not suffer from the substantial interlaboratory variability reported for the guinea pig methods, giving highly reproducible results both intra- and interlaboratory (Scholes et al. 1992; Kimber et al. 1995; Loveless et al. 1996). However, as the guinea pig methods, it is not a perfect assay: It can be less sensitive, certainly than the guinea pig maximization test, although this is not necessarily a disadvantage (Basketter et al. 1992). Also, as the guinea pig methods, it can yield false positive results (Montelius et al. 1995; Kligman and Basketter 1995; Loveless et al. 1996; Buehler 1996). The important consequence for all types of predictive skin sensitization assays is that the results require careful, scientific interpretation in the light of all available data (Kligman and Basketter 1995; Frankild et al. 1996; Basketter et al. 1996).

Test Results and the Estimation of Sensitizing Potency

In the initial evaluation, results from both guinea pig tests and the LLNA provide binary data, i.e. the test substance is, or is not, a skin sensitizer. This for example is essentially how the data are interpreted by European Union (EU) legislation (EC 1992). Interpretation of guinea pig data usually refers to the proportion of the test group that are judged to be sensitized when their skin reactions are compared to those of a sham-treated control group. In the EU a response rate of 30% in the maximization test or 15% in the Buehler test triggers classification as a skin sensitizer (EC 1993). In this context, the prediction model for the LLNA is that stimulation of proliferation in relation to controls of 3, together with a data which is not incompatible with a biological dose response, indicates the substance should be regarded as a skin sensitizer.

In any of these test types, the test concentrations and intensity of the positive response are not taken into account. Thus, neither of the above systems gives any idea of the relative potency of the skin sensitizer, which is a vital piece of information for safety assessment and risk management. Sensitizers of almost all potencies can be, and indeed are, used extensively without any significant adverse effects, but this relies absolutely on proper risk assessment (Basketter et al. 1996b). So how can these predictive models and the data they produce be used to assess skin sensitizing potency?

The guinea pig maximization test does not easily lend itself to the estimation of skin sensitizing potency; the use of Freund's complete adjuvant and intradermal injections coupled with test concentration selection which is based on the irritancy potential of the test substance are major complicating factors. The variety of vehicle(s) used and the absence, normally, of any dose response information create additional difficulties. Some of these problems arise also with the Buehler test. For both test types there is also the little investigated matter of interspecies differences. This whole subject has been extensively reviewed recently (Basketter et al. 1997). Nevertheless, the guinea pig maximization test and Buehler method have been used for more than two decades to assess inherent contact sensitizing potency. When properly conducted and interpreted, these tests have demonstrated the ability to detect chemicals with moderate to strong sensitization potential as well as those with relatively weak sensitization potential (Wahlberg and Boman 1985; Robinson et al. 1990; Botham et al. 1991; Basketter and Gerberick 1996). In practice they can address questions of sensitization potency and the data from such methods can be used in the development of a comparative risk assessment (Basketter et al. 1996b).

The process of risk assessment mentioned above compares the results obtained with an unknown material to those within a database of results of known contact allergens and nonallergens. Such an approach can be adopted only where the sensitivity and consistency of the sensitization method at the testing institution are well known and properly understood. The data must of course be interpreted in the context of the test concentrations, vehicles and the incidence and intensity of any sensitization reactions. Thus, it would be advisable to compare substances tested under similar conditions; for example, hexyl cinnamic aldehyde in the GPMT usually gives a result of about 70% positive, whereas at broadly similar test concentrations eugenol is hard to detect as a sensitizer, the usual rate of positives being 10%. So, eugenol might be regarded as distinctly less potent than hexyl cinnamic aldehyde in the GPMT, but without dose response data, it is difficult to quantify this difference. Furthermore, the injection of test substances in the GPMT means that the skin barrier is bypassed and differences in rates of skin penetration will have much less impact. This could lead to significantly misleading views on the relative potency of skin sensitizers.

This process of risk assessment is far from transparent to the outside observer and historically has proven subject to error (e.g. with certain preservatives). Thus one of the aspects of the LLNA that makes it particularly attractive as an alternative to the commonly employed guinea pig models is that it offers the prospect of a more soundly based assessment of sensitizing potency, although of course there is still the matter of interspecies differences. In recent intra and interlaboratory studies, the LLNA dose response data has been used in a novel way (Botham et al. 1991; Basketter et al. 1992; Kimber et al. 1995; Loveless et al. 1996). The data was plotted to enable determination of the concentration of test substance which would give a threshold sensitization response in the LLNA, the EC_3. This value can then be regarded as an index of relative sensitizing potency. A more detailed review of this is given in recent papers describing the use of the LLNA in risk assessment (Kimber and Basketter 1996; Basketter 1997).

For the purposes of demonstration, Table 1 contains the calculated values derived for a number of known sensitizing perfume ingredients. Such data could form an important part of a structured and defensible approach to the

Table 1. Threshold concentrations in the LLNA for a range of sensitizing fragrance chemicals

Chemical	Threshold LLNA concentration[a]	Reference to original publication	IFRA restriction related to contact sensitization
Cinnamic aldehyde	2.0%	Data from Table 3	Must be quenched
Citral	13%	Data from Table 3	Must be quenched
Dimethylisophthalate	NS[b]	Basketter and Scholes 1992	None
Eugenol	14.5%	Loveless et al. 1996	None
Geraniol	NS	Basketter et al. 1996	None
Hexylcinnamic aldehyde	7.6%	Loveless et al. 1996	None
Hydroxycitronellal	20%	Basketter and Scholes 1992	1% limit in product
Isoeugenol	3.3%	Loveless et al. 1996	0.2% limit in product
6-Methyl coumarin	NS	Basketter et al. 1993	None[c]
Musk ambrette	8.5%	Unpublished data from 4 studies	None[c]

[a] Concentration (%) required to give a stimulation index of 3.
[b] Not a sensitizer in the LLNA.
[c] IFRA has banned these due to their photoallergic properties.

definition of acceptable exposure limits for sensitizing fragrance ingredients. In particular it is noteworthy that generally those chemicals with the lowest EC_3 values are the ones which have IFRA restrictions. Furthermore, comparison of the figures for example for eugenol and isoeugenol clearly reflects the known human potencies of these fragrance materials. In human predictive sensitization tests, eugenol is a weaker sensitizer than isoeugenol (Marzulli and Maibach 1980) and this is borne out by clinical evidence (Johansen and Menné 1995). The rankings do not necessarily reflect elicitation dose response profiles in sensitized individuals though. For example, the elicitation threshold for isoeugenol is $< 0.02\%$, whereas for cinnamic aldehyde it is around 0.1 % (Basketter and Allenby 1991; Johansen et al. 1996). The LLNA EC_3 suggest the opposite order of potency, cinammic aldehyde > isoeugenol, a result which is in line with the evidence from human predictive tests (reviewed in Basketter 1997).

As expected, none of the weakest or nonsensitizing fragrance materials have IFRA restrictions. However, it is interesting to note that in the middle ground, some have limits (hydroxycitronellal), whilst others do not. It is tempting to speculate that this difference has arisen as a result of levels and extent of use of these fragrance materials in skin contact products. For example, citral is clearly a skin sensitizer (Basketter and Scholes 1992), but is rarely a cause of ACD perhaps simply because skin contact is fairly limited.

The Impact of Quenching Agents on Potency Estimations

A number of sensitizing fragrance chemicals have been reported to be "quenched" when skin contact occurs in the simultaneous presence of certain other fragrance materials (Opdyke 1976). For example, in predictive human skin sensitization testing, cinnamic aldehyde did not cause sensitization when in the presence of an equivalent amount of eugenol; citral did not cause sensitization when in the presence of limonene. Whilst there has been support for quenching phenomenon (Fisher and Dooms-Goossens 1976; Hanau et al. 1983), investigation of cinnamic aldehyde quenching by eugenol at the elicitation phase of allergic contact dermatitis in man was unsuccessful; only inhibition of nonimmunologicalurticarial reactions was demonstrated (Safford et al. 1990; Basketter and Allenby 1991).

This phenomenon of quenching provides an interesting opportunity to examine the evaluation of potency in various animals models and to see how this adds to the existing data. The results of investigations in guinea pig models have been reported (Basketter and Allenby 1991). The essential data from the GPMT and Buehler tests are reproduced in Table 2. In the GPMT, cinnamic aldehyde gave a 100 % positive response with a mean erythema score of 2.2 (scale 0 – 3). When the test was conducted with identical concen-

Table 2. Studies of the quenching phenomenon in the guinea pig: percentage of the test group with a positive sensitization reaction and mean erythema score of the positive reactions (simplified from Basketter and Allenby 1991)

Test type and substance	Results	
	% positive	Erythema score
GPMT, cinnamic aldehyde	100%	2.2
GPMT, cinnamic aldehyde + eugenol	100%	2.0
GPMT, citral	70%	1.2
GPMT, citral + limonene	90%	1.6
Buehler test, cinnamic aldehyde	40%	0.9
Buehler test, cinnamic aldehyde + eugenol	30%	0.8

trations of cinnamic aldehyde, but in the presence of an equal amount of eugenol, the response rate was still 100%, with a mean erythema score of 2.0. Whilst there is no dose response data, either from the induction or challenge phase, the similarity of the results, which are sub-maximal and therefore "on scale", provides no evidence for the quenching effect of eugenol. GPMT data for citral and citral/limonene also provided no evidence for quenching. Buehler tests carried out following the same principles led to a broadly similar conclusion; there was a 40% positive response with a mean erythema score of 0.9 to cinnamic aldehyde alone, and a 30% positive response with a mean erythema score of 0.8 to cinnamic aldehyde in the presence of eugenol.

As mentioned, none of the guinea pig data included dose response evaluations. Thus it is of particular interest to see whether quenching can be demonstrated in the LLNA, a predictive model which includes dose response data as a routine and from which the estimations of relative sensitizing potency appear to be meaningful (Kimber and Dearman 1991; Botham et al. 1991; Basketter et al. 1992; Kimber et al. 1995; Basketter and Chamberlain 1995; Loveless et al.

Table 3. Studies of the quenching phenomenon in the murine LLNA

Test substance	Test concentrations (%)	Stimulation indices	Threshold concentration (%)
Cinnamic aldehyde	1.0, 2.5, 5.0	2.2, 4.3, 4.8	2.0
Cinnamic aldehyde + eugenol (2.5%)	1.0, 2.5, 5.0	1.7, 3.6, 5.8[a]	2.1
Citral	5.0, 10.0, 25.0	1.2, 2.1 6.3	13
Citral + limonene (2.5%)	5.0, 10.0, 25.0	2.0, 3.1, 5.0	13

[a] Calculated after making allowance for the small contribution made by the quenching agent.

1996). The results of these investigations are presented in Table 3. In this case, the absence of the challenge phase necessitates a different approach, that of testing the sensitizing fragrance ingredient in the presence of a constant concentration of the quenching agent. The threshold concentration can then be determined and any shift in value caused by quenching can be quantified. Again, the quenching phenomenon could not be demonstrated; the dose responses are very similar in the presence and absence of the quenching agent. The EC_3 values derived by regression analysis were essentially identical.

Conclusions

Skin sensitization is unfortunately an fairly common phenomenon and once an individual is sensitized, the only sure way to eliminate the risk of allergic dermatitis is avoid contact with the causative allergen. It is the job of the toxicologist/safety evaluator to identify skin sensitizers and to define their safe use conditions; sensitizers cannot be banned – they represent a wide range of valuable chemicals. Indeed, probably the majority of small organic chemicals are sensitizers to some degree. When a skin sensitizer has been identified, the safety assessment depends heavily on an understanding of the degree of hazard present, the sensitizing potency. Traditional methods have served quite well for many years, but their use in determination of sensitizing potency is problematic. A new method, the LLNA offers an opportunity to define potency quantitatively in terms of the threshold concentration required to induce skin sensitization in the mouse. Such information cannot be directly translated to man, but does give a quantitative view of the relative sensitizing ability of chemicals.

The data presented herein give only a limited picture; they point to the need to assess a wider range of skin sensitizers whose ability to sensitize humans is well understood. The prize would be a much sounder assessment of sensitization potency offering the opportunity to more robust risk assessments and the consequent reduction in the incidence of allergic contact dermatitis.

References

Andersen KE, Maibach HI (1985) Guinea pig sensitization assays: an overview. In: Andersen KE, Maibach HI (eds) Contact allergy predictive tests in guinea pigs. Current problems in dermatology, vol 14. Karger, New York, pp 59–106

Basketter DA (1994) Guinea pig predictive tests for contact hypersensitivity. In: Dean J, Munson AE, Luster M, Kimber I (eds) Immunotoxicology and immunopharmacology. Raven, New York, pp 693–702

Basketter DA (1997) Current trends in the assessment of contact sensitizing potential. Toxicology (submitted)

Basketter DA, Allenby CF (1991) The quenching of contact hypersensitivity reactions. Contact Dermatitis 25:160–171

Basketter DA, Chamberlain M (1995) The validation of skin sensitization assays. Food Chem Toxicol 33:1057–1059

Basketter DA, Gerberick GF (1996) Interlaboratory evaluation of the Buehler test. Contact Dermatitis 35:146–151

Basketter DA, Scholes EW (1992) A comparison of the local lymph node assay with the guinea pig maximisation test for the detection of a range of contact allergens. Food Chem Toxicol 30:65–69

Basketter DA, Roberts DW, Cronin M, Scholes EW (1992a) The value of the local lymph node assay in quantitative structure activity investigations. Contact Dermatitis 27:137–142

Basketter DA, Scholes EW, Evans CD, Kimber I (1992b) Divergent responses to sulphanilic acid in the guinea pig maximization test and the local lymph node assay. Contact Dermatitis 27:209–213

Basketter DA, Scholes EW, Kimber I (1994) Performance of the local lymph node assay with chemicals identified as contact allergens in the human maximisation test. Food Chem Toxicol 32:543–547

Basketter DA, Cookman G, Gerberick GF, Hamaide N, Potokar M (1997) The identification of skin sensitization thresholds – a review. Food Chem Toxicol 35:417–425

Basketter DA, Gerberick GF, Kimber I, Loveless SE (1996b) The local lymph node assay – a viable alternative to currently accepted skin sensitization tests. Food Chem Toxicol 34:985–997

Basketter DA, Gerberick GF, Robinson M (1996c) Risk assessment. In: Kimber I, Maurer T (eds) The toxicology of contact hypersensitivity. Taylor and Francis, London, pp 152–164

Botham PA, Basketter DA, Maurer T, Mueller D, Potokar M, Bontinck W (1991) Skin sensitization – a critical review of predictive test methods in animals and man. Food Chem Toxicol 29:275–286

Boman A (1985) Guinea pig maximisation test. In Andersen KE, Maibach HI (eds) Current problems in dermatology, vol 14. Karger, New York, pp. 59–106

Buehler EV (1965) Delayed contact hypersensitivity in the guinea pig. Arch Dermatol 91:171–177

Buehler EV (1985) A rationale for the selection of occlusion to induce and elicit delayed contact hypersensitivity in the guinea pig. In: Andersen KE, Maibach HI (eds) Current problems in dermatology, vol 14. Karger, New York, pp 39–58

Chamberlain M, Basketter DA (1996) The local lymph node assay: status of validation. Food Chem Toxicol 34:999–1002

European Commission (1992) Annex V to the Dangerous Substances Directive 92/32/EC, ie Annex to the European Commission Directive 92/69/EEC of 31 July 1992 adapting to technical progress for the seventeenth time Council Directive 67/548/EEC on the Approximation of the Laws, Regulations and Administrative Provisions relating to the Classification, Packaging and Labelling of Dangerous Substances. Official Journal of the European Communities 35:L383A

European Commission (1993) Annex IV to Commission Directive 93/21/EEC of 27 April 1993 adapting to technical progress for the 18th time Council Directive 67/548/EEC on the approximation of the laws, regulations and administrative provisions relating to the classification, packaging and labelling of dangerous substances. Official Journal of the European Communities 36:59

Dooms-Goossens A (1976) The effect of perfume ageing on the allergenicity of individual perfume ingredients. Contact Dermatitis 2:155–159

Frankild S, Basketter DA, Andersen KE (1996) The value and limitation of rechallenge in the guinea pig maximisation test. Contact Dermatitis 35:135–140

Hanau D, Groshans E, Barbier P, Benezra C (1983) The influence of limonene on induced delayed hypersensitivity to citral in guinea pigs. Acta Dermatitis Venereol 63:1-7
Hilton J, Evans CD, Lees D, Hall TJ (1991) Assessment of the relative skin sensitizing potency of 3 biocides using the murine local lymph node assay. Contact Dermatitis 25:172-177
Hilton J, Dearman RJ, Gerberick GF, Ryan CA, Basketter DA, Scholes EW, Ladics, GS, Loveless SE, House RV, Guy A (1995) An international evaluation of the local lymph node assay and comparison of modified procedures. Toxicology 103:63-73
Johansen JD, Menné T (1995) The fragrance mix and its constituents: a 14 year material. Contact Dermatitis 32:18-23
Johansen JD, Andersen KE, Menné T (1996) Quantitative aspects of isoeugenol contact allergy assessed by use and patch tests. Contact Dermatitis 34:414-418
Kimber I, Basketter DA (1992) The murine local lymph node assay: a commentary on collaborative studies and new directions. Food Chem Toxicol 30:165-169
Kligman AM, Basketter DA (1995) A critical commentary and updating of the guinea pig maximisation test. Contact Dermatitis 32:129-134
Kimber I, Basketter DA (1997) Contact sensitization: A new approach to risk assessment. Hum Ecotoxicol Risk Assessment (in press)
Kimber I, Dearman RJ (1991) Investigation of lymph node cell proliferation as a possible immunological correlate of contact sensitizing potential. Food Chem Toxicol 29:125-129
Kimber I, Weisenberger C (1989) A murine local lymph node assay for the identification of contact allergens. Arch Toxicol 63:274-282
Kimber I, Dearman RJ, Scholes EW, Basketter DA (1994) The local lymph node assay: developments and applications. Toxicology 93:13-31
Loveless SE, Ladics GS, Gerberick GF, Ryan CA, Basketter DA, Scholes EW, House RV, Hilton J, Dearman RJ, Kimber I (1996) Further evaluation of the local lymph node assay in the final phase of an international collaborative trial. Toxicology 108:141-152
Magnusson B, Kligman AM (1970) Allergic contact dermatitis in the guinea pig. Identification of contact allergens. Springfield, Thomas
Marzulli F, Maibach HI (1980) Contact allergy predictive testing of fragrance ingredients in humans by Draize and maximization methods. J Environ Pathol Toxicol 3:235-245
Mauer T (1983) Contact and photocontact allergens. A manual of predictive test methods. Dekker, Basel
Montelius J, Wahlkvist H, Boman A, Fernstrom P, Grabergs L, Wahlberg JE (1994) Experience with the murine local lymph node assay: inability to discriminate between allergens and irritants. Contact Dermatitis 31:22-27
Organization for Economic Cooperation and Development (1993) Guideline 406: skin sensitization
Opdyke D (1976) Inhibition of sensitization reactions induced by certain aldehydes. Food Chem Toxicol 14:197-198
Robinson MK, Nusair TL, Fletcher ER, Ritz HL (1990) A review of the Buehler guinea pig skin sensitization test and its use in a risk assessment process for human skin sensitization. Toxicology 61:91-107
Safford RJ, Allenby CF, Basketter DA, Goodwin BFJ (1990) Immediate reactions to fragrance chemicals and a study of factors influencing contact urticaria to cinnamic aldehyde in humans and guinea pigs. Br J Derm. 123:595-606
Scholes EW, Basketter DA, Sarll AE, Kimber I, Evans CD, Miller K, Robbins MC, Harrison PTC, Waite SJ (1992) The local lymph node assay: results of a final interlaboratory validation under field conditions. J Appl Toxicol 12:217-222

In Vitro Phototoxicity Tests for Fragrances

W.W. Lovell

Introduction

Certain chemicals cause skin photoirritation or photoallergy. They include drugs (e.g. tetracyclines, 4-quinolones, nonsteroidal anti-inflammatories), skin germicides (e.g. tetrachlorosalicylanilide, bithionol), and tar ingredients (e.g. anthracene, acridine). Examples of fragrance materials causing such reactions include oil of Bergamot, which causes photoirritation via its content of a furocoumarin, 5-methoxypsoralen (Marzulli and Maibach 1970; Zaynoun 1978; Zaynoun et al. 1981). The oil is usually treated, prior to use in perfumery, to remove the furocoumarin which abolishes the photoirritancy (Forbes et al. 1977). Two ingredients which have been reported to cause photoallergy are musk ambrette and 6-methylcoumarin. Musk ambrette was used for many years at low levels in perfumes with no overt evidence of adverse reaction. But when it was introduced into after-shaves at high levels (1.5% in the product) clinical problems became evident (Raugi et al. 1979; Wojnarowska and Calnan 1986). Concentration of musk ambrette may not entirely account for the problems because other significant risk factors may be application to skin which is freshly shaved, relatively permeable and fully exposed to light. The number of people affected was not large and musk ambrette would not be regarded as a potent photoallergen for man. Nonetheless it is clearly unsuitable for unrestricted use in products applied to exposed areas of skin. The International Fragrance Association (IFRA) has recommended that musk ambrette should not be used as a fragrance ingredient (IFRA 1994).

6-Methylcoumarin was reported to cause photodermatitis in consumers following its inclusion in sunscreen products at levels regarded as high – up to 0.2% in the product (Kaidbey and Kligman 1978). The incident caused the Food and Drug Administration of the United States to request product withdrawal (Eiermann 1980). Use is again restricted by IFRA guidelines (IFRA 1978).

A consequence of the above is that fragrance materials should be assessed for adverse photoirritant and photoallergic potential.

Regulatory Guidelines

There are at present no regulatory guidelines for phototoxicity testing although a protocol for photoirritation testing in vivo has been submitted to the OECD (Nilsson et al. 1993). The European Cosmetic Toiletry and Perfumery Association (COLIPA) intend to submit to the OECD a validated in vitro cell-culture phototoxicity test guideline. The Scientific Committee for Cosmetology of the European Community has required sunscreen actives to be tested for phototoxicity (Loprieno 1992). In the absence of regulatory guidelines literature methods should be used. These are discussed below.

Safety Testing In Vitro

Safety tests for photoirritancy and photoallergy historically have used animal models but their use for testing purposes raises ethical issues. Legislation, notably in Europe, and public opinion has provided pressure to refine, reduce and replace animal testing. In addition, developments in cell culture and bio-analytical techniques have stimulated renewed interest in the use of in vitro methods for safety hazard evaluation. In vitro models for phototoxicity have been reviewed (Arlett et al. 1995; Johnson et al. 1986; Lovell 1994; Spielmann et al. 1994a) including mechanistic testing for photoallergy (Pendlington and Barratt 1990; Lovell 1993). A sequential approach to testing should be adopted.

Light absorption is essential for phototoxicity and as a first step in the testing process UV/visible absorption spectroscopy should be used, with care, as a preliminary screen (Lovell 1993). If the substance does not significantly absorb sunlight then it may be set aside as having no priority for phototoxicity testing. Absorbing substances (e.g. Fig. 1) should be tested further using in vitro techniques.

In vitro models for phototoxicity include yeast, erythrocytes, primary and cultured cells, and chemical substrates (Johnson et al. 1986). The yeast growth inhibition test has been used successfully to test perfume ingredients (Bagley et al. 1988; Weinberg and Springer 1981) but other workers, testing a variety of plant materials and drugs, have reported a high incidence of false-negative results (Johnson et al. 1986). The erythrocyte is useful for the study of cell membrane phototoxicity, but having no nucleus is negative to furocoumarins. It tends to be complementary to the yeast test but there are known phototoxic drugs which are negative in both systems. Use of a measure of haemoglobin photooxidation, in addition to haemolysis, can broaden the usefulness of the erythrocyte model (Pape et al. 1993).

Chemical tests include the use of histidine as a substrate for photooxidation (Johnson et al. 1986). Organic solvents may be used to ensure solubility of lipophilic materials, and photochemical efficiency may be computed (Lovell and

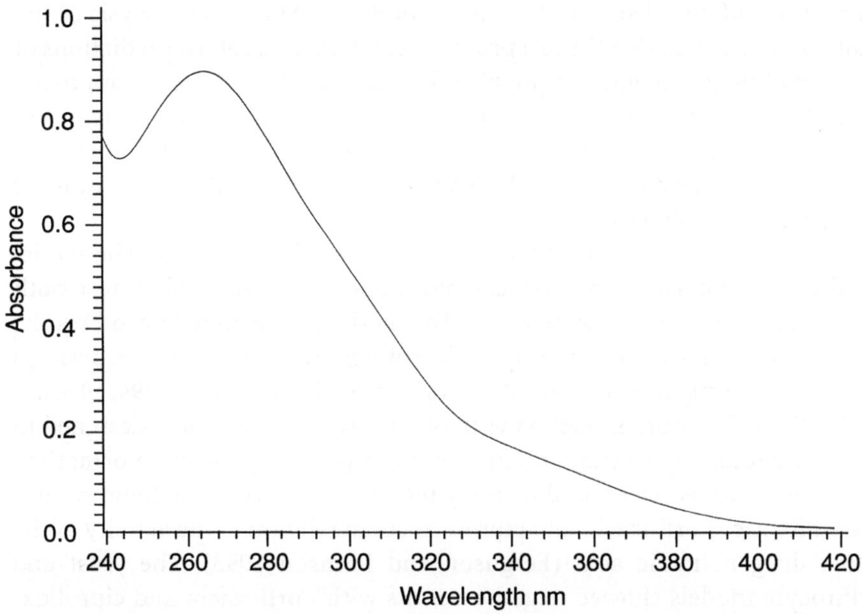

Fig. 1. Ultraviolet absorption spectrum of musk ambrette. The absorption spectrum of musk ambrette (0.004% w/v in ethanol) has a peak at 265 nm which is beyond the limit of sunlight. However the absorption edge extends past 300 nm into the sunlight region. Hence the substance absorbs sunlight and should be tested

Sanders 1990). Histidine is likely to react via the singlet oxygen pathway under most conditions and, for example, the test can usefully aid interpretation of the photobinding test or help in the prediction of phototoxic potency (see below). Histidine photooxidation may be assumed to parallel photohaemolysis but while some photohaemolytic substances photooxidize histidine others do not (Johnson et al. 1986). Two drugs, phototoxic in vivo, have been reported to photooxidize histidine without being photohaemolytic (Ferguson and Johnson 1993). Such differences may be ascribable to solubility properties of the phototoxin which affect localization rather than photochemical factors.

Primary lymphocytes have been used for phototoxicity testing (Morison et al. 1982). Variability of response is problematic and necessitates positive and negative controls concurrent with the test substance, but the majority of phototoxins tested were found positive (Johnson et al. 1986).

Cultured mammalian cell lines have been subject to relatively few studies of their utility for screening purposes (Duffy et al. 1987; Lasarow et al. 1992; Lock and Friend 1986; Maier et al. 1991). A 3T3 mouse fibroblast model has been developed and validated for toxicological purposes in a joint project of the European Union and the European Cosmetic Toiletry and Perfumery Association (EU/COLIPA; Spielmann et al. 1994b 1996). The model has been studied in a ring-test of 30 substances by nine laboratories. Statistical analysis of the results demonstrated that the test provided excellent and robust predictions of in vivo phototoxic potential. A possible drawback of the cell culture approach is that the cells must exist in aqueous media and that many phototoxins are hydrophobic. The 3T3 assay, however, performed remarkably well with hydrophobic materials and even oil of Bergamot was found phototoxic by most of the participating laboratories.

An alternative screening system used a skin equivalent, Skin^2. The model had dermal, epidermal and corneal layers and could be used to test both aqueous and lipid-soluble substances. The model gave generally good results in phototoxicity testing but a sample of oil of Bergamot was negative, perhaps because a relatively low concentration was tested (Liebsch et al. 1994, 1996).

The 3T3 cell culture model, as with other screening tests, was designed to predict phototoxic potential. In vitro tests can provide potency information. Five in vitro models were used to study the phototoxicity of the fluoroquinolone antibiotics norfloxacin and ciprofloxacin in relation to the activity of the related drug nalidixic acid (Ferguson and Johnson 1993). The yeast and erythrocyte models showed negative results with norfloxacin and ciprofloxacin compared with positive results using nalidixic acid. Histidine photooxidation, the lymphocyte test and a macrophage model demonstrated lesser activity of norfloxacin and ciprofloxacin compared with nalidixic acid. The prediction from the in vitro tests, that norfloxacin and ciprofloxacin are likely to be much less phototoxic for man than nalidixic acid, was born out by controlled clinical tests. The use of in vitro tests to predict potency deserves greater attention and development.

Photoallergy is considered to be a delayed-type hypersensitivity reaction mediated by the formation of a test substance-protein photoconjugate. In vitro photobinding of test substance to human serum albumin has been proposed as a screening test for photoallergens (Barratt and Brown 1985; Pendlington and Barratt 1990; Lovell 1993). All known photoallergens which have been tested show photobinding to HSA. Thus the level of false-negative results from this test is expected to be low. Chemicals which are not phototoxic have been negative in this assay. Some photoirritants, however, have given false-positive results in the standard photobinding test (e.g. by the photooxidation of tryptophan to UVA-absorbing products; such reaction cannot be discriminated from photobinding when UV absorbance is used to detect bound ligand). The histidine test for photooxidation proved useful in this regard since efficient photooxidation is a property of many photoirritants which allowed them to be discriminated from photoallergens. A test battery consisting of the photobinding and photooxidation models was useful both for the identification of phototoxicity (corroborating the 3T3 cell model) and for the discrimination of photoallergens from photoirritants (Lovell and Pendlington 1996).

Photomutagenicity testing has been required for sunscreen actives (Loprieno 1992). Test protocols suitable for screening purposes have been considered and may commence using bacterial or yeast strains. Use of a single tester strain (Dean et al. 1991) or a limited number of strains (Chetelat et al. 1993a) has been recommended. Other workers have recommended a more comprehensive approach (Henderson et al. 1994). These tests could be followed where required by mammalian cell tests. Protocols using Chinese hamster ovary cells in chromosome aberration assays have been reported (Dean et al. 1992; Chetelat et al. 1993b).

Conclusions

A sequential approach has long been adopted in photobiology with ultraviolet and visible absorption spectroscopy being used as a pre-screen prior to animal studies. Advances in science and technology now allow an extension of the in vitro approach. Cell culture or skin equivalent models can be used to screen substances which absorb sunlight for photobiological hazard. The photobinding test may be used to identify potential photoallergens, and protocols for photomutagenicity testing are available. These tests enable the predictive identification of photoirritant, photoallergenic and photogenotoxic fragrance materials. Thus substantial progress has been made in the achievement of the 3R principles (reduction, refinement and replacement of animals). The major challenge of in vitro toxicology is now the development and validation of procedures to predict potency and estimate risk.

References

Arlett C, Earl L, Ferguson J, Gibbs N, Hawk J, Henderson L, Johnson B, Lovell W, Menage H, Navaratnam S. Proby C, Steer S, Young A (1995) British Photodermatology Group workshop on predictive in vitro methods for identifying photosensitizing drugs: a report. Br J Dermatol 132:271–274

Bagley DM, Blankson J, Kong BM, De Salva SJ (1988) Optimisation and evaluation of an in vitro yeast assay to predict phototoxicity. J Toxicol Cut Occular Toxicol 7:295–397

Barratt MD, Brown KR (1985) Photochemical binding of photoallergens to human serum albumin: a simple in vitro method for screening potential photoallergens. Toxic Lett 24:1–6

Chetalat A, Albertini S, Dresp JH, Strobel R, Gocke E (1993a) Photomutagenesis test development. I. 8-methoxypsoralen, chlorpromazine and sunscreen compounds in bacterial and yeast assays. Mutat Res 292:241–250

Chetalat A, Dresp JH, Gocke E (1993b) Photomutagenesis test development. II. 8-Methoxypsoralen, chlorpromazine and sunscreen compounds in chromosomal aberration assays using CHO cells. Mutat Res 292:251–258

Dean SW, Lane M, Dunmoor RH, Ruddock SP, Martin CN, Kirkland DJ, Loprieno N (1991) Development of assays for the detection of photomutagenicity of chemicals during exposure to UV light. I. Assay development. Mutagenesis 6:335–341

Dean SW, Dunmoor RH, Ruddock SP, Dean JC, Martin CN, Kirkland DJ (1992) Development of assays for the detection of photomutagenicity of chemicals during exposure to UV light. II. Results of testing photomutagenic chemicals. Mutagenesis 7:179–182

Duffy PA, Bennett A, Roberts M (1987) Prediction of phototoxic potential using human A431 cells and mouse 3T3 cells. Mol Toxic 1:579–587

Eiermann HJ (1980) Regulatory issues concerning AETT and 6-methylcoumarin. Contact Dermatitis 6:120–122

Ferguson J, Johnson BE (1993) Clinical and laboratory studies of the photosensitizing potential of norfloxacin, a 4-quinolone broard-spectrum antibiotic. Br J Dermatol 128:285–295

Forbes PD, Urbach F, Davies RE (1977) Phototoxicity testing of fragrance raw materials. Food Cosmet Toxicol 15:55–60

Henderson L, Fedyk J, Bourner C, Windebank S, Fletcher S, Lovell W (1994) Photomutagenicity assays in bacteria: factors affecting assay design and assessment of photomutagenic potential of para-aminobenzoic acid. Mutagenesis 9:459–465

IFRA (1978) Code of practice. International Fragrance Association, Geneva

IFRA (1994) Code of practice. International Fragrance Association, Geneva

Johnson BJ, Walker EM, Hetherington AM (1986) In vitro models for cutaneous phototoxicity. In: Marks R, Plewig G (eds) Skin models. Springer, Berlin Heidelberg New York, pp 264–281

Kaidbey KH, Kligman AM (1978) Contact photoallergy to 6-methylcoumarin in proprietary sunscreens. Arch Dermatol 114:1709–1710

Lasarow RM, Isseroff RR, Gomez EC (1992) Quantitative in vitro assessment of phototoxicity by a fibroblast-neutral red assay. J Invest Dermatol 98:725–729

Liebsch M, Doring B, Donally TA, Logemann P, Rheins LA, Spielmann H (1994) Application of the human dermal model Skin^2 ZK 1350 to phototoxicity and skin corrosivity testing. Toxic In Vitro 9:557–562

Liebsch M, Doring B, Donally T, Logemann P, Demetrulias J, Spielmann H (1996) Assessment of Skin^2 ZK 1351: a test using a human cutaneous model for testing photoirritancy potential. ATLA 24:327

Lock SO, Friend JV (1986) Phototoxicity testing in vitro. Evaluation of mammalian cell culture techniques. Food Chem Toxicol 24:789

Loprieno N (1992) Guidelines for safety evaluation of cosmetics ingredients in the EC countries. Food Chem Toxicol 30:809–815

Lovell WW (1993) A scheme for in vitro screening of substances for photoallergenic potential. Toxic in Vitro 7:95–102

Lovell WW (1994) Assessing phototoxicity by in vitro methods: a review. In: A Rougier, AS Goldberg, HI Maibach (eds) In vitro skin toxicology. Irritation, phototoxicity, sensitization. Liebert, New York, pp 195–202

Lovell WW, Pendlington RU (1996) A strategy for phototoxicity testing in vitro. ATLA 24:267

Lovell WW, Sanders DJ (1990) Screening-test for phototoxins using solutions of simple biochemicals. Toxic In Vitro 4:318

Maier K, Schmitt-Landgraf R, Siegemund B (1991) Development of an in vitro test system with human skin cells for evaluation of phototoxicity. Toxic In Vitro 5:457–461

Marzulli FN, Maibach HI (1970) Perfume phototoxicity. J Soc Cosmetic Chemists 21:695–715

Morison WL, McAuliffe DJ, Parrish JA, Bloch KJ (1982) In vitro assay for phototoxic chemicals. J Invest Dermatitis 78:460–463

Nilsson R, Maurer T, Redmond N (1993) A standard protocol for phototoxicity testing. Contact Dermatitis 28:285–290

Pape WJW, Brandt M, Pfannenbecker U, Hoppe U (1993) Photohaemolysis and Hb-oxidation combined as part of phototoxicity testing in vitro examined with different phototoxic substances. Toxic in vitro 8:755–757

Pendlington RU, Barratt MD (1990) Molecular basis of photocontact allergy. Int J Cosmet Sci 2:91–103

Raugi GJ, Storrs FJ, Larson WG (1979) Photoallergic contact dermatitis to men's perfumes. Contact Dermatitis 5:251–260

Spielmann H, Lovell WW, Holzle E, Johnson BE, Maurer T, Miranda MA, Pape WJW, Sapora O, Sladowski D (1994a) In vitro phototoxicity testing. The report and recommendations of ECVAM workshop 2. ATLA 22:314–348

Spielmann H, Balls M, Holzhutter H, Kalweit S, Liebsch M, l'Eplattenier H, Lovell WW, Maurer T, Moldenhauer F, Moore L, Pape WJW, Potthast J, de Silva O, Steiling W, Willshaw A (1994b) EEC/COLIPA project on in vitro photoirritancy testing. Toxic In Vitro 8:793–796

Spielmann H, Balls M, Clothier R, Dupuis J, de Silva O, Pape WJW, Holzhutter H, Lovell WW, Maurer T, Potthast J, Sladowski D, Steiling W (1996) Validation study of in vitro phototoxicity tests in a joint EU/COLIPA project. ATLA 24:140

Weinberg EH, Springer ST (1981) The evaluation in vitro of fragrance materials for phototoxic activity. J Soc Cosmet Chem 32:303–315

Wojnarowska F, Calnan CD (1986) Contact and photocontact allergy to musk ambrette. Br J Dermatol 114:667–675

Zaynoun ST (1978) The quantitative analysis of bergapten in perfumes. J Soc Cosmet Chem 29:247–263

Zaynoun ST, Aftimos BA, Tenekjian KK, Kurban AK (1981) Berloque dermatitis – a continuing cosmetic problem. Contact Dermatitis 7:111–116

RIFM Activities in the Safety Assessment of the Dermal Effects of Fragrance Materials

R. A. Ford

RIFM Background

RIFM Charter

The Research Institute for Fragrance Materials (RIFM) was established thirty years ago, chartered as a nonprofit international organization to:

- Gather and analyze available scientific data and other information on fragrance ingredients and to engage in a testing and evaluation program related to such materials.
- Distribute descriptions and other information relating to the uniform standards of testing and evaluation and the results thereof.
- Cooperate with governmental agencies in connection with any testing or evaluation program related to the use of fragrance ingredients or end products containing such ingredients.
- Encourage members of RIFM and others to adopt and adhere to uniform standards in the testing and evaluation of fragrance ingredients.

RIFM Expert Panel

From its inception RIFM has accepted and discharged this responsibility utilizing expert and independent consultation in the form of an expert panel made up of toxicologists, pharmacologists and dermatologists from around the world. Requirements for becoming a member of this panel include not only an established reputation in a relevant field of expertise, but also an independence of the fragrance industry demonstrated by having no connection to a fragrance or cosmetic manufacturer. This panel serves as the ultimate scientific authority of RIFM and directs all of the testing and evaluation undertaken by RIFM. The current members of the Panel are:

- Dr. Donald Birmingham, Wayne State University Medical School
- Dr. Adrianne Rogers, Boston University School of Medicine
- Dr. David Bickers, Columbia-Presbyterian Medical Center

- Dr. I. Glen Sipes, University of Arizona
- Dr. Helmut Greim, GSF Forschungszentrum für Umwelt und Gesundheit
- Dr. Robert Smith, Imperial College, University of London
- Dr. John Hanifin, Oregon Health Sciences
- Dr. Raymond Suskind, University of Cincinnati
- Dr. Paul Newberne, Boston University School of Medicine
- Dr. Kunihiko Yoshikawa, Osaka University School of Medicine

Early Days at RIFM

In the early days of RIFM, these experts focused on the obvious target organ, the skin. As such, they designed a program to assure the existence of a basic battery of tests on all fragrance ingredients in common use in other than trivial quantities. This battery consisted of at least skin irritation and sensitization testing and, as a screen for systemic toxicity, oral and dermal limit tests (generally at 5 g/kg) or LD_{50} tests. To round out the basic battery, where the chemical nature of the ingredient indicated, phototoxicity and photosensitization tests were conducted. Over the years RIFM has subjected about 1300 substances to this battery resulting in recommendations by the International Fragrance Association (IFRA) for the restriction of use level, prohibition of use or use only with certain specifications of approximately 70 fragrance ingredients (see the chapter by F. Grundschober, this volume).

In keeping with the purpose of RIFM, the results of our testing along with other available data were published in the peer reviewed journal, Food and Chemical Toxicology, where we have published approximately 1200 monographs on fragrance ingredients. We fully recognize that many of these monographs are very badly out of date and we are currently designing a program to review and update all of these along with reviewing and evaluating the additional approximately 1400 materials on the European Fragrance inventory. This formidable job will take several years to complete and will be directed by a priority scheme based on the principles mentioned by E. A. Pfitzer (see his chapter, this volume).

In the late 1970s the RIFM experts recognized the growing evidence that materials applied to the skin may be absorbed and available systemically. RIFM then expanded its program to include research and testing for dermal absorption and possible systemic effects on selected fragrance ingredients chosen by priority determined by consideration of structure, exposure and available data either from the literature or from the test programs of member companies. Some of the results of this expanded program are discussed in more detail by Pfitzer (this volume).

Over the approximately 30 years since its inception, RIFM has tested virtually all important fragrance materials in common use. (It has always been the policy of RIFM that if a material is used only by one company, it is that company's responsibility to see that the material is adequately tested and evaluated.)

Originally RIFM used the Kligman (1966) human maximization test as a screening test for potential sensitization, generally using petrolatum as a solvent. A panel of industry experts was asked to determine the maximum use level in consumer products and then the material was tested at ten times this level. This was done for two purposes. First, it was considered a safety factor to allow for some uncertainty in the use levels reported by industry. Second, it tended to make the screening test more stringent since it was routinely conducted on only 25 volunteers. Although, it was well recognized that the severity of the maximization test provided a significant exaggeration in exposure because of the irritation required at the patch site and the fact that the material was applied under semi-occlusion.

Current RIFM Activities Concerning Dermal Sensitization

RIFM continues its program of testing and evaluating fragrance ingredients for irritation and sensitization potential with substances chosen based on 3 criteria, increased use levels, reports from dermatologists and newly reported materials. In about 1985 RIFM switched from the maximization test to the modified (Draize 1959) Human Repeat Insult Patch Test (HRIPT) as a screening test for sensitization. This procedure involves treating volunteers with a 24-h patch on Mondays, Wednesdays and Fridays for a three week period followed by a 2-week rest period and then by a single 24-h challenge patch. Total occlusion is achieved by using a 25-mm Hill Top Chamber.

While RIFM looks to the results from the human screening test for a final decision as to whether a fragrance material has the potential for induction of sensitization, materials are screened in a Buehler (1965) guinea pig sensitization test. This test, while not the most stringent, seems to predict the results in an HRIPT better than other protocols. It is important to note here that RIFM only screens fragrance materials for potential for induction of sensitization not for elicitation or cross reactions with other materials which may have caused sensitization.

Considerable effort was put into deciding the most appropriate solvent to use. In brief, it was determined that 95% ethanol caused too many irritant reactions and sometimes resulted in what seemed to be sensitization to the alcohol. A solvent that was representative of actual use, 70% ethanol, proved to be not very useful because many fragrance materials are not soluble enough to allow for solutions 10 times higher than reported use levels. In other words, it seems that many fragrance materials may, in some cases, be used at levels up to close to their limit of solubility. The ideal solvent in many cases has turned out to be 75% ethanol, to represent commercial use with 25% diethyl phthalate, to simulate the rest of the perfume compound and to increase solubility. In some cases where high concentrations are required pure diethyl phthalate is used to prevent irritation and increase solubility.

Of course, whatever solvent is used, it is included in the challenge patching as a control. Likewise, RIFM always includes a negative control, in most cases ethylene brassylate.

While RIFM has screened all of the large volume fragrance ingredients in general use, the sensitization studies continue with substances chosen as follows.

When data become available that the use levels in consumer products have increased since the original screening test, a review of the material is undertaken by the expert panel. After consideration of the available data from the original studies and from any other sources, along with consideration of the chemical structure and current reported use levels, the panel decides whether additional testing is required. On this basis, dihydromyrcenol was chosen for further testing as described below.

Of course, RIFM monitors the literature, especially reports by dermatologists of diagnostic patch tests. While a few reports of isolated positive patch tests generally do not trigger action, as these reports become more common, the substance in question is again reviewed by the expert panel along with all other relevant data. It was this that triggered additional testing of α-amylcinnamaldehyde and α-hexylcinnamaldehyde in 1976 and 1977. More recently, as described below, reported increased use levels triggered still more testing. Of course, in cases such as these where it is known that some potential for sensitization exists, tests are started at either a low concentration working up to the desired concentration or on a small panel gradually expanding to the desired size. These substances are tested on exclusive panels with no other substances other than the solvent and negative controls.

RIFM also continues, although at a much slower pace than historically, to test newly reported materials and to work through the lesser used previously reported materials. In these cases, where there is no evidence of sensitization from other sources, several substances, up to eight, may be tested simultaneously on the same panel as long as these substances are not chemically related so as to decrease the likelihood of cross-reactions.

Some examples of recent studies not previously reported, are as follows:

Dihydromyrcenol

Dihydromyrcenol was originally tested in a human maximization test at 4% in petrolatum with 0/25 reactions in an all male panel (Opdyke 1974a). This test level was based on a reported maximum use level in consumer products of

Table 1. Human repeat insult patch test: dihydromyrcenol

Substance	Test conc.	Challenge results[a]
Dihydromyrcenol	20.0%	0/109
Ethylene brassylate[b]	10.0%	0/109
Diethyl phthalate[c]	100%	0/109

[a] Induction and challenge concentrations were the same.
[b] Negative control.
[c] Solvent control.

0.4% in a perfume. Over the years the use levels have increased to almost 10 times that level. Although there was no evidence of problems with consumers, it was decided to test dihydromyrcenol at a higher level. An initial screen in a Buehler guinea pig test, gave no reactions when tested at 100% on 20 guinea pigs. RIFM has long had the principle of testing on humans only up to a maximum of 20% and so this level was selected. An HIRPT at 20% caused no reactions in a panel of 109 (see Table 1).

α-Substituted Cinnamaldehydes

α-Amylcinnamaldehyde (ACA) and α-hexylcinnamaldehyde (HCA) are well known for their weak sensitization potential. ACA was originally tested in a human maximization test at 6% (Opdyke 1973). No reactions were seen in a panel of 25. HCA was originally tested at 12% in a human maximization test based on reports of uses up to 1.2% in perfumes (Opdyke 1974b). Because of the appearance of reports from dermatologists of a significant number of patch test positives to these materials, RIFM, undertook to retest both materials in human maximization tests. In these tests, ACA produced no reactions at 6% in petrolatum in three separate tests (Kligman 1973a; Epstein 1977a) on panels of 25, 25 and 21, respectively. Similarly HCA produced no reactions at 12% in petrolatum in three separate tests (Kligman 1973b; Epstein 1977b) on panels of 25, 30 and 26, respectively.

RIFM has recently become aware of significantly higher use levels for both HCA and ACA. Thus HRIPTs were undertaken on both materials at the maximum RIFM level of 20%. Because of potential solubility and irritation problems, the solvent chosen was diethyl phthalate. Consideration of the possibility of cross reactions led to decisions to test these materials on separate panels with only solvent control and ethylene brassylate as a negative control and to include a cross challenge patch with both materials. Because of the potential for sensitization at that level, testing was started on small separate panels of approximately 20. These were expanded first to approximately 50 and finally to 95 after no reactions were seen (see Table 2).

Table 2. Human repeat insult patch test: α-amylcinnamaldehyde and α-hexylcinnamaldehyde

Substance	Test conc.	Challenge results
α-Amylcinnamaldehyde (panel A)	20%	0/95
α-Hexylcinnamaldehyde (panel B)	20%	0/95
Ethylene brassylate[a]	10%	0/95
Diethyl phthalate[b]	100%	0/95

[a] Negative control.
[b] Solvent control.

Thus, no sensitization induction potential under test conditions has been demonstrated to date for either HCA or ACA. While this appears to be in conflict with the dermatologists reports of positive reactions to these materials, at least to HCA, several explanations can be hypothesized.

It could be that sensitization arises from exposure to these materials from sources other than fragrance use. This seems unlikely since the only other uses known to RIFM are as flavor materials at very low levels, less than 20 ppm.

It is possible, that the reactions seen are as a result of cross reactions, that is, the patients that reacted positively were actually sensitized to some other material. The most likely suspect would be cinnamaldehyde. However, this should have been detected by the dermatologists since cinnamaldehyde is also in the test tray. Furthermore, there was no evidence of cross sensitization with cinnamaldehyde in a limited study (Ishihara et al. 1981).

The most likely explanation is that these materials are very weak sensitizers in humans and the predictive screening tests have not been sensitive enough to detect them. It is possible, that using an alcoholic, or at least the alcohol/DEP solvent mentioned above would enhance penetration to the point that some reaction would be seen. Also, testing at a level higher than 20% might have an effect. On the other hand, these tests indicate that induction of sensitization to these materials on humans does not occur readily.

Low Volume and New Materials

Of course, it is recognized that the approximately 1300 fragrance materials that RIFM has tested and evaluated over the years is only a portion of those materials in use in the industry. (The recently reported European indicative inventory lists approximately 2650 materials.) On the other hand, it has been reported to RIFM that most of the materials used by the industry are used in very small volumes with a resulting low exposure. While these materials are considered of relatively low priority, the RIFM program involves a review of all materials known to be in use and to develop test data as needed.

Table 3. Human repeat insult patch test: low volume and new materials

Substance	Test conc.	Challenge results
Bay oil, terpeneless	3.0%	0/99
Labdanum resinoid	4.0%	0/99
Methyl *N*-acetyl anthranilate	0.4%	0/99
Olibanum oil	9.0%	0/99
Rose crystals	13.0%	0/99
Ethylene brassylate [a]	10%	0/99
Diethyl phthalate [b]	100%	0/99

[a] Negative control.
[b] Solvent control.

Additionally, the industry is continually developing new materials. The RIFM program also involves review and evaluation of such materials as they become into general use. It is generally expected, however, that the company that has developed such materials will provide the necessary test data for proper evaluation.

Some results of the RIFM program of sensitization testing of low volume and newly developed materials are shown in Table 3.

Future Activities

As mentioned above, RIFM has undertaken a program to review and evaluate all of the fragrance materials on the European indicative inventory. This includes all of the previously reviewed "RIFM materials" on which monographs have been published as well as the approximately 1400 additional materials not previously reported to be in general use. This huge task will be undertaken using a priority scheme which takes into consideration quantity used, use levels on the skin and consideration of structural alerts for dermal effects, systemic effects and genotoxicity/carcinogenicity potential. This task will require cooperation of the fragrance industry in supplying exposure data and, of course, any unpublished safety data they might have.

The first phase of this project has already begun with a world wide survey of volume of usage of all materials on the inventory. In order to obtain the cooperation of industry, RIFM has agreed to keep the results of this survey confidential with composite data only made available on an as needed basis. However, these data will play a very important role in our priority setting.

These data will be combined with level of use data, which the industry will be asked to supply, as well as a weighting based on chemical structure. After a material is chosen by the priority system, literature searches will be conducted and the industry solicited for any unpublished safety data. The RIFM expert panel will then, in order of priority, undertake a review of each material to assure that adequate data are available to assess the safety under the conditions of use. The results of this review will, of course, be transmitted to IFRA for consideration of any possible action and will be published in the open literature.

The outcome of this project will be updated monographs as well as new monographs on those materials previously published. This should provide a necessary and comprehensive database for the safety evaluation of all commonly used fragrance materials.

Reference

Buehler EV (1965) Delayed contact sensitivity in guinea pigs. Arch Dermatitis 91:171–177

Draize JH (1959) Dermal toxicity. In: Staff of the Division of Pharmacology of the Federal Food and Drug Administration (eds) Appraisal of the safety of chemical in foods, drugs and cosmetics. Editorial Committee of the Association of Food and Drug Officials of the United States, Texas State Health Department, Austin, p 52

Epstein WL (1977a) Report on human maximization studies. Report to RIFM. 25 February, 21 March, 19 April

Epstein WL (1977b) Report on human maximization studies. Report to RIFM. 21 March, 31 May

Ishihara M, Itoh M, Hosono K, Nishimura M (1981) Some problems with patch testing using fragrance materials. Skin Res 23(6) 808–817

Kligman AM (1966) The identification of contact allergens by the human assay. III. The maximization test. A procedure for screening and rating sensitizers. J Invest Dermatitis 47:393–409

Kligman AM (1973a) Report on human maximization studies. Report to RIFM. 23 July

Kligman AM (1973b) Report on human maximization studies. Report to RIFM. 9 October

Opdyke DL (1973) Monographs on fragrance raw materials – amyl cinnamic aldehyde. Food Cosmet Toxicol 11:855–856

Opdyke DL (1974a) Monographs on fragrance raw materials – dihydromyrcenol. Food Cosmet Toxicol 12:430

Opdyke DL (1974b) Monographs on fragrance raw materials – hexyl cinnamic aldehyde. Food Cosmet Toxicol 12:125

Part V
The Producer's View

The Producer's View: Do We Worry About Adverse Effects?

P. CADBY

In answer to the question in the title: producers of fragrances are indeed concerned about the effects of their products. The association of allergic contact dermatitis with the use of fragrances gave the initial impetus to the founding of the Research Institute for Fragrance Materials (RIFM) as an independent research institute 30 years ago. It also led to the creation of the International Fragrance Association (IFRA) as an autoregulatory body which would implement the findings of RIFM into clear guidelines on ingredient use.

The main focus of this Institute has been on detecting unacceptably allergenic fragrance ingredients. The real effectiveness of this programme may be questioned by some dermatologists today, but our industry's concern has involved considerable expense. In today's terms the cost of just the dermatological testing in this programme is well in excess of U.K. £8 million. The costs of running RIFM and maintaining a distinguished panel of experts is also far from negligible.

As could be anticipated, the results of the tests have not been without consequence. RIFM findings have led to IFRA restrictions which have clearly caused great but necessary pain to perfumers by limiting their full creative scope. This has, we hope, all been in a good cause.

It is an appropriate time to ask whether the approach of the fragrance industry has been correct and effective. It has been based on detecting the possible inducers of contact allergy using so-called predictive testing under maximized conditions followed by the voluntary restriction of whatever showed allergenicitiy in these studies. Although our knowledge of the causes and control of allergy is still in its infancy, IFRA has always attempted to base its Guidelines on sound science.

The IFRA Guidelines will be constantly up-dated to take account of new findings, and this demonstrates that the fragrance industry is most attentive to developments in clinical dermatology.

By necessity, clinical dermatology approaches this problem from a different angle. Instead of examining the potential of substances to induce allergy, it is based on the detection and etiology of allergies which have already been acquired. As such, it relies on the elicitation of the allergy. The fragrance industry is clearly aware of the value of this approach. At the same time, the fragrance industry is highly concerned about the apparent discrepancies between the findings of the two approaches. RIFM has repeatedly investigated whether some frequent clinical elicitors such as geraniol and amylcinnamic aldehyde will induce allergy under its standard experimental conditions. Repeated insult patch tests on these substances using human volunteers failed to detect any allergenicity. As with most chemicals, they apparently have a finite potential to sensitize, but they do not seem to be as potent as some of the other fragrance ingredients restricted by IFRA such as citral and methyl octine carbonate which, on the other hand, do not seem to be frequent clinical elicitors.

In some cases it is possible to determine with some degree of certainty the fragrance ingredient which is the causative agent for a specific case of allergy to a cosmetic product in a patient who is referred to a dermatological clinic. This usually involves patch testing to increasingly smaller fractions of incriminated cosmetic product, and its component fragrance until only the causative agent gives a reaction. In an ideal world it would be possible to do this for all cases of allergy. If it could then be possible to refer back to each patient's apparent exposure to the causative agent and to the number of people exposed in the population at large, we could obtain good epidemiological evidence of the relative potency of different allergens.

I have enjoyed collaborating with dermatologists in breaking fragrances down in this way to find the ultimate causative allergen. We have had some very interesting successes over the past few years, with unexpected results. We do not, however, live in an ideal world, and in some cases our attempts to split a formula have led to more than one eliciting fraction. In other cases there has been no reaction to any of the fractions. More frequently still, the patient has been unwilling to continue patch testing. The fragrance industry is very conscious of the practical problems facing the clinical dermatologist.

Lack of cooperation from the fragrance manufacturer should never be an obstacle. IFRA requires fragrance manufacturers to cooperate with dermatologists. It also encourages dermatologists to report cases where fragrance manufacturers do not cooperate satisfactorily. IFRA encourages anyone to report cases of noncompliance to its Code of Practice.

The fragrance industry is particularly interested in knowing what the true frequency of allergy to fragrances is and just how effective the IFRA Guidelines have been in reducing this. We would hope that it is decreasing in response to the implementation of the IFRA Guidelines. However, some clinical data indicates that this may not be the case (Johansen and Menné 1995).

There have been a number of patch-test studies that have been carried out on the population at large. One study on nurses (Guin and Berry 1980), showed that almost 18% reacted to the Fragrance Mix. Another (Nielsen and

Menné 1992) gave a figure of 1.1%. Interviews with members of the population regarding past experience with perfume-sensitivity, indicate a higher frequency of 12.2% (De Groot 1988) and even 32% (Guin and Berry 1980). Numerous studies from dermatological clinics indicate that 4%–11% of patients react to the Fragrance Mix (Frosch et al. 1995). An earlier and quite different North American study (Adams et al. 1985) showed that out of more than 280,000 patients examined, of which only 5.4% were diagnosed as having allergic contact dermatitis, only 51 patients (that is less than 0.02%) reacted to specific individual fragrance ingredients whereas an equivalent number (67) reacted to unspecified fragrance. On this basis, our industry's enthusiasm to participate in a complete survey of the frequency of fragrance sensitivity was dampened by an epidemiologist's warning that an extemely large sample of the population would be needed for statistically meaningful results.

It is difficult to interpret what these figures mean. By necessity, patch tests are performed on patients who are referred to dermatological clinics, and this in itself is a form of epidemiological "gerrymandering". Although it is possible that this procedure concentrates potential sufferers from perfume allergy in an unquantifiable way, many sufferers from fragrance-allergy may never be referred to these clinics. The similarities between the frequency of reactions to the fragrance mix in healthy people, on the one hand, and in patients, on the other, is very surprising.

The difference between the proportion of patients who react to the eight-component fragrance mix and those who reacted to individual fragrance ingredients, albeit in quite different studies in different continents, is also perplexing. There is probably substantial uncertainty over the clinical relevance of a positive patch test to the fragrance mix, and it is possible that the fragrance mix is some kind of fortuitous super-elicitor. It is difficult to know just how much cross-reactivity occurs from the real causative allergen to the fragrance mix or to its constituents if these are subsequently patch tested.

On the other hand, however, it is also quite conceivable that these eight components do not adequately represent the thousands of chemical structures found in fragrances. The fragrance mix may consequently be missing cases of real fragrance sensitivity and leading to under-estimates of the true frequency of allergy to fragrance ingredients.

All in all, perhaps the only thing we can be certain about here is the uncertainty associated with using clinical patch test data for statistical purposes. This, coupled with uncertainty over the clinical significance of each positive patch test, means that dermatologists, through no fault of their own, are dealing with a rather inadequate epidemiological instrument. It is difficult to exclude the possibility that fragrance sensitivity is in reality much lower or even much higher than the patch tests would indicate. It is therefore unlikely that the frequency of reactions to the fragrance mix could detect any upward or downward trends of allergy to fragrance in general.

This symposium represents a meeting of two quite different philosophical and experimental approaches. Our industry has focused its attention on reducing the causes of allergy in the not-yet-sensitized. Clinical dermatology has obviously concentrated on the elicitation of reactions in the already-sensitized. There is little doubt that most persons who suffer reactions to fragrances would consider irrelevant whether the original root cause of their allergy is responsible for their latest reaction. IFRA could possibly attribute more importance not only to the inducers but also to the most frequent elicitors among cosmetics users. Before doing so we must be certain that we know what the main elicitors are. It is therefore necessary that the fragrance industry work even more closely with dermatologists to detect and quantify the relative importance of these eliciting fragrance ingredients.

The fragrance industry is concerned about this problem and is willing to cooperate with dermatologists in this extremely complex and technically difficult area.

References

Adams RM, Maibach HI, Clendenning WE, Fisher AA, Jordan WJ, Kanof N, Larsen W, Mitchell JC, Rudner EJ, Schorr W, Storrs F, Taylor JS (1985) A five-year study of cosmetic reactions. J Am Acad Dermatol 13:1062–1069

De Groot AC (1988) Adverse reactions to cosmetics. Thesis, University of Groningen

Frosch PJ, Pilz B, Andersen KE, Burrows D, Camarasa JG, Dooms-Goosens A, Ducombs G, Fuchs T, Hannuksela M, Lachapelle JM, Lahti A, Maibach HI, Menné T, Rycroft RJG, Shaw S, Wahlberg JE, White IR, Wilkinson JD (1995) Patch testing with fragrances: results of a multicenter study of the European Environmental and Contact Dermatitis Research Group with 48 frequently used constituents of perfumes. Contact Dermatitis 33:333–342

Guin JD, Berry VK (1980) Perfume sensitivity in adult females. A study of contact sensitivity to a perfume mix in two groups of student nurses. J Am Assoc Dermatol 3:299–302

Johansen JD, Menné T (1995) The fragrance mix and its constituents: a 14-year material. Contact Dermatitis 32:18–23

Nielsen NH, Menné T (1992) Allergic contact sensitization in an unselected Danish population. The Glostrup Allergy Study, Denmark. Acta Dermato-venereologica 72:456–460

The IFRA Guidelines

F. Grundschober

The International Fragrance Association (IFRA) was created in 1973 to ensure the safe use of fragrance ingredients by establishing a system of self-regulation for the fragrance industry. The members of IFRA are the national associations of fragrance manufacturers from France, Germany, Italy, the Netherlands, Spain, Switzerland, the United Kingdom, Australia, Brazil, Canada, Japan, Mexico, Singapore and the United States. The member associations have adopted the IFRA Code of Practice and Guidelines (copies available at the IFRA, 8 rue Charles-Humbert, 1205 Geneva, Switzerland). The Code and the Guidelines are published in the format of a loose-leaf binder in English, French, and German and are regularly updated. The Guidelines and its amendments are also published in the journal *Perfumer & Flavorist.*

IFRA collaborates closely with the Research Institute for Fragrance Materials (RIFM). RIFM collects and generates data for risk analysis and risk assessment, whereas IFRA deals with risk management. It is the task of IFRA to translate the results of the safety evaluation made by RIFM into practical recommendations for perfumers and fragrance manufacturers. These recommendations are published as IFRA Guidelines.

Fragrance manufacturers are members of their national association and they must follow the Code of Practice and Guidelines of IFRA. Adherence to the IFRA Guidelines is requested as a basis for commercial transactions between fragrance manufacturers and fragrance users. Fragrance manufacturers also respect the restrictions for reasons of product liability. Many governmental authorities have recognized the IFRA Guidelines as valid expert opinion, and it is known that they control by analysis whether certain restrictions of IFRA are indeed respected.

The IFRA Code of Practice applies to the manufacturing and handling of all fragrance materials. The most important part of the Code is that dealing with the use of fragrance materials. Since thousands of different fragrance ingredients are used by the various manufacturers, a special system for their regulation has been implemented. All fragrance ingredients can be divided in two groups: (a) those which are in general use by the industry and (b) those which are only used by one manufacturer or which are newly introduced.

Fragrance ingredients in general use have been used for many years by several manufacturers. These materials therefore have in-use experience, and the low number of reported adverse reactions is an additional indication of their safety. Since this would not be enough to assure their safe use, they have also been included in the continuing safety evaluation program of RIFM.

Fragrance ingredients recently introduced by one manufacturer have no in-use experience. Since the identity of these substances is not always known and since they are marketed only by one manufacturer, it is not possible for RIFM to undertake their testing and their evaluation. These fragrance ingredients must satisfy standards established in Annex 1 of the IFRA Code, and the evaluation which has been made of their safety for the intended use is the responsibility of the manufacturer.

IFRA requires that fragrance ingredients always conform to the relevant legislation and regulations of the countries in which they are to be used. Data enabling a proper evaluation to be made may be obtained from: (a) literature sources or available data bases, (b) information required for conformity to chemical or health and safety at work legislation, and (c) a consideration of structure-activity relationships based on known effects of other substances.

If there is inadequate data from the above sources, a properly designed toxicological program should provide data on: (a) acute toxicity, (b) skin irritation, (c) skin contact sensitization, and (d) phototoxicity and photosensitization, if the ingredient shows significant absorption in the UV region.

Before embarking upon any toxicological programme consideration should always be given to the use of properly validated and accepted alternatives to animal experimentations. Systemic toxicity should be considered in relation to the quantities used and likely to enter the body. Possible environmental effects should be considered in relation to the quantities used and released into the environment.

All the volumewise important fragrance ingredients have already been evaluated and most of them have been found suitable for use without restrictions. Only a relatively small number has shown some adverse reactions. These materials have been included in IFRA Guidelines.

The Guidelines of IFRA are elaborated in close cooperation by RIFM and IFRA and lead to recommendations made by the Technical Advisory Committee (TAC) of IFRA. This Committee is composed of perfumers as well as technical and scientific experts nominated by the member associations. It represents the expertise of the fragrance industry worldwide. The recommendations of IFRA are based on scientific evidence, very often provided by RIFM as a result of its testing program, as well as additional data, for example, reports of dermatologists in the literature or unpublished data provided by manufacturers or users as a result of their research. All this information is taken into consideration in formulating a new Guideline or amending an existing Guideline.

Up to now 91 Guidelines have been published; 26 deal with natural materials. An explanation is given for every recommendation. As can be expected for materials coming in contact with the skin, the most important reason for restrictions is skin sensitization, mentioned in 65 Guidelines, followed by 14 cases of phototoxicity, 6 of photosensitization and 10 of systemic toxicity. Some materials show more than one of these adverse findings.

The Guidelines contain recommendations either not to use an ingredient or to limit its use by a quantitative restriction. At present 35 ingredients should not be used and at least 16 other materials are not used (see "Appendix 1"). An example of an ingredient that should not be used is musk ambrette. The use of 12 phototoxic ingredients is limited (see "Appendix 1"); an example is bergamot oil expressed. Twenty-eight fragrance ingredients showing a sensitizing potential are limited (see "Appendix 1"). Examples of restricted sensitizing ingredients are *trans*-2-hexenal and isoeugenol (see "Appendix 2").

Currently most restrictions in the IFRA Guidelines are the result of skin sensitization potential of individual ingredients. Fragrance ingredients are tested in a human repeat insult patch test (HRIPT) at ten times the use concentration in leave-on-skin products. If there is evidence of sensitization, the no-effect concentration for induction of sensitization is determined and one-tenth of the no-effect level is taken as the maximum permitted level in the IFRA Guideline. The decision on whether a substance should not be used or should be restricted depends on the scientific evidence as well as on its perfumery value and its olfactive potency. A powerful fragrance ingredient can be restricted to, for example, 0.01 % in a consumer product and may still have a useful function without presenting a health risk. A less powerful fragrance ingredient would be useless at such a level and can therefore no longer be used.

Specific purity criteria or use instructions are recommended for 14 materials. The use instructions may require the addition of antioxidants to prevent peroxide formation or the use of a material in the presence of other materials (see "Appendix 1"). Examples are the recommendations for Pinacea derivatives and for citral. Safrole, isosafrole, dihydrosafrole and *cis*- and *trans*-asarone are limited for reasons of systemic toxicity.

The system of self-regulation based on the IFRA Guidelines has been well accepted by governments and by the customers of the fragrance industry. IFRA is also willing to make sure that the Guidelines are adapted to new evidence. A new provision of the Code of Practice is requesting fragrance manufacturers to cooperate closely with dermatologists.

The formula of fragrance compounds is a valuable intellectual property of the fragrance manufacturers. They have invested time, effort, creativity and the know-how of perfumers in a development which often cannot be protected by patents. This explains why manufacturers keep confidential the formulae of the perfumes. It is recognized by legislators that fragrance formulae need adequate protection. The label declaration "perfume" on finished cosmetic products has recently been endorsed by the European Union and will inform consumers about the presence of fragrances.

There is, however, also a need for transparency and the last amendment of the European Cosmetics Directive requires the establishment of a fragrance inventory (European Commission 1996a). It is recognized that this inventory is not exhaustive but is merely indicative of what the European fragrance industry is currently using. The fragrance industry has submitted a draft inventory, comprising fragrance ingredients in the RIFM evaluation program as well as fragrance ingredients notified by manufacturers. The list has already been published in the *Official Journal* of the European Union (EU) (European Commission 1996b). The list has not the legal meaning of a positive list and fragrance ingredients used as captive materials are not necessarily listed. But it is certain that the inventory contains the great majority of fragrance ingredients presently in use.

According to the self-regulatory practice of the fragrance industry some kind of evaluation must be undertaken either by RIFM or by the manufacturers. The basis for the RIFM evaluations are the data published in the RIFM monographs. The long-term aim should be to prepare a monograph for every fragrance ingredient in the inventory. This is a considerable task considering that over a thousand substances must be added to this program.

This work has already started since IFRA invited fragrance manufacturers who have notified materials for the inventory to provide their safety data. RIFM will review these data, and inquires will be made to collect other safety-related information such as use levels and volume of use. The aim of the self-regulation of the fragrance industry is not to determine the potential hazard of a fragrance ingredient but rather to find safe conditions for its use.

The crucial question remains of whether any effects of this self-regulation can be seen in practice. Banning 35 fragrance materials and restricting the use of 54 materials which were in unrestricted use in cosmetics 20 years ago should have reduced the number of adverse reactions. During the same period there was an increase in the use of consumer products containing fragrances. Additionally, the awareness of consumers and reporting by dermatologists increased. This makes it difficult to establish a clear relationship between cause and effect.

At least one example has been reported in the literature (Schauder 1995) that cases of berloque dermatitis are markedly reduced or have even disappeared in recent years. This is a clear result of the IFRA recommendation to limit bergapten at 15 ppm in cosmetic products. The limitation of bergapten has no official regulatory status: nevertheless an effect has been seen, and it can be concluded that self-regulation works.

The self-regulation of the fragrance industry must ensure the safe use of fragrance ingredients. IFRA and RIFM will continue their work and cooperate with authorities as well as with the medical profession.

Appendix 1

Fragrance Ingredients Not To Be Used (December 1995)

- Acetyl ethyl tetramethyl tetralin
- Acetyl isovaleryl
- Allantroot oil
- Anisylidene acetone
- Benzylidene acetone
- *p-tert*-Butylphenol
- Colophony
- Costus root oil, absolute and concrete
- Diethyl maleate
- Dihydrocoumarin
- 2,4-Dihydroxy-3-methyl-benzaldehyde
- 4,6-Dimethyl-8-*tert* butyl coumarin
- Dimethylcitraconate
- Ethyl acrylate
- Fig leaf absolute
- *trans*-2-Heptenal
- Hexahydrocoumarin
- *trans*-2-Hexenal diethyl acetal
- *trans*-2-Hexenal dimethyl acetal
- Hydroabietyl alcohol
- Hydroquinone monoethylether
- Hydroquinone monomethylether
- 6-Isopropyl-2-decalol
- 7-Methoxycoumarin
- α-Methylanisylidene acetone
- 6-Methylcoumarin
- 7-Methylcoumarin
- Methyl crotonate
- 4-Methyl-7-ethoxycoumarin
- Musk ambrette
- Nitrobenzene
- Pentylidene cyclohexanone

- Pseudoionone
- Pseudomethylionones
- Verbena oil
- Other materials not used as or in fragrance ingredients
  - Allylisothiocyanate
  - Chenopodium oil
  - Cinnamylidene acetone
  - Ethylene glycol monoethyl ether and its acetate
  - Ethylene glycol monomethyl ether and its acetate
  - 3,7-Dimethyl-2-octen-1-ol
  - Diphenylamine
  - Furfurylideneacetone
  - Methyl methacrylate
  - Phenylacetone
  - Phenyl benzoate
  - Esters of 2-octynoic acid, except methyl and allyl heptine carbonate
  - Esters of 2-nonynoic acid, except methyl octine carbonate
  - Thea sinensis absolute

Phototoxic Fragrance Ingredients, Use Limited (December 1995)

- 5-Acetyl- 1,1,2,3,3,6-hexamethyl indan
- Angelica root oil
- Bergamot oil expressed
- Bitter orange oil expressed
- Citrus oils
- Cumin oil
- Grapefruit oil expressed
- Lemon oil cold pressed
- Lime oil expressed
- Marigold oil and absolute
- Methyl *N*-methyl anthranilate
- Rue oil

Fragrance Ingredients with Sensitizing Potential, Use Limited (December 1995)

- Allyl heptine carbonate
- Amyl cyclopentenone
- *p-tert*-Butyl-dihydrocinnamaldeyde
- Cassia oil
- Cinnamic alcohol
- Cinnamon bark oil, Ceylon
- Cyclamen alcohol
- *trans*-2-Hexenal
- α-Hexylidene cyclopentanone

- Hydroxycitronellal
- Isocyclogeraniol
- Isoeugenol
- Menthadienyl formate
- Methyl heptadienone
- Methyl heptine carbonate
- *p*-Methylhydrocinnamic aldehyde
- 3-Methyl-2(3)-nonenenitrile
- Methyl octine carbonate
- Oak moss extracts
- 1-Octen-2-yl acetate
- Opoponax
- Perilla aldehyde
- Peru balsam
- Propylidene phthalide
- Styrax
- Tree moss extracts
- 1-(Trimethylcyclohexenyl/hexadienyl)-2-buten-1-ones (Rose ketones)
- Verbena absolute

Fragrance Ingredients with Specific Purity Criteria or Use Restrictions (December 1995)

- Acetylated Vetiver oil
- Allyl esters
- Cade oil
- Carvone oxide
- Cinnamic aldehyde
- Cinnamic aldehyde–methyl anthranilate Schiff base
- Citral
- Farnesol
- Limonene
- Nootkatone
- Phenylacetaldeyde
- Pinacea derivatives
- Savin oil
- Sclareol

Appendix 2

Musk Ambrette. The Committee recommends that musk ambrette should not be used as fragrance ingredient. This recommendation is based on photosensitivity (Cronin 1984), neurotoxic effects (Spencer et al. 1984) and on accumulated evidence that musk ambrette can penetrate human skin and is only slowly excreted (private communication to IFRA). (June 1981, last amendment July 1994; replacement sheet, December 1995)

Bergamot Oil Expressed. The Committee recommends that for applications on areas of skin exposed to sunshine, excluding bath preparations, soaps and other products which are washed off the skin, bergamot oil expressed should not be used such that the level in the consumer product exceeds 0.4%. This is equivalent to 2% in a fragrance compound used at 20% in the consumer product (see remark on phototoxic ingredients in the "Introduction" and the Guideline on citrus oils). The Committee further recommends that for qualities of the expressed oil in which the less volatile components have been concentrated by partial or total removal of the terpene fraction, this limit should be reduced in proportion to the degree of concentration. These recommendations are based on the published literature on the phototoxicity of this material, summarized by Opdyke 1973) and other investigations (Zaynoun et al. 1977). (October 1974; last amendment, June 1992)

trans-2-Hexenal. The Committee recommends that *trans*-2-hexenal should not be used such that the level in consumer products exceeds 0.002%. This is equivalent to 0.01% in a fragrance compound used at 20% in the consumer product. For use in consumer products for which no skin contact is foreseeable under normal conditions of use, for example, closed system air fresheners, toilet blocks but not rinse off products and household cleaning products, the Committee recommends that the level in the consumer product should not exceed 0.02%. This recommendation is based on test results of RIFM showing sensitization reactions at 0.2% and no sensitization reaction when tested at 0.02% (private communication to IFRA). (April 1989; last amendment, June 1992)

Isoeugenol. The Committee recommends that isoeugenol should not be used such that the level in consumer products exceeds 0.2%. This is equivalent to 1% in a fragrance compound used at 20% in the consumer product. For use in consumer products for which no skin contact in foreseeable under normal conditions of use, for example, closed system air fresheners, toilet blocks but not rinse off products and household cleaning products, the Committee recommends that the level in the consumer product should not exceed 0.5%. This recommendation is based on an evaluation of the test results of RIFM at 8% and 10% showing the sensitizing potentials of the material, and many other RIFM and other data on consumer products, fragrances and the materials itself at lower dosages (private communication to IFRA; Thompson et al. 1983). (May 1980; last amendment, June 1992)

Pinacea Derivates. The Committee recommends that essential oils (e.g. turpentine oil) and isolates (e.g. Δ^3-carene) derived from the Pinacea family, including Pinus and Abies genera, should be used only when the level of peroxides is kept to the lowest practicable level, for instance, by adding antioxidants at the time of production. Such products should have a peroxide value of less than 10 mmol/l, determined according to the EOA method. This recommendation is based on the published literature, mentioning sensitizing properties when containing peroxides (Opdyke 1973; Opdyke 1978; Opdyke 1978). This Guideline does not permit the use of colophony. (May 1976; last amendment, July 1994)

Citral. The Committee recommends the use of citral as a fragrance ingredient in conjunction with substances preventing sensitization, for example, 25% *d*-limonene, mixed citrus terpenes, and α-pinene. This recommendation is based on results showing sensitizing potential for the individual ingredient, but absence of sensitizing reactions in a number of compounds (private communication IFRA), with lemongrass oil as well as in mixtures of 80 parts of citral to 20 parts of *d*-limonene, or mixed citrus terpenes, or α-pinene. (Opdyke 1976, 1979). (October 1975; replacement sheet, February 1980)

References

Cronin E (1984) Photosensitivity to musk ambrette. Contact Dermatitis 11:88

European Commission (1996a) Commission Decision of 8 May 1996 establishing an inventory and a common nomenclature of ingredients employed in cosmetic products (96/335/EC). Official J European Communities L 132/1–4 (1 June 1996)

European Commission (1996b) Perfume and aromatic raw materials, sect II. Official J European Communities L 132/526–679 (1 June 1996)

Obdyke DLJ (1973) Bergamot oil expressed. Food Cosmet Toxicol 11:1031

Opdyke DLJ (1973) Δ^3Carene. Food Cosmet Toxicol 11:1053

Opdyke DLJ (1976) Inhibition of sensitization reactions induced by certain aldehydes. Food Cosmet Toxicol 14:197

Opdyke DLJ (1978) α-Phellandrene. Food Cosmet Toxicol 16:843

Opdyke DLJ (1978) α-Pinene. Food Cosmet Toxicol 16:853

Opdyke DLJ (1979) Citral. Food Cosmet Toxicol 17:259–266

Schauder S (1996) Basiswissen Photoallergie. Allergologie 19:556–559

Spencer PS, Bischoff-Fenton MC, Moreno OM, Opdyke DLJ, Ford RA (1984) Neurotoxic properties of musk ambrette. Toxicol Appl Pharmacol 75:571

Thompson GR, Booman KA, Dorsky J et al. (1983) Isoeugenol: A survey of consumer patch-test sensitization. Food Chem Toxicol 21:735–740

Zaynoun ST, Johnson BE, Frain-Bell W (1977) A study of oil of bergamot and its importance as a phototoxic agent. II. Factors which affect the phototoxic reaction induced by bergamot oil and psoralen derivatives. Contact Dermatitis 3:325

Fragrances and Environmental Issues: A Case Example of Environmental Risk Assessments of Ingredients

W. de Wolf and P. J. Kloepper-Sams

Introduction

Fragrances are made up of many individual ingredients, each of which may have a range of differing physical and chemical properties. Indeed, it is this range that provides the creative perfumer with the ability to impart desirable fragrance characteristics across a variety of consumer products and across the "lifespan" of the aroma following product use. This range of physico-chemical properties also gives each ingredient characteristic behaviour in the environment (fate). Finally, it will also influence the (eco)toxicological properties (effect) of the material. This provides the rationale why in environmental sciences the focus is not on fragrances but on the fragrance ingredients.

Recent publications indicate an increased interest in the environmental fate and effects of perfume ingredients, such as nitromusks (Geyer et al. 1994; Rimkus and Wolf 1995; Gatermann et al. 1995; Fernandez et al. 1996; Boleas et al. 1996). Due to extensive use in consumer products such as detergents and surface cleaners, these materials may be disposed down the drain and may end up in the environment. To assess the environmental risks for any general chemical associated with these practices, a risk assessment strategy has been developed by the scientific community with recent European Union (EU; 1995) guidelines reflecting current practices (EU 1995). The main objective of this paper is to introduce an understanding of the critical steps in the tiered approach used in environmental risk assessments (ERA; e.g. exposure assessment, effects assessment, and risk characterization) and then provide a case-example of an ERA of musk xylene and musk toluene in the Dutch environment (Tas and van de Plassche 1996). This example will clearly indicate the reduction in uncertainty which is achieved when a tiered approach is used. The reduction in uncertainty proceeds to the point where one is sufficiently confident that release of an ingredient does not pose a risk to the environment, or where risk management decisions must be taken.

Environmental Risk Assessment Methodology

To accommodate the tiered data availability within the context of the environmental risk assessment, a stepwise or iterative modelling approach is adopted (EU 1995). The principal decision points involve a comparison of the predicted environmental concentration (PEC) with the predicted no-effect concentration (PNEC). Figure 1 shows that the PEC is calculated in the exposure assessment phase, and the PNEC in the effects assessment phase. The PEC is compared with the PNEC to obtain PEC/PNEC ratios or risk quotients in the risk characterization phase.

Exposure Assessment

The calculation of a predicted environmental concentration (PEC) is the ultimate goal of an environmental fate assessment. A step-wise approach to the PEC calculation is used with increased refinement of the exposure models and exposure parameters. More information on use, partitioning in sludge and soil, and physico-chemical parameters will refine the assessment. At the highest tier, the PEC can be compared with actual measured environmental concentrations (monitoring data). The tiered approach provides an iterative

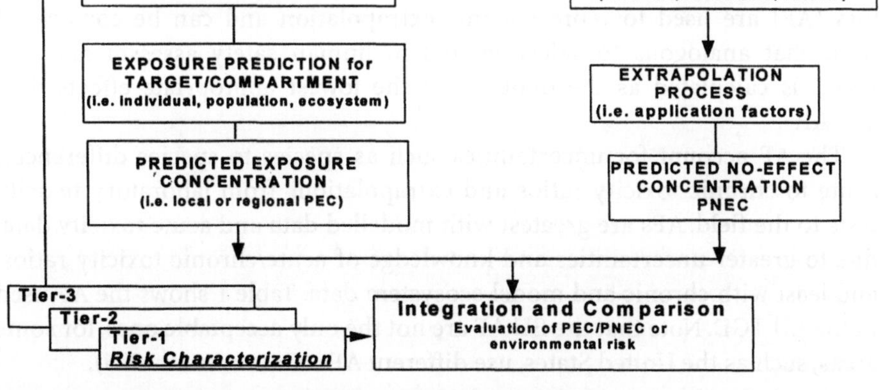

Fig. 1. Tiered approach used in the EU TGD (1995) with calculation of the PEC in the exposure assessment phase, and the PNEC in the effects assessment phase, and a final comparison of PEC/PNEC ratios or risk quotients in the risk characterization phase

process of refinement with additional or improved data at each step, allowing the risk assessor to focus the correct level of resources on the materials of greatest interest.

Effects Assessment

The primary objective of effects assessment is to derive a predicted no effect concentration (PNEC) for receiving environmental compartments relevant to the material of interest. There are three environmental compartments that are traditionally assessed: aquatic, sediment and terrestrial.

Aquatic and sediment effects assessments can be divided into four tiers. Consistent with the fate assessment, early tiers rely on modelled and acute toxicity data to estimate the PNEC. Later tiers use chronic and ecosystem-level data to derive PNECs. Though not used in the EU, other areas, including the United States, do use quantitative structure activity relationships (QSAR) as a first tier. In the second tier, acute toxicity data are generated for organisms representing three important trophic levels in the environment, for example, an algae, an invertebrate, such as *Daphnia magna*, and a fish. It is important to recognize that in contrast to human safety assessments, the ERA does not aim to protect one species, but aims to protecting the multiple species present in the environment, as well as ecosystem function.

In the third tier, chronic toxicity data are generated which are expressed as "no observed effect concentrations" (NOECs). An NOEC is similar to a no observed effect level or NOEL. Finally, field data can be generated if needed. Note that to date few chemicals have proceeded to this tier.

As a consequence of the step-wise approach, environmental realism increases with each tier such that the uncertainty of extrapolating from experimental results to the PNEC decreases concomitantly. Assessment factors (AF) are used to represent this extrapolation and can be considered somewhat analogous to safety factors in human safety assessments. The PNEC is calculated as the quotient of the lowest appropriate effects data and AF.

The AF account for uncertainties such as species to species differences, acute to chronic toxicity ratios and extrapolations from laboratory toxicity tests to the field. AFs are greatest with modelled data and acute toxicity data, due to greater uncertainties and knowledge of acute/chronic toxicity ratios, and least with chronic and model ecosystem data. Table 1 shows the AF used in the EU TGD. Note that the EU AF are not the only acceptable ones, for some areas, such as the United States, use different AFs (Cowan et al. 1995).

Table 1. Assessment factors used in the EU (1995) to extrapolate from effects data to a predicted no effect concentration (PNEC) for the environment

Tier	Available data on chemical	EU assessment factors
1	QSAR estimates	Does not use SAR/QSAR data alone
2	Base set acute toxicity data [a]	1000
3	One chronic NOEC	100
	Two chronic NOECs	50
	Three chronic NOECs	10
4	Field or mesocosm data	Case by case

[a] The base set refers to the amount of aquatic toxicity data needed for notification of new chemicals at base set level (> 1 ton/year) according to EU (1992), e.g. 3 acute LC (EC)50's for algae, invertebrates and fish.

Risk Characterization

To characterize the risk of use of a material the PEC/PNEC ratio or risk quotient is used. A risk quotient greater than 1 indicates a potential for adverse effect. For a PEC/PNEC outcome less than 1, no additional testing or refinement is required (EU 1995), and the material can be considered safe.

The tiered ERA proceeds until a risk quotient is obtained that provides sufficient confidence no risk to the environment exist. In those cases where all practical tiers in the ERA have been exhausted and the PEC/PNEC ratio still indicates some risk to the environment, a risk management decision must be taken. Professional judgement plays an important role at the risk characterization stage.

Environmental Risk Assessment: A Case Example with Musk Xylene and Musk Ketone

The Dutch National Institute of Public Health and the Environment published an initial ERA of Musk Ketone and Musk Xylene in the Netherlands in accordance with the EU guidance (Tas and van de Plassche 1996). The ERA is based on information and results provided by the fragrance industry (NEA, RIFM) and international open literature.

Background Information and Test Methods

Structures, important physico-chemical properties and estimated Dutch use volumes for musk xylene and musk ketone are presented in Table 2. Estimated values for physico-chemical properties were obtained by reducing the 2 dimensional structure to SMILES notation and executing the appropriate QSAR

Table 2. Identification, some physico-chemical properties and estimated use volumes for musk xylene and musk ketone

	Musk ketone	Musk xylene
Identification		
CAS no.	81-14-1	81-15-2
Structure	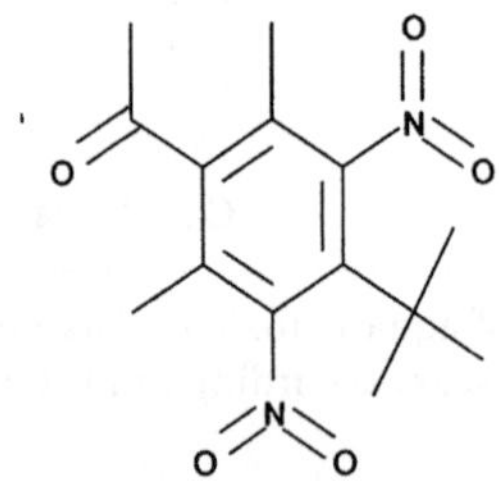	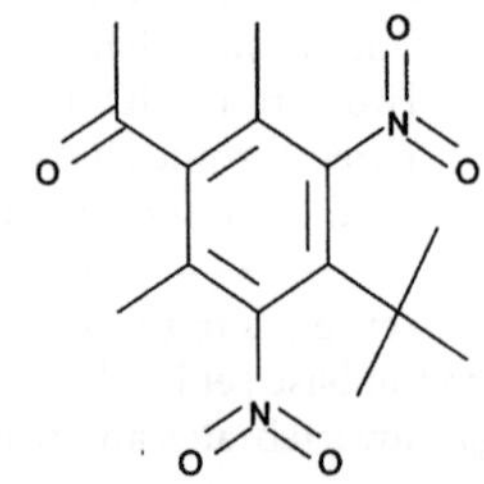
SMILES	O=C(c(c(c(N(=O)=O)c(c1 N(=O)=O)C(C)/ C)C)C)c1C)C	O=N(=O)c(c(c(N(=O)=O)c(c1 N(=O)=O)C(C)/ C)C)C)c1C
Physico-chemical properties		
Octanol/water partition	4.3	4.9
coefficient (log Kow)	4.31 (est.)	4.45 (est.)
Solubility in water (mg/l)	1.9 (est.)	0.49 (est.)
Use volume		
Tonnage in the Netherlands (ton/y)	5	3
Environmental fate		
Biodegradation	Not inherently	Not readily

modules produced by the Syracuse Research Corporation. Measured values for the Log Kow were obtained using the HPLC retention method outlined in OECD Guideline 117. Biodegradation data were from results in an OECD 301C "readily biodegradable" test (musk xylene) or an OECD 302C "inherently biodegradable" test (musk ketone).

Toxicity tests were conducted on algae, daphnia and fish according to OECD Guidelines 201, 202 and 204, respectively (Tables 3, 4). A bioconcentration study was performed with bluegill sunfish under flow-through conditions according to OECD Guideline 305. Bioconcentration factors (BCFs) were calculated from steady-state residue concentrations and average measured water concentrations.

Estimates of surface water concentrations in Dutch rivers were obtained via execution of the Uniform System for Evaluation of Substances (USES 1.0) computer model developed in the Netherlands (RIVM, VROM and WVC 1994).

ERA: Aquatic Environment

For the PEC calculations it is assumed 100% of material used enters the aquatic environment through a sewage treatment plant with no musks remaining on the fabric, skin or surfaces. In this 'worst-case' scenario, the PEC for local situations can be estimated as 0.00051 and 0.00011 mg/l for musk ketone and musk xylene, respectively.

Table 3 presents the first tier in the risk assessment. If we have data only on acute toxicity, the AF is a 1000, and the PNECs are then 0.000118 mg/l and 0.0004 mg/l. The risk quotient, PEC/PNEC, for musk ketone is above 1 which indicates we need a further refinement of the ERA. The PEC/PNEC for musk xylene is below 1, which indicates that this nitromusk does not pose a risk to the Dutch aquatic environment. For illustrative purposes we keep musk xylene in the subsequent tiers.

Table 4 presents the second tier in the risk assessment. Chronic toxicity data are available. The lowest NOEC value of the two accepted chronic toxicity values (daphnia and algae) in the ecotoxicity dataset of musk xylene was divided by an application factor of 50 to derive a PNEC of 0.0011 mg/l. The lowest NOEC value of the three accepted chronic toxicity values (fish, daphnia and algae) in the ecotoxicity dataset of musk ketone was divided by an application factor of 10 to derive a PNEC of 0.063. The final PEC/PNEC risk quotients are then 0.081 and 0.098, respectively. These numbers indicate that both nitromusks do not pose a risk to the Dutch aquatic environment. Since monitoring date are available, the risk quotient can also be determined using real-world concentrations instead of predicted ones.

The use of these real world concentrations confirms that the model predictions are conservative, as these concentrations are below the model predicted

Table 3. First tier in the aquatic risk assessment for musk xylene and musk ketone which makes use of modelled fate and acute toxicity data only

	Musk ketone	Musk xylene
Exposure		
PEC (mg/l)	0.00051	0.00011
Effects		
Algae (mg/l)	3d $EC_{50} = 0.118$	5d $EC_{50} > 5.6$
Daphnids (mg/l)	No data	2d $EC_{50} > 5.6$
Fish (mg/l)	21d $LC_{50} > 0.5$	4d $LC_{50} = 1.2$ 14d LC50 = 0.4
Assessment Factor	1000	1000
PNEC (mg/l)	0.000118	0.0004
Risk characterization		
PEC/PNEC	4.3	0.275

Table 4. Second tier in the aquatic risk assessment for musk xylene and musk ketone which makes use of modelled fate and chronic toxicity data

	Musk ketone	Musk xylene
Exposure		
PEC (mg/l)	0.00051	0.00011
Effects		
Algae (mg/l)	3d NOEC = 0.088	5d NOEC > 5.6
Daphnids (mg/l)	21d NOEC = 0.169	21d NOEC = 0.056
Fish (mg/l)	21d NOEC = 0.063	No data
Assessment Factor	10	50
PNEC (mg/l)	0.0063	0.00112
Risk characterization		
PEC/PNEC	0.081	0.098

Table 5. Third tier in the aquatic risk assessment for musk xylene and musk ketone which makes use of environmental monitored concentrations and chronic toxicity data

	Musk ketone	Musk xylene
Exposure		
PEC (mg/l)	0.00003	0.00001
Effects		
Algae (mg/l)	3d NOEC = 0.088	5d NOEC > 5.6
Daphnids (mg/l)	21d NOEC = 0.169	21d NOEC = 0.056
Fish (mg/l)	21d NOEC = 0.063	No data
Assessment Factor	10	50
PNEC (mg/l)	0.0063	0.00112
Risk characterization		
PEC/PNEC	0.0047	0.0089

ones. Using the real world date, the risk quotients are further reduced to 0.0047 and 0.0089 (Table 5).

In summary, using the tiered approach in the risk assessment of the nitromusks the uncertainty in the predicted values was reduced and the environmental realism increased. The PEC/PNEC ratios reflect the increased realism with a decrease in the risk quotient.

ERA: Soil Environmental

For other environmental compartments such as sludge-amended soils (terrestrial environment) and for secondary poisoning of predators a similar tiered approach can be used.

A fraction of musk ketone and musk xylene in the waste water treatment plant partitions into the sludge. In the EU TGD (1995) a scenario is available to determine the risk for the soil ecosystem when the sludge is applied to agricultural soil. The PEC in the soil environment is estimated as 0.34 mg musk ketone/kg soil and 0.29 mg musk xylene/kg soil. Few data are available on soil toxicity of musk ketone and musk xylene. Thus, the PNEC was calculated from the PNEC for the aquatic environment using the equilibrium partitioning theory. This theory assumes that the test organisms are exposed only through the pore water, and that material bound to soil matter is not bioavailable. The reliability of such a PNEC in soil is less than one based on experimental data from soil organisms, hence it should be considered as an indication only (Tas and van de Plassche 1996). The calculated PNEC values for soil are 0.43 musk ketone/kg soil, and 0.23 musk xylene/kg soil. The corresponding PEC/PNEC ratios are 0.80 and 1.3 for musk ketone and musk xylene respectively. The availability of one experimental data point for musk xylene shows that the equilibrium partitioning theory probably overestimates the PNEC calculated in this manner for this substance.

Due to the limited amount of data available regards the soil environment, the ERA indicates that additional data could be used to refine the PEC/PNEC for this compartment. However, in contrast to some other countries in Europe, sludge application to soil is not a common practice in the Netherlands. The fragrance industry (RIFM) is currently generating additional experimental effects data from soil organisms to further refine the soil assessment for other EU countries where use of sludge on agricultural land is a common practice.

ERA: Secondary Poisoning

Secondary poisoning is concerned with toxic effects in organisms at higher levels in the food chain, which may result from ingestion of organisms that contain accumulated substances. The hazard connected to bioaccumulation is taken into account when assessing secondary poisoning. Both nitromusks bioaccumulate to some extent in fish tissue. They have total body bioconcentration factors of approximately 1400 and 1600 (Tas and van de Plassche 1996). The ERA indicates that these compounds do not pose a risk of secondary poisoning of predators in the Dutch environment, as the PEC/PNEC ratios are well below 1 (Table 5).

Summary

The aim of this paper is to provide an introduction to ERA methods, the use of predictive screening models and a series of tests which progressively

Table 6. Summary of the PEC/PNEC risk quotients obtained in the environmental risk assessments of musk xylene and musk ketone

	Musk ketone	Musk xylene
PEC/PNEC aquatic environment		
Tier 1	4.3	0.275
Tier 2	0.081	0.098
Tier 3	0.0047	0.0089
PEC/PNEC terrestrial environment		
Tier 1	0.80	1.3
PEC/PNEC secondary poisoning of predators		
Tier 1	0.015	0.011
Tier 2	<0.0008	<0.0038

provide more data on an ingredient's potential to bioaccumulate, its partitioning and fate in relevant environmental compartments, and its toxicity to environmental organisms. As an example of how the ERA approach can be applied to perfume ingredients, we have presented an EU TGD style assessment of the nitromusks musk xylene and musk ketone in the Dutch environment. This case example clearly illustrates the increased refinement which results from increasing environmental realism for both the fate and effects portions of the assessment, thus improving the overall risk characterization (Table 6).

References

Boleas S, Fernandez C, Tarazona JV (1996) Toxicological and kinetic study of musk xylene in rainbow trout, Oncorhynchus mykiss. Bull Environ Contam Toxicol 57:217–222

Cowan CE et al. (1995) Integrated approach for environmental assessment of new and existing substances. Regul Toxicol Pharmacol 21

EU (1992) EC Council directive of 30 April 1992 amending for the 7th time directive 67/548 EEC on the approximation of laws, regulation and administrative provisions relating to the classification, packaging and labeling of dangerous substances (92/32/EEC). Official Journal L154/35 5-6–92

European Union (1995) Technical guidance document environmental risk assessment of new and existing substances. October 1995

Fernandez C, Caballo M, Tarazona JV (1996) A new method to determine musk xylene in water sewages, fish and related products. Chemosphere 32:1805–1811

Gatermann R, Hühnerfuss H, Rimkus G, Wolf M, Franke S (1995) The distribution of nitrobenzene and other nitroaromatic compounds in the North Sea. Marine Pollution Bull 30:221–227

Geyer HJ, Rimkus G, Wolf M, Attar A, Steinberg C, Kettrup A (1994) Synthetische Nitromoschus-Duftstoffe und Bromocyclen. UWSF-Z Umweltchem Ökotox 6:9–17

Rimkus GR, Wolf M (1995) Nitro musk fragrances in biota from freshwater and marine environment. Chemosphere 30:641–651

RIVM, VROM and WVC (1994) Uniform System for the Evaluation of Substances (USES), version 1.0. National Institute of Public Health and Environmental Protections (RIVM), Ministry of Housing, Spatial Planning and the Environment (VROM), Ministry of Welfare, Health and Cultural Affairs (WVC). VROM, the Hague, the Netherlands, distribution no 11144/150

Tas JW, van de Plassche EJ (1996) Initial environmental risk assessment of musk ketone and musk xylene in the Netherlands in accordance with the EU-TGD, report 601503002, National Institute of Public Health and Environmental Protections (RIVM), Bilthoven,. the Netherlands, pp. 44

Fragrances – Future Aspects

I. R. White

The Present Situation

The Sixth Amendment to the Cosmetics Directive (Council Directive 93/35/ EEC of June 14th 1993), which came into force in 1997, is an important and powerful piece of legislation. It will have an enormous impact on the safety of cosmetics, provide necessary information to the consumer and enable a better evaluation of adverse reactions to cosmetics. Ultimately, the consumer will benefit from enhanced protection and this will cause significant savings in costs to health care.

It is accepted by those who investigate adverse reactions that the most common allergens in cosmetic products are in fragrance compounds. It is salutary to note that some fragrance compound manufacturers do not consider that fragrances are important allergens. This may be because they themselves receive no or little 'feedback' about reactions to the particular compounds which they supply or doubt the clinical relevance of diagnostic patch test investigations.

In an initial draft of the Sixth Amendment of the Cosmetics Directive there was a proposal that greater information on the composition of fragrance compounds be provided. This was omitted from the final document. This omission resulted from the lobbying activities of the fragrance compound manufacturers as represented by EFFA (European Fragrance and Flavour Association) [RIFM (Research Institute for Fragrance Materials) 7th International Information Exchange, 1995]. Because of such manoeuvres, fragrances are exempt from meaningful regulation in Europe and elsewhere.

The fragrance industry remains self-regulated. The International Fragrance Association (IFRA) has a code of practice and produces guidelines on the use of certain fragrance ingredients. Although the larger manufacturers may be members of the association and adhere to the code and guidelines, others may not. It is unknown what proportion of fragrance compounds are provided by non-IFRA members and what proportion of compounds comply with the IFRA guidelines.

There remains an absence of information, which IFRA justifies in its 1984 statements on confidentiality:

1. *The task of the fragrance industry is to provide a key contribution necessary for many cosmetic and household products.*
2. *Fragrances are products obtained by combining numerous raw materials of natural or synthetic origin in a well balanced ratio. Genuine research efforts have been invested in identifying and synthesizing the most appropriate fragrance ingredients as well as in combining them in the most efficient way.*
3. *The products of the fragrance industry are based on intensive and large scale scientific research, as well as on creative skill. The development of a fragrance formula is very expensive and it constitutes a valuable intellectual property.*
   The protection of the intellectual property of the fragrance industry is of vital importance for this industry.
   The extent of secrecy maintained for formula files is fully commensurate with this investment. Stringent precautions are taken to safeguard the confidential nature of the formulas and only a few employees are allowed access to an entire formulation.
4. *The protection of the intellectual property of the fragrance industry is only possible by maintaining this secrecy, since in most cases patent protection cannot be obtained.*
   It may be argued that persons within government authorities who receive confidential information, are bound to observe secrecy with regard to any confidential and proprietary information they might learn during this work. In our view, this obligation, notwithstanding the best of intentions, provides an insufficient guarantee against such information leaking out. Individuals may change positions, carrying their experience with them. Moreover a breach of confidence may be practically impossible to prove.
5. *The disclosure of the intellectual property of the fragrance industry contributes nothing to the protection of consumers. Consumer protection can only be achieved by adhering to certain specific rules. Detailed legislation on fragrances does not exist even in the highly industrialized countries. Fragrances are only covered in general terms by the cosmetic regulations of many countries. None of these regulations require the disclosure of fragrance formulas. In some countries, e.g. France, the law recognizes that the secrecy of fragrance formulas should be safeguarded.*
6. *The Guidelines of the IFRA Code of Practice set standards for the safe use of fragrance ingredients. These Guidelines are established following a review by the Technical Advisory Committee of IFRA of all safety data obtained from RIFM, the fragrance industry and from the scientific literature.*

Adherence to the Guidelines protects the consumer against known hazards which might arise from the use of fragrances. The fragrance industry observes the Guidelines in the interest of consumer protection; they are widely accepted throughout the world.

7. *At present no country requires formula disclosure. If however this should be required, it is possible that very simple inadequate fragrances will be offered for sale, below the actual state of the art, leading to inferior finished products. This is not only detrimental to the interest of consumers, who would not enjoy the best fragrances available, but may also be harmful to the cosmetic and household products industry and its export capability.*

Formula disclosure will not improve the safety of fragrances. In the absence of an overriding and substantial benefit, such a regulation will bring serious loss not only to the cosmetic and household products industry, but also to the consumer. Research and development will be adversely affected so that product development will come to a standstill.

Under the current legislation a certificate of conformity must be provided by the fragrance compound supplier for each compound it provides for cosmetic use. This certificate contains statements certifying that the compound conforms to the IFRA guidelines and to the Cosmetics Directive. *Manufacturers have, however, no obligation to respect guidelines in the absence of possible health risk* (RIFM 7th International Information Exchange, 1995). It also gives the maximum concentration that the compound may be used in within a particular product. The blanket secrecy remains in that there is no information on the presence of particular substances which may be of concern regarding health or other issues.

The safety evaluation of fragrance ingredients is not legally required (RIFM 7th International Information Exchange, 1995). IFRA guidelines provide inadequate and insufficient toxicological information. *So far the main objective of RIFM and IFRA has been to assure product safety for skin contact* (RIFM 7th International Information Exchange, 1995). Although the skin reactions induced by certain ingredients are well known, the same is not true of the toxicological data concerning systemic effects, and this is a serious matter. The great majority of fragrance ingredients placed on the market have not been evaluated at all or poorly so.

A Wider Opinion on Fragrance Ingredient Safety and Regulation

The fragrance industry knows the law and has been careful to act within it. It is a damning indictment that the most important cosmetic allergens have escaped adequate legislation. What can be done to change this unsatisfactory situation?

The Scientific Committee on Cosmetology (SCC) is an independent 'expert' committee which advises the general directorate, DGXXIV, at the European Commission. It is this directorate which is concerned with consumer policy. The SCC produces guidelines for the safety evaluation of cosmetic ingredients as well as assessing the safety of particular cosmetic ingredients. At the plenary of the SCC on 5 February 1997 the following was adopted:

According to the Code of Practice for the fragrance industry:

Fragrance manufacturers should provide customers with all available information to ensure that fragrance materials are used in accordance with standards of good practice.

In its guidelines for communicating the IFRA status of a fragrance compound, IFRA recommends consideration – in particular – on:

- *a statement that the fragrance complies with the IFRA guidelines for the mentioned application and used concentration,*
- *a reference to the bases of the IFRA guidelines, RIFM data and other available sources ....*

Without questioning the principle of intellectual property underlying the derogation concerning the qualitative and quantitative formula of fragrance compounds [dir. 93/35/EEC, art. 7a, I(a)], ***several measures should be considered with a view to providing something more than a safety guarantee of a purely legal nature*** *and to informing the person responsible for safety with regard to human health.*

3.1. Certificate of conformity

The existing certificate of conformity with IFRA standards attached to a fragrance compound should be systematically supplemented by

- *a semi-quantitative declaration which also highlights those fragrance ingredients which have been subject to restrictions in the IFRA code of practice and, in a more general way, those which have an established potential to cause contact sensitization and (or) phototoxic reactions (e.g. F.I. listed in the European Standard Fragrance Mix)*

  e.g. Essential oil from the bark of cinnamonum zeylanicum < 1 %
  Evernia prunasti concrete (oak moss extract) < 3 %
  Methyl oct-2-ynoate < 0,01 %
  Geraniol.... %
  Eugenol... %
  a-amyl-cinnamaldehyde .... %

- *an indication of the cosmetic product types in which it may be used.*

While safeguarding the formula's confidentiality, the safety assessment should be confirmed on the fragrance compound considered as a whole, and the data and the scientific reasoning should be included in the conformity certificate.

3.2. Safety assessment of perfumed cosmetics

The exact concentration of the perfume composition (=fragrance compound) in the cosmetic product should be indicated [art. 7a, 1,(a) Dir. 93/35/EEC].

In the safety assessment of the cosmetic product for human health (art 7a, I (d), Dir. 93/35/EEC),

- *reference should be made to semi-quantitative formula of the fragrance compound naming the fragrance ingredients declared in the certificate of conformity (see 3.1 above) and consideration should be taken to their toxic potential.*
- *reference should be made to the safety assessment of the fragrance compound considered as a whole.*

The aim of self-regulation of the fragrance industry is not to determine the potential hazard of fragrance ingredients, but rather to find safe conditions for their use (RIFM 7th International Information Exchange, 1995). This opinion of the SCC permits an independent evaluation of fragrance compound safety over any which a supplier may provide.

About 10% of individuals with eczema investigated by diagnostic patch test investigations are found to be allergic to one or more of the standard indicators for fragrance allergy. The prevalence of fragrance allergy in the general population is not known but may be about 2%. The fact that fragrance allergy is important is seen in the simultaneity of fragrance allergy and cosmetic dermatitis. The IFRA guidelines have obviously failed to provide protection for this enormous cohort of individuals. It could be argued that but for the guidelines the situation would have been worse. Some companies have fragrance ingredient restrictions which are tighter than in the IFRA guidelines.

Whilst in-depth toxicological evaluation of fragrance ingredients is desirable in the long term, in the short term it is possible to take measures on the basis of currently available information. These data exist for the 70 or so perfume ingredients which have been subject to internal recommendations by the industry. *The self-regulation of the fragrance industry is still ahead of govern-*

mental regulations. Several fragrance ingredients restricted by IFRA have been regulated years later by the European Cosmetics Directive (RIFM 7th International Information Exchange, 1995).

Legislation already exists to provide more control and information on fragrance ingredient use than has hitherto been available. Annex 2 of the Cosmetics Directive is a listing of those substances which must not be present in cosmetic products. The IFRA guidelines provides tables of a series of substances which the association recommends should not be used. Although the photoallergic property of musk ambrette was known in 1979 and several years later the IFRA guidelines recommended that this ingredient should not be used, the substance was slowly removed from some existing fragrance compounds over a number of years by incrementally decreasing the concentration whilst other compounds remained unmodified. There was a legal prohibition in 1993 when it was included in Annex 2. Substances to be included in Annex 2 must be assessed first by the SCC. Those ingredients which IFRA recommends should not be used need to be added to Annex 2 and such an action could not be seen by the industry to be controversial.

It is clearly advisable to inform consumers of the presence of allergy inducing ingredients (on the basis of information in monographs drafted by the fragrance manufacturers themselves and on published data from clinical studies) and to propose measures designed to provide this information to the consumer.

Annex 3 of the Cosmetics Directive provides a way of controlling the use of certain substances in regards to the type of product in which they may be used and the concentration maximum which may be present in the finished product. It also provides a means of including information on a cosmetic products label. Those substances for which the IFRA guidelines provide restriction on use should be included in Annex 3, again after review by the SCC. It is curious that all the ingredients in the standard fragrance mix used in diagnostic patch test investigations are not present in the IFRA guidelines. Therefore, also to be included in Annex 3 should be those other substances which have a well recognised potential to cause skin sensitization, other cutaneous toxic effects, or for which there is concern about other aspects of toxicity.

Under current legislation all ingredients in a cosmetic product must be identified on the product label and the internationally agreed INCI terminology is obligatory for this use.

The exception is that fragrance compounds are identified merely by the word 'parfum'. Inclusion of a substance in Annex 3 allows a means of providing more information in that it can require that the presence of that ingredient be identified as such on the product. Hence, following the word 'parfum' the caution could be added *'contains isoeugenol'*. It would also be possible to extend the caution to *'contains isoeugenol – risk of sensitization'*. The latter would be controversial and of dubious benefit.

Using the cautions available through Annex 3 could provide information on those fragrance compounds which contain the well-recognised allergens. This would permit a greater understanding of the sources of exposure to these substances, information which is notable for its absence presently. The epidemiological data generated could have an important impact on consumer protection and preventative medicine. A possible sequel to Annex 3 inclusion is that the fragrance manufacturers will then omit those substances present in Annex 3 to avoid label identification. If such allergen substitution is performed wisely, using substances which have been demonstrated to be safe, the important fragrance allergens could be removed from the cosmetic market.

Individuals are exposed to fragrance substances in household, industrial and other products and in cosmetics. The regulation of fragrance ingredients in these non-cosmetic products does not exist and manoeuvres to provide control and information above the IFRA guidelines will be difficult. However, in a reorganisation of the European Commission, all those scientific committees which advise the Commission on aspects relevant to consumer health are now under DGXXIV. This will create a better transfer of information and opinion between the different divisions of consumer policy.

The Fragrance Ingredient Inventory

An inventory of fragrance ingredients has been published by the European Commission on the basis of a listing produced by industry. This is an indicative but not exhaustive list of the chemical substances which the fragrance industry may be using. In itself this inventory is purely a catalogue and provides no information on the quantities of these substances used or for what purposes. This inventory is remarkable for its lack of practical purpose.

Information should be provided on the most widely used fragrance ingredients in terms of the quantities used and for what purposes. The fragrance industry has been very reluctant to communicate this information, although the number of individuals with allergies caused by perfume ingredients justifies requests for such information and the provision of such relevant information to consumers.

The inventory of fragrance ingredients needs to be modified to provide useful information on the quantities of the ingredients used and for what purpose. EFFA has promised that during 1997 it will provide some details about the quantities used of the most common fragrance ingredients and it is hoped that the association will also provide information as to the types of products they are used in. Only with such basic detail will it be possible to assess population exposure and the possible risks to the consumer.

A Change in Philosophy

The fragrance industry has maintained a protectionist stance which is now archaic and out of tune with the ethos of the consumer's right to know and need to be protected. It has and remains a powerful lobby which has persuaded legislators that its self-regulation is satisfactory for consumer protection. The enormous problem of fragrance sensitivity is a clear demonstration that self-regulation has failed. By forceful moral pressure on the industry and by controlled use of the Annexes in the Cosmetics Directive it will be possible to improve on the present sorry and unsatisfactory situation.

A 'think tank' has been set up consisting of a balanced representation of dermatologists, fragrance-compound manufacturers and users to address aspects of the 'problems' and 'needs'. It is hoped that with goodwill and sincerity discussions will take place which will answer the present difficulties and provide better understanding and protection for the consumer.

Subject Index

A
abbalide 139
absorption 125 ff.
- benzyl acetate 129
- cinnamic
- - acid 129
- - alcohol 129
- - aldehyde 129
- cinnamyl anthranilate 129
- coumarin 129
- dibutyl phthalate 129
- diethyl phthalate 129, 185, 188
- dimethyl phthalate 129
- diphenyl ether 129
- dose 130
- eugenol 129
- δ-limonene 129
- 1-menthol 129
- 2-methoxynapththalene 129
- 2-phanoxyethyl isobutyrate 129
- 2-phenylethanol 129
- vehicle 130
ACA (α-amylcinnamic aldehyde) 114, 115, 186, 194
acetyl cedrene 82, 94
acetyl ethyl tetramethyl tetralin 201
5-acetyl-1,1,2,3,3,6-hexamethyl indan 202
acetyl isovaleryl 201
acetylated vetiver oil 203
acetylethyltetramethyltetralin (AETT, Versalide) 122
ACS (allergen control system) 87
actinic dermatitis, chronic 72
activity-structure relationships 126
AETT ("Acetyl-Ethyl-Tetramethyl-Tetralin") 122
aftershave lotions 69
alarm pheromone 39
aldehydes 44
allantroot oil 201
allelochemicals 36
allergen
- controlled system (ACS) 73, 87
- hypoallergenic jasmine oil 88
- hypoallergenic ylang-ylang oil 88
allergy/allergic reactions 94
- fragrance allergy 69
- perfume allergy 100
- photoallergy 175, 178
allomones 37
allylesters 203
allylheptine
- carbonate 202
- carboxylatea 60
allylisothiocyanate 202
α-amylcinnamic alcohol 53
amylcinnamic aldehyde/α-amylcinnamic aldehyde (ACA) 79, 114, 115, 186, 194, 95
amylcyclopentenone 202
amylsalicylate 78, 94, 95
amylcyclopentenone 60
5-α-androst-16 en-3-α-one 32
androstenol 22, 28, 29
androstenone 22, 28, 33
androsterol 28
androsterone 29
Angelica root oil 202
angry back phenomenon 154
animal methods/tests 166, 179
- alternative methods 179
- for skin sensitization 166
anisyl alcohol 79
anisylidene acetone 60, 201
anosmia 16
antifungal agent 107
antiperspirants 71

aphid 36
apocrine
- ASOB 1 and 2 („Apocrine Secretion or Binding Proteins" 1 and 2) 23
- glands 22
aquatic risk assessments 211
armoise oil 85, 87
asthma 73
atranorin 71
attractiveness 29
axillary odours 21 ff.

B
balm 114
balsam of Peru 72, 79
bay oil 85, 87, 188
- terpeneless 188
bees 43 ff.
benzoyl peroxide 157
benzyl
- acetate 94, 129, 132
- alcohol 72, 73, 79, 87, 115
- benzoate 72
- dimethylcarbinol 60
- propionate 87
- salicylate 73, 79, 80, 87, 94
benzylidene acetone 60, 201
benzylsalicylate 60, 62
Bergamot oil of 76, 175, 199, 202, 204
- expressed 76, 199, 202
Berloque dermatitis 73, 200
BMHCA (para-tertiary „Butyl-Methyl-Hydro-Cinnam-Aldehyde") 123
- reproductive effects 123
body odour 21
Buehler test 166, 184, 186
- *Buehler* guinea pig sensitization test 184, 186
- occluded application test of *Buehler* 166
Butyl-dihydrocinnamaldehyde, *p-tert* 202
Butyl-methylhydrocinnamaldehyde, *p-tert* (*see* BMHCA) 123
Butyl-phenol, *p-tert* 201

C
C_9- and C_{10} acid, unsaturated 23
cade oil 203
camomile 114
cananga oil 73, 87
carcinogenicity 122
δ^3-carene 205
carvone 106, 110
- oxide 203
cashmeran 79, 140
cassia oil 202
cedar wood oil 96
cedramber 79
celstolide 139
chenopodium oil 202
cinnamaldehyde 132
cinnamic
- acid 72, 129
- alcohol 53, 59, 79, 114, 129, 202
- aldehyde/cinnamaldehyde 53, 59, 72, 73, 78, 79, 101, 114, 118, 129, 169, 171, 187, 203
- aldehyde-methyl anthranilate schiff base 203
cinnamon bark oil, Ceylon 202
cinnamyl
- anthranilate 129
- cinnamate 72
cinnamylidene acetone 202
cis-asarone 199
citral 44, 45, 59, 77, 95, 114, 118, 169, 171, 194, 199, 203, 205
citronellal 114, 118
- hydroxycitronellal (*see there*) 53, 59, 62, 79, 87, 94, 98, 114, 115, 132, 133, 159, 162, 169
- methoxycitronellal 73, 87
citronellol 78, 94, 95
citrus 106, 202, 205
- oil 202
- terpenes 205
civet 4
cleaning 107
clove bud oil 80
coal tar dyes 72
COLIPA („European Cosmetic Toiletry and Perfumery Association") 176
colophony 109, 201
conformity certificate 220
connubial contact dermatitis 67
contact dermatitis 67, 69, 71, 73
- connubial 67
- depigmented airborn 73
- photocontact dermatitis 69, 71
- phototoxic (*see there*) 76
contact urticaria 72
cosmetics 69, 72, 104, 113 ff., 136, 220, 221

- European cosmetics directive/cosmetics directive 220, 221
- - annex-2 221
- - annex-3 221
- - sixth amendment 216 ff.
- "European Cosmetic Toiletry and Perfumery Association" (COLIPA) 176
- pigmented cosmetic dermatitis 69, 72, 73
costus root oil 85, 87, 201
- absolute 201
- concrete 201
coumarin 71, 79, 95, 114, 115, 129, 132
- dihydro coumarin 59, 77, 114, 118, 201
- 4,6-dimethyl-8-*tert* butyl coumarin 201
- hexahydro coumarin 60, 201
- 7-methoxy coumarin 60, 201
- 6-methyl coumarin 71, 76, 169, 175, 201
- 7-methyl coumarin 201
- 4-methyl-7-ethoxycoumarin 201
cream 114
crysolide 139
cumin oil 76, 202
cutaneous toxicity 132
cyclacet 78, 94, 96
cyclamen alcohol/cyclamen alcohol[b] 59, 202

D

D&C yellow no.11 85
damacenone 85
damascone 85
9-decenoic acid 23
deodorant 66, 71, 114
depigmented airborn contact dermatitis 73
DEREK ("Deductive Estimation of Risk from Existing Knowledge") 58
dermatitis 67, 69, 73
- actinic dermatitis, chronic 72
- *Berloque* dermatitis 73, 200
- contact dermatitis (*see there*) 67, 69, 71, 73, 76
- irritant dermatitis 69, 71
- pigmented cosmetic dermatitis 69, 72, 73
dibutyl phthalate 128, 129, 132
diethyl
- maleate 60, 201
- phthalate 129, 132, 185, 188
dihydrocoumarin/dihydrocoumarin[b] 59, 77, 114, 118, 201
dihydromyrcenol 185
dihydrosafrole 199
2,4-dihydroxy-3-methyl-benzaldehyde 201
3,7-dimethyl-2-octen-1-ol 202
4,6-dimethyl-8-*tert* butyl coumarin 201
dimethylcitraconate 60, 201
dimethylisophthalate 169
dimethylphthalate 128, 129, 132
diphenylamine 202
diphenylether 129
dipropylene glycol 115
DMBCA 78, 96

E

(*E*)-β-farnesene 37
E-3M2H (*E*-3-methyl-2-hexenonic acid) 22, 23
ECDs (equivalent current dipoles) 10
eczema, hands 70
EFFA ("European Fragance and Flavour Association") 216
environmental
- contaminants 138
- risk assessments 206 ff.
enzyme reaction 53
erotic effect 28
erythema multiforme 73
erythrocyte membrane phototoxicity 176
essential oils 205
esters
- allylesters 203
- ethylesters 45
- of 2-nonynoic acid, exept methyl octine carbonate 202
- of 2-octynoic acid, exept methyl and allyl heptine carbonate 202
ethanol 185
- 2-phenylethanol (48 h) 129
ethylacrylate 201
ethylesters 45
ethyloctadecadienoate 45
ethyloctadecenoate 45
ethylenebrassylate 188
ethyleneglycol
- monoethyl ether and its acetate 202
- monomethyl ether and its acetate 202
4-ethylheptanoic acid 23

4-ethylnonanoic acid 23
4-ethyloctanoic acid 23
4-ethylpentanoic acid 23
ethylvanillin 96
eucalyptus oil 87
eugenol 53, 54, 66, 78, 79, 94, 114, 115, 129, 169, 171
- eugenol derivatives 54
- isoeugenol 53, 78, 79, 80, 102, 114, 169, 199, 204, 221
"European"
- "Cosmetic Toiletry and Perfumery Association" (COLIPA) 176
- directive (*see also* cosmetics) 220, 221
- "Fragance and Flavour Association" (EFFA) 216
evernic acid 71

F
fabric softeners 132
face water 114
farnesol 203
Fenn materials 97
fig leaf absolute 201
fixolide 60, 139
floropal 79
folione 60
fragrances
- absorption (*see there*) 125 ff.
- allergy 69
- class A 90
- class B 90
- class C 90, 91
- class D 91
- epidemiology 67, 98
- exposure assessment 103
- fine fragrances 93
- fragrance-free products 66
- fragrance mix (FM) 52, 67, 77, 79, 80, 92, 194, 195
- history 92
- - patch testing 92
- ingredients 202, 203, 222
- - inventory 222
- - with sensitizing potential (*see* IFRA) 202, 203
- - with specific purity criteria (*see* IFRA) 203
- psychological effects 28
- systemic effects 121 ff.
- threshold responses 100
- toxicological program 198
furfurylideneacetone 202

G
galaxolide 95, 139
galbanum resin 79
gas chromatography (GC) method 114
gel 114
geraniol 53, 59, 60, 73, 78, 79, 95, 114, 169, 194
- geraniol [14] 59
geranium
- geranium o.b. 95
- geranium oil 73, 87, 95
grapefruit oil expressed 202
guidelines 89
guinea pig
- *Buehler* guinea pig sensitization test 184, 186
- maximization test 58, 153 ff.

H
hand
- cleansers 107
- eczema 70
haptens 51
- pro-haptens 51
HCA (α-hexylcinnamic aldehyde) 87, 115, 186
hedione 95
helional 79
heliotropine 95
trans-2-heptanal 201
n-heptanoic acid 23
hexahydrocoumarin 60, 201
trans-2-hexenal 201, 202, 204
- diethyl acetal 201
- dimethyl acetal 201
hexanonic acid 23
hexylcinnamic aldehyde 95, 114, 168, 169
- HCA (α-hexylcinnamic aldehyde) 87, 114, 115, 186
α-hexylidene cyclopentanone 202
hexylsalicylate 59
histidine 176
household cleaning products 132
houshold products 93
HRIPT (human repetivitve insult patch test) 161, 184
human maximization test 153 ff., 160, 184

hydroabietyl alcohol 60, 62, 201
hydrogen sulfide 7
hydroquinone 201
- monoethylether 201
- monomethylether 201
hydroxycitronellal/hydroxycitronellal[a] 53, 59, 62, 79, 87, 94, 98, 114, 115, 132, 133, 159, 162, 169, 202
- 7-hydroxy-3,7-dimethyloctan-1-al 159
- metabolism 132
- use test 162
hymenoptera 39, 43 ff.
hyperirritable skin 154
hyperparasitoids 39
hyperpigmentation 83
hyposmia 16

I
IFRA ("International Fragrance Research Association") 59, 175, 183, 193, 197, 201–203, 216, 220
- fragrance ingredients not to be used 201, 202
- - acetyl ethyl tetramethyl tetralin 201
- - acetyl isovaleryl 201
- - allantroot oil 201
- - anisylidene acetone 201
- - benzylidene acetone 201
- - butylphenol, *p-tert* 201
- - colophony 201
- - costus root oil (*see there*) 201
- - diethyl meleate 201
- - dihydrocoumarin 201
- - 2,4-dihydroxy-3-methyl-benzaldehyde 201
- - 4,6-dimethyl-8-*tert* butyl coumarin 201
- - dimethylcitraconate 201
- - ethyl acrylate 201
- - fig leaf absolute 201
- - *trans*-2-heptanal 201
- - hexahydrocoumarin 201
- - *trans*-2-hexenal diethyl acetal 201
- - *trans*-2-hexenal dimethyl acetal 201
- - hydroabietyl alcohol 201
- - hydroquinone monoethylether 201
- - hydroquinone monomethylether 201
- - 6-isopropyl-2-decalol 201
- - 7-methoxycoumarin 201
- - α-methylanisylidene acetone 201
- - 6-methylcoumarin 201
- - 7-methylcoumarin 201
- - methyl crotonate 201
- - 4-methyl-7-ethoxycoumarin 201
- - moss extracts 203
- - musk ambrette 201
- - nitrobenzene 201
- - pentylidene cyclohexanone 201
- - pseudoionone 201
- - pseudomethylionones 202
- - verbena oil 202
- fragrance ingredients with sensitizing potential 202, 203
- - allyl heptine carbonate 202
- - amyl cyclopentenone 202
- - *p-tert*-butyl-dihydrocinnamaldehyde 202
- - cassia oil 202
- - cinnamic alcohol 202
- - cyclamen alcohol 202
- - cinnamon bark oil, Ceylon 202
- - cyclamen alcohol 202
- - *trans*-2-hexenal 202
- - α-hexylidene cyclopentanone 202
- - hydroxycitronellal 202
- - isocyclogeraniol 203
- - isoeugenol 203
- - menthadienyl formate 203
- - methyl heptadienone 203
- - methyl heptine carbonate 203
- - *p*-methylhydrocinnamic aldehyde 203
- - 3-methyl-2(3)-nonenenitrile 203
- - methyl octine carbonate 203
- - oak moss extracts 203
- - 1-octen-2-yl acetate 203
- - opoponax 203
- - perilla aldehyde 203
- - Peru balsam 203
- - propylidene phthalide 203
- - rose ketones 203
- - styrax 203
- - 1-trimethylcyclohexenyl(hexadienyl)-2-buten-1-ones 203
- - verbena absolute 203
- fragrance ingredients with specific purity criteria 203
- - acetylated vetiver oil 203
- - allyl esters 203
- - cade oil 203
- - carvone oxide 203

IFRA
- - cinnamic aldehyde 203
- - cinnamic aldehyde-methyl anthranilate schiff base 203
- - citral 203
- - farnesol 203
- - limonene 203
- - nootkatone 203
- - phenylacetaldehyde 203
- - pinacea derivates 203
- - savin oil 203
- - sclareol 203
- guidelines 193, 197, 220
- other materials not used as or in fragrance ingredients 202
- - allylisothiocyanate 202
- - chenopodium oil 202
- - cinnamylidene acetone 202
- - esters of 2-nonynoic acid, exept methyl octine carbonate 202
- - esters of 2-octynoic acid, exept methyl and allyl heptine carbonate 202
- - ethylene glycol monoethyl ether and its acetate 202
- - ethylene glycol monomethyl ether and its acetate 202
- - 3,7-dimethyl-2-octen-1-ol 202
- - diphenylamine 202
- - furfurylideneacetone 202
- - methyl methacrylate 202
- - phenylacetone 202
- - phenyl benzoate 202
- - thea sinensis absolute 202
- phototoxic fragrance ingredients 202
- - 5-acetyl-1,1,2,3,3,6-hexamethyl indan 202
- - *Angelica* root oil 202
- - *Bergamot* oil expressed 202
- - bitter orange oil expressed 202
- - citrus oil 202
- - cumin oil 202
- - grapefruit oil expressed 202
- - lemon oil cold expressed 202
- - lime oil expressed 202
- - marigold oil and absolute 202
- - methyl-*N*-methyl anthranilate 202
- - rue oil (*see there*) 202
- restriction 193
insecticide 107
insects 25
"International Fragrance Research Association" (*see* IFRA) 59, 175, 183, 193, 197, 201–203, 216, 220
ionone 95, 96
- ionone α 95, 96
- ionone β 95, 96
irritant dermatitis 69, 71
Iso E super 78, 85, 94
isoamyl salicylate 96
isobornyl acetate 95
isocyclogeraniol 203
isoeugenol 53, 78, 79, 80, 102, 114, 169, 199, 203, 221
α-isomethyl-ionone 95
6-isopropyl-2-decalol 60, 62, 201
isosafrole 199

J
jasmine 73, 87, 88, 96, 114
- absolute 73, 96
- oil 87, 88
- - hypoallergenic 88

K
kairomones 37

L
labdanum resinoid 188
lanolin 79
laundry detergents 132
lavandin oil 95, 96
lavender 114
lemon
- oil 76, 95, 96, 202
- - cold presses 76, 202
- - lemon grass oil 95, 96
- perfume 71
light reactions, persistent 71
ligustral 79
lilial 59, 60, 79, 95
- lilial [15] 59
lime oil, expressed 77, 202
limonene 59, 95, 96, 110, 171, 203, 205
- δ-limonene 106, 107, 129, 205
- l. dipentene 59, 95, 96
- l. hydroperoxide 110
- l. oxide/oxidation 107, 110
linalool 94, 115
linalyl acetate 95
lipocalin 24
LLNA (local lymph node assay) 167

lotion 69, 114
- aftershave 69
lupus erythemathosus (SLE) 85, 86
lymph node assay, local (LLNA) 167
lyral 78, 82, 94, 98

M
machines 107
magnetometer 8
majantol 79
malodor 21
marigold oil and absolute 202
mass spectrometic (MS) method 114
massage oil 114
maximization test, human 153 ff., 160, 184
melanosis, *Riehl's* 72
menstrual cycle 25, 29, 31
- odour 25
menthadienyl formate 203
1-menthol (48 h) 129
metabolism 132
- benzyl acetate 132
- cinnamaldehyde 132
- coumarin 132
- dibutylphthalate 132
- diethylphthalate 132
- dimethylphthalate 132
- hydroxycitronellal 132
4-methoxyacetophenone 59
methoxycitronellal 73, 87
7-methoxycoumarin 60, 201
2-methoxynapththalene 129
1-(4-methoxyphenyl)-1-penten-3-one[b] 60
5-methoxypsoralen 73, 175
α-methylanisylidene acetone 201
methylbenzoate 115
6-methylcoumarin 71, 76, 169, 175, 201
7-methylcoumarin 201
methylcrotonate 59, 201
4-methyl-7-ethoxycoumarin 201
methylheptadienone 203
- 6-methylheptadienone 60
2-methylheptanoic acid 23
6-methyl-5-hepten-2-one (MHO) 44, 45
methylheptine carbonate 85, 87, 203
3-methylhexanoic acid 23
- (*Z*)-3-methyl-2-hexonic acid 23
4-methyl-3,5-hydrocinnamaldehyde[a] 60
p-methylhydrocinnamic aldehyde 203
methylionone γ 95
methylmethacrylate 202
methyl-*N*-acetylanthranilate 188
methyl *N*-methylanthranilate 60
3-methyl-2(3)-nonenenitrile 60, 203
methyloctine carbonate 95, 96, 194, 203
methylsalicylate 87
MHO (6-methyl-5-hepten-2-one) 44, 45
microorganisms 21
mouse fibroblast model 177
musks 4, 60, 71–73, 79, 95, 96, 122, 123, 136–139, 142, 169, 175, 177, 199, 201, 203, 209
- m. ambrette 71–73, 79, 95, 96, 122, 137, 169, 175, 177, 199, 201, 203
- m. ketone 60, 137, 209
- m. moskene 136
- m. tibetene 136
- m. xylene 60, 95, 123, 136, 137, 142, 209
- - human adipositas tissue 142
- - human blood 142
- - human milk 142
- - liver tumor 123
- nitro musk (*see there*) 138
- polycyclic musks 138, 139
- resorption 136 ff.
- synthetic musk fragrances 136
mutagenicity 122

N
narcissus absolute 79, 85, 87
nepetalactol 37
nepetalactone 37
neurotoxicity 123
nitro musk 138
- fish 138
- mussels 138
- shrimps 138
nitrobenzene 201
NOAEL ("No Observed Adverse Effect Level") 122
nootkatone 203
nucleophilic sites 52

O
oak moss 52, 71, 78, 79, 80, 203
- absolute 79, 80
- extracts 203
occluded application test of *Buehler* 166
occlusion 128
n-octanoic acid 23

1-octene-2-yl acetate 203
1-octene-3-yl acetate 60, 62
7-octenoic acid 23
odours
- ASOB 1 23
- ASOB 2 23
- axillary 21 ff.
- body 21, 28
- menstrual cycle 25
OECD 176
OERMF ("Olfactory Event Related Magnetic Fields") 9
OERP ("Olfactory Event Related Potentials") 9
oil
- acetylated vetiver oil 203
- allantroot oil 201
- *Angelica* root oil 76, 202
- armoise oil 85, 87
- bay oil (*see there*) 85, 87, 188
- of *Bergamot* (*see there*) 76, 175, 199, 202, 204
- cade oil 203
- canango oil 73, 87
- cassia oil 202
- cedar wood oil 96
- chenopodium oil 202
- cinnamon bark oil, Ceylon 202
- citrus oil 202
- clove bud oil 80
- costus root oil (*see there*) 85, 87, 201
- cumin oil 76, 202
- essential oils 205
- eucalyptus oil 87
- geranium oil 73, 87, 95
- grapefruit oil expressed 202
- jasmine oil (*see there*) 87, 88
- lavandin oil 95, 96
- lemon oil (*see there*) 76, 95, 96, 202
- lime oil, expressed 77, 202
- marigold oil and absolute 202
- massage oil 114
- olibanum oil 188
- orange oil (*see there*) 77, 96, 202
- *Patchouli* oil 73, 87
- rue oil 77, 202
- sandal wood oil 73, 79, 87
- savin oil 203
- spearmint oil 80, 85, 87
- tagetes oil 77
- turpentine oil 205
- verbena oil 77, 201
- ylang-ylang oil (*see there*) 73, 79, 86–88
olfactometer 8, 38
olfactory
- bioresponses 16
- cortical areas 13
- OERMF („"Olfactory Event Related Magnetic Fields") 9
- OERP ("Olfactory Event Related Potentials") 9
- stimulation 6
- structure 6
olibanum oil 188
opoponax 203
orange oil 96, 77, 202
- bitter orange oil expressed 202
- bitter orange peel oil 77

P

paint, solvent in 107
parasitoids 36, 38
para-tertiary butyl-methylhydrocinnamaldehyde (*see* BMHCA) 123
Patchouli oil 73, 79, 87
PCBs (polychlorinated bihphenyls) 141
pearlide 139
PEC (predicted environmental concentration) 207
penetration 51, 107
- enhancer 107
- skin penetration 51
pentyl cyclopentanone propanone 60
pentylidene cyclohexanone 201
- 2-*n*-pentylidene cyclohexanone 60
perfume allergy 100
perfumers 3
perillaaldehyde/perillaldehyde 60, 203
persistent light reactions 71
Peru balsam 72, 79, 203
pesticide 141
petrolatum 79
2-phanoxyethyl isobutyrate 129
phantolide 139
phenylacetaldehyde 60, 203
phenylacetic acid 23
phenylacetone 202
phenylbenzoate 202
2-phenylethanol 129
phenylethyl alcohol 7, 95, 115, 123
- 2-phenylethyl alcohol 60
pheromones 21, 24, 28, 36, 38, 39

- alarm pheromone 39
- sex pheromone 38
photoallergy 175, 178
photocontact dermatitis 69, 71
photohaemolysis 177
photoirritation 175
photomutagenicity 179
photosensitization 199
phototoxic/phototoxicity 76, 77, 176, 199, 202
- contact dermatitis (*see there*) 76, 77
- - 5-acetyl-1,1,2,3,3,6-hexamethylindane 76
- - *Angelica* root oil 76
- - *Bergamot* oil expressed (*see there*) 76, 199, 202, 204
- - cumin oil 76
- - fig leaf absolute 76
- - lemon oil cold presses 76
- - lime oil, expressed 77
- - methyl *N*-methylanthrailate 77
- - orange peel oil, bitter 77
- - rue oil 77
- - tagetes absolute 77
- - tagetes minute absolute 77
- - tagetes oil 77
- - verbena oil 77
- erythrocyte membrane phototoxicity 176
- fragrance integredients (*see* IFRA) 203
phthalate
- dibutyl 129, 132
- diethyl 129, 132
- dimethyl 129, 132
- dimethylisophthalate 169
pigmentary incontinence 83
pigmented cosmetic dermatitis 69, 72, 73
pinacea derivates 199, 203, 204
α-pinene 205
plants 38
p-methylhydrocinnamic aldehyde 203
PNEC (predicted no-effect concentration) 207
polychlorinated bihphenyls (PCBs) 141
polycyclic musks 138, 139
predicted
- environmental concentration (PEC) 207
- no-effect concentration (PNEC) 207
predictive assays/tests 62, 166, 193
primrose 114
pro-haptens 51
propylidenephthalide 203
- 3-propylidenephthalide 60
pseudoionone 201
pseudomethylionones 59, 202
psychological effects, fragrances 28
p-tert-Butylphenol 59, 201
p-tert-Butyl-dihydrocinnamaldehyde 202
pthalate 128
- dibutyl 128
- diethyl 128, 185
- dimethyl 128

Q

QSAR ("Quantitative Structure Activity Relationship") 57, 208
quenching phenomenon 166 ff.

R

3R principles 179
RED-219 87
rhinitis 73
Riehl's melanosis 72
RIFM ("Research Institute for Fragrance Materials") 121, 182, 197, 216
risk assessments 156, 168, 211
- aquatic 211
rose
- crystals 188
- ketones 203
rue oil 77, 202

S

safrole 199
- dihydrosafrole 199
- isosafrole 199
salicylaldehyde 96
salicylate 59
sandalore 79
sandalwood 114
sandalwood 85
- oil 73, 79, 87
sandela 79
santalol 73
savin oil 203
sclareol 203
semiochemicals 36
sensor array 13
sesquiterpene lactone mix 72
sex pheromone 38
sexual partners 29

shampoo 114
shaving foams 69
skin
- animal tests for skin sensitization 166
- equivalent 178
- hyper-irritable 154
- metabolism 131
- penetration 51
- reservoir 127
SLE (lupus erythemathosus) 85, 86
soaps 69, 93, 136
solvent 106, 107, 184
- for testing 184
- in paint 107
sorbitan sesquioleate 78, 79
spearmint oil 80, 85, 87
spices 70
standards in testing 182
strawberry 114
stress buffer 114
structure-activity relationships 126
styrax 203
sunscreen 76
systemic toxicity 199

T
terpenes 44
terpenoid 37
terpineol 95
terpinyl acetate 95
tests
- animal tests for skin sensitization 166
- *Buehler* test 166, 184, 186
- guinea pig maximization test 58, 153 ff.
- human maximization test 153 ff., 160, 184
- human repetivitve insult patch test (HRIPT) 161, 169
- patch testing 92
- predictive tests 62, 193
- solvent for testing 184
- standards in testing 182
- usage tests/use test 102, 162
- yeast growth inhibition test 176
thea sinensis absolute 202
three moss extracts 203
tonalide 95, 139
toxic/toxicity
- chronic toxicity data 208
- cutaneous toxicity 132
- neurotoxicity 123
- phototoxicity (*see there*) 76, 77, 176, 199
- systemic toxicity 199
- toxicological program 198
trans-asarone 199
trans-2-heptanal 60, 201
trans-2-hexenal 59, 199, 202
- diethylacetal 59, 201
- dimethylacetal/dimethylacetalb 60, 202
traseolide 140
trimethylaminuria 21
1-trimethylcyclohexenyl(hexadienyl)-2-buten-1-ones 203
3,5,5-trimethylhexyl acetate 59
turpentine 154
- oil 205

U
10-undecenoic acid 23
unsaturated C_9- and C_{10} acid 23
urticaria 72, 73
- contact urticaria 72
usage tests/use test 102, 162
UV/visible absorption spectroscopy 176

V
vanilla 114
vanillin 7, 11, 13
vanoris 95, 96
verbena
- absolute 203
- oil 77, 201
verdox 96
versalide 60
- (acetylethyltetramethyltetralin/AETT) 122, 140
vertofix 78, 94, 95
vetivers 87
violet leaves absolute 79
volatile
- bouquet 44
- signals 36
Y
yeast growth inhibition test 176
ylang-ylang oil 73, 79, 86–88
- hypoallergenic 88

Z
(*Z*)-3-methyl-2-hexonic acid 23

MIX
Papier aus verantwortungsvollen Quellen
Paper from responsible sources
FSC® C105338

If you have any concerns about our products,
you can contact us on
ProductSafety@springernature.com

In case Publisher is established outside the EU,
the EU authorized representative is:
Springer Nature Customer Service Center GmbH
Europaplatz 3, 69115 Heidelberg, Germany

Printed by Libri Plureos GmbH
in Hamburg, Germany